SPORTS MEDICINE HANDBOOK

The editors would like to dedicate this book to their wives, Gillian Hackney and Jackie Wallace, and their children.

SPORTS MEDICINE HANDBOOK

Edited by
Roger G Hackney

*Consultant Orthopaedic Surgeon, Royal Hospital, Haslar,
Hampshire, UK*

and

W Angus Wallace

*Professor of Orthopaedic and Accident Surgery, University of
Nottingham, Queen's Medical Centre, UK*

First published in 1999
by the BMJ Publishing Group, BMA House, Tavistock Square,
London WC1H 9JR

British Library Cataloguing in Publication Data

A catalogue record for this book is available from the
British Library

ISBN 0-7279-1031-0

Typeset by Latimer Trend & Company Ltd, Plymouth
Printed and bound by Craft Print, Singapore

Contents

Contributors

Nicholas Barton Emeritus Consultant Hand Surgeon, Queen's Medical Centre, Nottingham, UK

Steven R Bollen Consultant Orthopaedic Surgeon, The Yorkshire Clinic, Bingley, West Yorkshire, UK

Richard Budgett Director of Medical Services, British Olympic Association, London, UK

Louise Burke Head of Department of Sports Medicine, Australian Institute of Sport, Belconnen, Australia

Neil Buxton Department of Neurosurgery, University of Nottingham, Queen's Medical Centre, Nottingham, UK

Roslyn Carbon Senior Lecturer/Sports Physician, Academic Department of Sports Medicine, The Royal London Hospital (Mile End), London, UK

Tom Crisp Sports Physician, The Royal London Hospital, London, UK

John Firth Department of Neurosurgery, University of Nottingham, Queen's Medical Centre, Nottingham, UK

Michael Gleeson Senior Lecturer in Exercise Biochemistry, School of Sport and Exercise Sciences, University of Birmingham, UK

Roger G Hackney Consultant Orthopaedic Surgeon, Orthopaedic Division, Royal Hospital, Haslar, UK

W Stewart Hillis Professor of Cardiovascular and Exercise Medicine, Glasgow University, Western Infirmary, Glasgow, UK

Graham MN Holloway Consultant in Orthopaedic Surgery, Sports Injury Clinic, Ridgeway Hospital, Wroughton, Swindon, UK

D Glenn Hunter   Senior Lecturer, Biomechanics, Sports Medicine and Rehabilitation, Department of Allied Health Sciences, Faculty of Health and Social Care, University of the West of England, Bristol, UK

Timothy E Kilmartin   Consultant Podiatrist, South Derbyshire and Nottingham Community Trusts, Ilkeston Hospital, Derbyshire, UK

Pirkko Korkia   Senior Lecturer in Sport and Exercise Science, University of Luton, Bedfordshire, UK

Nancy Laurenson   Director, National PACE Association, San Francisco, California, USA

Rose Macdonald   Former Director, Sports Injury Centre, Crystal Palace National Sports Centre, London, UK

Donald AD Macleod   Consultant General Surgeon, Honorary Professor of Sports Medicine, University of Aberdeen, Foresterhill, Aberdeen, UK

Nicola Maffulli   Senior Lecturer and Consultant in Orthopaedic Surgery, University of Aberdeen, Foresterhill, Aberdeen, UK

Ron Maughan   Professor, Department of Biomedical Sciences, University of Aberdeen, Foresterhill, Aberdeen, UK

Lars Neumann   Consultant Orthopaedic Surgeon, Nottingham Shoulder and Elbow Unit, Nottingham City Hospital, Nottingham, UK

Malcolm TF Read   Consultant in Orthopaedic and Sports Medicine, Barbican Health, The Barbican, London, and Guildford, Surrey, UK

NC Craig Sharp   Professor of Sports Science, Brunel University, Isleworth, Middlesex, UK; Former Director of Physiological Services, British Olympic Medical Centre

W Angus Wallace   Professor of Orthopaedic and Accident Surgery, University of Nottingham, Queen's Medical Centre, Nottingham, UK

Preface

Participation in sport is an important part of life for millions of people, the benefits are beyond question. Athletes at all levels probe the limits of their own physical and mental capabilities. Sports medicine practitioners require a thorough understanding of the demands of sport. This understanding must include knowledge of training technique and methods, equipment and footwear, rules of the sport, physiology of exercise, as well as the injuries unique to sport. Sports medicine demands a truly holistic approach. The practitioner must search for the underlying cause of an injury. Simply treating the pain and then allowing the athlete to return to the same training habits, using the same footwear, and so on will lead to recurrence of injury.

Sports medicine has been recognised as a specialty in its own right for a long time in the USA and much of Europe. Progress in gaining the recognition deserved for sports medicine from those who control medicine in the UK is being made, but is long overdue. Despite this, there exists a huge wealth of experience in sports medicine in this country.

There are many books on sports medicine on the bookshelves. This book seeks to provide a practical insight from a different viewpoint. There is an extra perceptiveness gained from experience. This book brings together chapter authors who have practical experience and expertise in their field. There are many details and insights to be gained from direct involvement. Authors were asked to contribute their specialist knowledge. For example, Roger Hackney travelled worldwide in his career as an athlete, Tom Crisp has been team doctor for several major championship teams, hence the chapter on travel contains information gained from direct experience, and not found elsewhere. The list of banned drugs and substances is widely available; of more practical use is advice on how one does treat an athlete with asthma, a cold etc. Richard Budgett, an Olympic gold medallist and British Olympic team doctor and Roslyn Carbon provide that practical advice.

This book should be of use to everyone from the lay coach, the physiotherapist, and the doctor with a passing interest through to those involved in care of the athlete at the highest level.

Roger Hackney spent 12 years as an international athlete for Great Britain. He competed in three Olympic Games, travelling widely. He still trains daily. He is a Consultant Orthopaedic Surgeon who has a unique experience of sports medicine from both sides of the couch. He is active in both the British Association of Sport and Medicine and the British Orthopaedic Sports Trauma Association.

Angus Wallace is a Professor of Orthopaedic Surgery with a special interest in shoulder surgery. Since 1991 he has developed the Centre for Sports Medicine in Nottingham into a thriving department which offers higher degrees in sports medicine. He is currently President of the British Orthopaedic Sports Trauma Association.

RH
AW

1 Principles of training

NC CRAIG SHARP

Introduction

Overall preparation of an individual or a team for sports competition involves some eight different areas of expertise, embracing collectively:

- **Physical fitness** – with its cluster of different items, each varying markedly between sports, and being very highly sports-specific.
- **Techniques and motor skills** – some of which may need biomechanical analysis, either relatively intuitively by the analytical skills of the expert coach (as in gymnastics or athletics field events or racket sports) or by formal biomechanical recording techniques.
- **Tactics** – more appropriate in some sports (team games, racket sports) than others (500 m sprint canoe, athletics 100 m, swimming 100 m).
- **Nutrition** – including fluid and electrolyte balance – important in all sports, but more so in those, including team games, of longer duration, i.e. over about 10 minutes.
- **Sports medicine** – appropriate physiotherapy, podiatry, massage, medical and surgical back-up.
- **Sports psychology** – increasingly useful and important, and encompassing a very broad spectrum of topics from motivation and determination, i.e. the "will to win", to modes of stress reduction before or during competition.
- **Squad and team selection** and **team management** – if these are badly performed, all the above may count for very little.

At the level of a school team, the staff member in charge might expect to embrace virtually all of the above aspects, whereas for an Olympic or national squad, separate experts in each of the eight areas may well be the norm. Of the above, "training" would mainly embrace the first three areas, namely physical fitness, technical skills, and tactics. The current chapter will deal briefly with the physical fitness side of training, which itself comprises a menu of some five items, differently and specifically selected for each sport or discipline. The five physical fitness items are:

1

- **Cardiorespiratory fitness**, often referred to as "aerobic fitness".
- **Local muscle endurance**, often referred to as "anaerobic fitness". These first two items are often collectively included in the term "stamina".
- **Muscle speed** and
- **Muscle strength**, which collectively account for muscle power.
- **Flexibility**, which may range from the hypermobility of the gymnast to its possible contraindication in the distance runner. Flexibility training will be discussed in the next chapter.

Body composition, in terms of percentage body fat and lean body mass, may be said to represent a sixth fitness item, but it is not a quality that many competitors consciously strive to change. For most highly trained competitors, for example marathon runners, body fat is appropriately low as a spin-off from training. In some high skill sports, such as women's badminton, this may not necessarily be the case, while in weight-categorised sports competitors *should* attain the appropriate weight by body fat adjustment, but in practice often resort to fluid loss techniques.

Items of physical fitness

The fitness items will be discussed as aerobic fitness, local muscle endurance, and muscle strength, speed, and power. A difficulty in physical training is to know what proportion of each fitness item is required for a particular sport, and what levels of each item are possessed at a given time by the individual competitor. Ideally, these may be determined by physiological analysis of the sport and of the competitor.

For training purposes, the sporting year may be divided into a number of major periods, or macrocyles, of which the minimum number would be three, comprising the pre-season, the competition season, and the post-season. The pre-season macrocycle may be further divided into three lesser periods or mesocycles: an aerobic-base mesocycle, which may also include muscle power training and some flexibility work; a subsequent anaerobic mesocycle, which would still contain power and flexibility work; and a power and speed mesocycle which would carry the competitor into the early season competitions. Figure 1.1 represents a macrocycle of 12 weeks such as one might work through in preparation for the start of the season in a "multiple-sprint sport" such as football, hockey, squash, badminton etc. We have found that, for many sports, basic levels of fitness deteriorate throughout the competition season,[1] so would strongly advise maintenance programmes. Roughly, what has taken three sessions a week to gain, may be maintained by one such session per week.

During the competition season, the important factor is to target the few vital competitions, and to peak and taper for them.

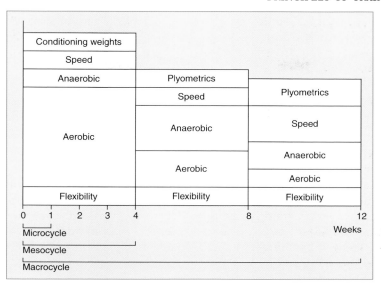

Figure 1.1 Schematic example of a 12-week macrocycle physical conditioning programme, containing three 4-week mesocycles, each with four 1-week microcycles. In this instance the programme is for pre-season training for a multiple-sprint sport. The overall macrocycle leads into the playing season. Each of the three mesocycles targets a major fitness parameter, namely aerobic fitness, anaerobic fitness and speed and power respectively, although all three are represented in each mesocycle. Flexibility work is a constant throughout, and the first mesocycle conditioning weights programme gives way to two following mesocycles of plyometric training. Each microcycle consists of a week's work in a particular training mode, which will tend to increase in intensity and decrease in volume as the microcycle proceeds, and this pattern will be reflected throughout the mesocycle. The programme will, of course, run in parallel to appropriate skill and practice training for the specific sport. For a much fuller version of such a programme, see the chapter by NCC Sharp in: McKenzie I, ed. The squash workshop, The Crowood Press, *1992*

Training principles

All programmes should be flexible enough to cope with illness, injury, weather, and individual timetables.

It is important to note some general principles which apply to all training regimes.

- **Specificity** The effect of training is fairly specific to its type, which means that it should be geared to the relevant energy systems, and to the relevant muscle groups, and to their relevant ranges of movement.
- **Reversibility** Training effects are reversible, either by injury or illness and bed rest, or too infrequent or insufficiently intensive training, as may occur during the competition season. A competition edge lost by a week's injury or bed rest should be recovered in 2–3 weeks.

3

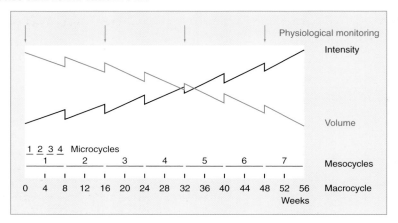

Figure 1.2   Diagram of a periodisation pattern of a training programme for a single-discipline sport such as running, race-walking, cycling, swimming, rowing or sprint canoeing. Here the macrocycle is just over a year, leading up to a major competition. The one-year macrocycle is divided into seven mesocycles each of 8 weeks, and these in turn consist of four 2-week microcycles. Note that intensity rises (and volume drops) towards the end of each mesocycle, and that throughout the macrocycle the volume decreases as the intensity increases. The programme allows for four sessions of laboratory or field physiological monitoring, of which the first two might be in the laboratory and the next two in the field

- **Overload** Adaptation to the training is dependent on overload, thus training quality (intensity and/or duration) progressively increases, often on a weekly basis. As fitness increases, a higher quality of exercise stress is needed to create the overload. Figure 1.2 represents this basic principle behind most training – the art of reducing the volume of work while stepping up the quality or intensity.
- **Monitoring** This is part of progression; the programme should be quantitatively sampled, possibly by simple appropriate fitness tests, to assess progress and to reset training goals and intensity.

A training programme will comprise a number of elements such as:

- **Reps (repetitions)** Specific exercises which are repeated a fixed number of times.
- **Sets** A number of repetitions, for example, "two sets of 15 reps".
- **Intensity** The rate of effort, or the weight lifted, or the degree of joint stretch.
- **Duration** The length of time of the exercise set, including rest intervals where appropriate.
- **Rests** The time interval between reps or sets. Often, such a rest would be an "active" rest, where the activity is continued but at about 50% of the rep effort.
- **Training type** Continuous and interval are the main types, each containing a wide variety of training modes, ranging from long steady

4

runs to plyometrics or proprioceptive neuromuscular facilitation flexibility work.

Aerobic fitness

This has the following elements.

1. A *central delivery* of oxygen, involving lungs, blood, heart, and circulation. Following long periods of intensive aerobic training, little change is noted in lung parameters; the haemoglobin may drop to the low end of the normal range (the so-called "sports anaemia") due to relative plasma hypervolaemia; the cardiac output may increase by some 25–30% through an increase in stroke volume; the vascular shunt may supervene more quickly at the commencement of exercise and there may be a more rapid increase in blood flow to the active muscles.
2. A *peripheral uptake* of oxygen, involving the muscle capillary bed, myoglobin and mitochondria. Following similar training, the capillary density may increase by 50% or more, myoglobin may show a similar increase, as may the mitochondria which both multiply and increase their internal enzyme density. The importance of the peripheral aspect may easily be seen following, for example, one-legged training on a cycle ergometer for a month, followed by a $\dot{V}o_2$max test with the trained and untrained legs respectively;[2] the trained leg would be of the order of 10% or more higher.

The above central and peripheral factors provide the maximum oxygen uptake or $\dot{V}o_2$max (which may increase by up to about 25%), and they also determine the anaerobic threshold, which is the proportion of the $\dot{V}o_2$max that may be utilised continuously throughout the duration of the sport (from the few minutes of the rower, canoeist or middle distance runner, to the much longer periods of the team games and squash and badminton, or of the long distance walks, swims, runs, and triathlon). As a rough guide, $\dot{V}o_2$max is an indication of potential, but the anaerobic threshold (lactate threshold, OBLA point) is more a guide to current *aerobic* fitness status. The anaerobic threshold may be increased by some 30% or more. Following 2 weeks of bed rest, it is not uncommon for $\dot{V}o_2$max to decline by some 20%, which may take 4–5 weeks of appropriate training to restore. During bed rest, of course, there is a degree of loss of lean body mass, and possibly an increase in body fat.

The intensity of aerobic training for sport varies with the initial fitness, but roughly the exercise heart rate (HR) should just exceed the sum of the resting heart rate and 60% of the difference between resting and maximal heart rates, with age-related HR maxima being estimated from 220 minus

5

age in years. In general, for the younger age groups, a training HR of around 150 bpm is appropriate.

For general sports fitness, the duration at this intensity should not normally be below 15 or above 40 minutes of continuous effort. It is sometimes preferable to do *interval aerobic* training, for example by running three repetition miles each in 6 minutes, with a 5 minute rest between, during which the heart rate should drop back to around 100–120 bpm, otherwise the rest may need to be longer. In these interval runs, it is most important that each rep is *not* ended with a sprint; the runs should be done

Table 1.1 Programmes for aerobic endurance training by running

Exercise mode	Reps	Sets	Intensity	Rest or warm-down
600 metres	8	1	2 min	2 min jog
800 metres	6	1	3 min	3 min jog
1 mile run	3	1	6 min	5 min jog
3 miles run	1	1	20 min	6 min jog or walk
5 miles run	1	1	38 min	8 min jog or walk

at constant pace from three to five times per week. Table 1.1 shows examples of aerobic endurance training by running.

For health-related fitness of the general population, some of the above could be adapted, to give approximately 20 minutes of exercise, at a pace that just makes talking difficult, about three times per week. It is worth noting that the energy cost of brisk walking may well be greater than that of slow jogging. Also, it is probable that two 10 minute sessions in a day are as effective as one 20 minute session. In terms of paramenopausal women, swimming and cycling, because they are *not weight-bearing*, are probably not as effective against osteoporosis as running (and aerobics, dance, badminton, squash, and tennis). In such women, the upper body skeleton should not be neglected, and here rowing (land- or water-based), canoeing, weights, or Multigym work are suitable forms of exercise.

Anaerobic fitness

This refers to local muscle endurance, which, strictly, is a mix of both aerobic and anaerobic endurance. Anaerobic energy sytems act to deliver higher rates of energy supply than mitochondria can produce. For example, on a cycle ergometer, a subject may only be able to maintain an output of 300 W aerobically, but may well increase this to upwards of 900 W with the addition of the muscles' anaerobic energy supply. Glycolysis supervenes far more to keep up to the demands of high power, than as a response to relative hypoxia.

Thus, for anaerobic training, the intensity must be around 80–95% of maximum in each rep (lower for the more anaerobic subjects, who may be higher in fast twitch fibre %; higher for the more aerobic, possibly lower in fast twitch fibre %), and the rep length should normally be between 20 and 40 seconds. Reps which are too short rely too much on creatine phosphate; those which are too long begin to over-involve aerobic energy supply.

Anaerobic training is almost invariably done in an interval mode, with appropriate active rest periods, which may occur in a time ratio of about 1:3 work to rest at the beginning of the anaerobic mesocycle, going down perhaps to 1:1 a few weeks later. The training mode is usually shuttle running on court, pitch, gym, or track; but it may involve skipping, or even step-ups – or appropriate reps of swimming, rowing, canoeing, or cycling. Specialised sports such as dinghy sailing or skiing have their own dry-land hiking benches or ski-agitators respectively, and wrestlers work with weighted leather manikins, on all of which interval work is done on similar principles. It is important that the *quality* of the work is not allowed to drop off, through attempts to achieve an overoptimistic target number. It is better to do less work of high quality. Table 1.2 gives examples.

Table 1.2 Examples of anaerobic interval conditioning training

Exercise mode	Reps	Sets	Intensity	Rest
200 m run	6	2	35 sec	2 min jog between reps[a] 10 min jog/walk between sets
Skipping	10 × 30 sec	1	180 skips/min	2 min jog between reps
Step-ups	5 × 1 min	1	60 steps/min	2 min jog between reps
Weights	40–70	1	40–60% max	Perform to a rhythm, about one lift every 2 sec

[a] A 1500 m track competitor of national standard would run 26–27 sec reps, with 30 sec recovery.

Anaerobic endurance may be improved by at least 20–50%, depending on initial levels and the severity of the training regime.

Muscle strength and speed

In weight-lifting and power-lifting, the prime requirement is sheer strength, "the greatest force possible in a single maximum voluntary contraction". Nevertheless, a degree of power is required to overcome the inertia of the load and impart momentum. Apart from the weight-lifters, most competitors in the weights room desire increments in *power* – to run faster, or jump higher or longer, or throw further, or kick harder, or pull the paddle or sweep through the water faster. The coach would refer to "speed power" for these, and to "strength power" for the rugby scrum and some

7

aspects of wrestling. To be more specific, strength-power is more important in the shot and hammer, and speed-power in the javelin and discus. The smaller the resistance, the greater the requirement for the speed component of power.

On a strength programme, the initial third of the mesocycle should be spent in developing general strength; thereafter the emphasis should gradually shift to the sport-specific requirements – which will differ between, for example, canoeing and long jumping.

Especially with free weights, safety is very important and expert instruction should be sought regarding techniques and equipment used. Free weights are claimed to be better for developing three-dimensional control in terms of proprioception. However, there are many other different modes of applying resistance to muscle, including: fixed weights (Multigym); exercise machines (Nautilus, Cybex, Universal); isokinetic dynamometers (Lido, Kincom, Cybex, Merac); accommodating resistances (Minigym); accelerating resistance devices (Biokinetics); body resistance (press-ups, pull-ups); circuit training (involving weights, body resistance, ropes); elastic bands, springs and pulleys; medicine ball work (throws); and isometric exercise. A fixed weight system, such as a Multigym, is safer than free weights; it is also much easier for novice weight-trainers, as the different stations, equating to different muscle groups, are clearly distinguishable, for example, the quadriceps station, or that for wrist extensors. Most sports centres and virtually all fitness clubs have Multigyms or similar, or other varieties of strength machinery.

Such resistance equipment and free weights can be used to develop *strength*, *speed*, or *endurance*, depending on the loading and number of reps, and the speed of the lifts. An important concept is that of the Single Repetition Maximum load or lift (1-RM), that is, the maximum weight that can be lifted, or force generated, by a particular muscle group in a particular position.

For strength, loading of the order of 85–95% of 1-RM is used, obviously with a small number of reps. This may be done simply as 5–8 lifts of 95% of 1-RM, or as a pyramid, with a progression such as 85%, 90%, 93%, 95% of 1-RM and back down, in reps of 5,4,3,1,3,4,5 respectively. The timing should be a steady rhythm and left to the subject, but would be around one lift per 1 or 2 seconds. The above would constitute a set followed by a 2 minute rest, and it could be followed by other sets working on entirely different muscle groups, before returning to the original to start a second series of sets. For example, quadriceps and gluteal exercise could be followed by pectorals, then from triceps to lower lumbar, then from hamstrings to triceps surae, then shoulders with posterior deltoids, then abdomen and finally, the trio of biceps, brachialis, and brachioradialis. The sequence of sets could then be repeated. Larger muscle groups should be

8

worked before smaller in the same limb, for example, quadriceps before triceps surae, or wrist flexors before finger flexors.

It is important in weight or force training that the full range of muscle movement be utilised. It was through athletes (mainly body-builders) working over months in the inner range of movement that the concept of being "muscle bound" arose, namely a marked loss of flexibility as strength increased. That this is by no means inevitable is easily seen from the male artistic gymnasts, who demonstrate their strength on the rings and their flexibility in the floor discipline, as do the women on the vault and floor respectively. Male dancers demonstrate similar qualities, as do platform divers of both sexes. There should normally be two or three strength sessions per week (one for beginners), each lasting between 45 and 90 minutes, preceded by a warm-up including "pulse-warmers", stretches, and rehearsals of the movements with relatively light loads. Warm-down would include a general stretching sequence, and a short jog of a few minutes. Those new to weight training should start very gradually, that is, with small numbers of reps, and only one series of sets. Delayed onset muscle soreness is a feature of the novice weight-trainer, probably due to the eccentric component inherent in most of the work.

The overall rate of strength improvement is relatively slow, but there is often a relatively fast (around $5–10+$ %) improvement in the first two or three weeks, which is mainly due to neurogenic factors. By about the third week, muscle protein synthesis will be appropriately under way, but improvements take months rather than weeks. Nevertheless, it is within the capability of most people, of whatever age, to double the strength of the major muscle groups. For an excellent introduction to strength training and its regimens, see Hazeldine.[3]

Muscle speed

In weight training for speed, loading of the order of 70% of the 1-RM is appropriate. This is heavy enough to force recruitment right through the fibre bed, but light enough to be moved relatively fast. The number of reps in a set would be of the order of 20, and the lifts would be done as fast as possible, rhythmically, with up to 5 seconds in between.

For running speed, apart from leg muscle speed work in the weights room, there are various forms of interval sprint training, best done on a running track, or firm smooth grass, or as appropriate to the sport, e.g. hockey, camogie, lacrosse, hurling, shinty, soccer, Gaelic football, and rugby, or on the court for squash, badminton, and tennis.

The run periods should last for a minimum of 5 seconds, but not more than 10. Adequate rest is extremely important, as speed demands the highest quality of muscle output. Thus a 1:5 or 1:6 ratio of work to rest is

Table 1.3 A speed schedule

Exercise mode	Reps	Sets	Intensity	Rest
50 m run	6	3	Maximal – e.g. 7 sec	45 sec walk between reps 5 min jog between sets
Court ghosting	10 × 10 sec	2	Maximal	50 sec jog between reps 5 min jog between sets

advised, with a 5–10 minute gently active recovery period between sets. The mode may be track or grass running, or shuttle running in a sports hall, or shadow running on-court for squash or badminton. Table 1.3 gives two examples.

Other speed training methods for the legs involve speed drills, such as running on the spot with a high knee lift and exaggerated arm movements: 50% effort for 20 sec with 1 minute active recovery; then 20 sec of 75% effort, with 1 minute recovery and finally 20 sec of maximal effort with 90 sec recovery. This forms one set, which may be repeated two to five times according to fatigue level.

Downhill running, on a moderate gradient, similar to the sprint schedule given above (although faster, of course) is also useful. Throughout these drills, it is important to maintain a good technique, with good use of the arms.

Speed work should always be done when the athlete is *fresh*. So, after a thorough warm-up, speed training is usually the first work done in a mixed session, as the whole emphasis in speed training is on *quality*. This is the reason for its relatively long rests after very short work periods, and the reason also why a speed session should be terminated as soon as the quality (that is, the pace) begins to fall off. Improvements in speed are not dramatic, being of the order of 10–20%, but this can lead to an important increase in muscle power. Speed is one of the fitness qualities that diminishes first, following injury or lay-off, but it can also be restored relatively quickly – within weeks. It should be noted that it is generally agreed that a block of general strength training should occur before speed training. It is particularly important that a general strength training block be undertaken *before* plyometrics is introduced. The latter is a particularly forceful training mode, and it is important that muscle, tendon, and bone–tendon junction are all capable of coping with the forces generated by plyometric work.

Muscle power: plyometrics

Plyometrics is a conditioning system geared specifically to *power*. It involves stretching the appropriate muscles immediately prior to contraction, as when the forwards in a rugby line-out, or volleyball spikers, crouch or bounce down immediately before leaping up, thus inducing the spindle-mediated myotactic or stretch reflex, and a stretch–contraction cycle for the muscle. As a result of plyometric training, it is proposed that neuromuscular adaptations involve a faster spindle response;[4] also, it is a method of fast-weight training which ensures both that the whole fibre bed is engaged, and works at speed. Finally, plyometrics may well alter the energy storage characteristics of tendon, ligament, and fascia, through its effects on collagen.[5]

Plyometric training methods include depth jumping from boxes, bounding, hopping, and fast catching and throwing exercises, usually with various weights of medicine ball. The important factors are *maximum speed and effort* (i.e. maximum intensity). There should be up to 10 reps in a set, with two to five sets, and three minutes between sets, with usually two plyometric sessions per week. A thorough warm-up is essential, and the whole plyometrics training cycle should be increased very gradually week by week. Good technique must be observed in the jumps. Good quality trainers should be worn, and landing should be on the ball of the foot with the ankle locked, while holding the hands in the "thumbs-up" position helps counteract the tendency of the shoulders to drop forward during jumps, hops, and leaps.[3] As plyometrics involves considerable negative or eccentric work on landing, it produces disproportionate amounts of delayed-onset muscle soreness, hence the need to take it very easy to begin with, and for the gradual progression.

Details of plyometric exercises for all body regions may be found in appropriate texts.[6] The classic plyometric exercise is the depth jump. Place two to five boxes about one metre apart and stand on the first one with the knees slightly flexed, and arms down. Jump down to the floor (a sprung, matted, or carpeted floor), absorb the shock and immediately jump up onto the next box, with a strong arm swing. Pause briefly and repeat over the successive boxes, or turn and jump back to the original one. To estimate the ideal height for depth jumping, do an accurate vertical jump-and-reach measure, that is, stand sideways on to a wall, wet your finger, crouch down and immediately jump up to make a mark on the wall as high as you can. Then repeat this on jumping down, and immediately rebounding up, from a 40 cm height. If you achieve the same height or higher on the wall, then increase the height of the box by 15 cm. Continue to increase the height until you fail to reach your original standing jump-and-reach mark. The previous height is then the correct box height. If you cannot reach the standing jump height from a 40 cm box, you are probably not ready in musculoskeletal terms for plyometrics work; you need more individual strength and speed training.

There are a number of one- and two-legged hopping and bounding plyometric variations, an example of which involves standing with feet

11

together on a low gymnastics bench. Jump down astride it, then immediately up onto it, and continue to bound up and down to the end of the bench.

For the arms, stand facing a partner about one to two metres apart, holding a medicine ball, which should be thrown either as a soccer throw in, or by a strong push from the chest. The partner catches the ball, either overhead or on the chest, and immediately propels it back.

For the trunk, stand beside a partner, about one metre away. Hold the medicine ball on the opposite side from the partner, then swing round hard and release the ball fast; the partner should catch it and turn away from you then immediately swing back and release the ball.

Physiological laboratory and field testing

It is appropriate to finish with discussions regarding physiological testing. Ideally, in elite sport, one wants to know the answers to three questions: What are the fitness requirements for the *sport* in question? What are the fitness levels of a sample of the world's *best* practitioners of the sport? and what are the current fitness levels of one's *own squad*? With this knowledge, one can plan training schedules appropriately and individually, concentrating on improving fitness areas of relative weakness.[7] The importance of laboratory and field fitness tests is to measure progress and to motivate the competitor in training. An excellent guide to laboratory aspects of exercise and fitness testing is that of Eston and Reilly.[8]

The fitness testing has to be performed on equipment which simulates the sport as well as is reasonably practicable. For example, Canadian-style canoeists should be tested on a canoe ergometer, not a kayak ergometer. Cyclists should be tested on their own bicycles on a "King-cycle" apparatus or equivalent, and not on an ordinary cycle ergometer. Swimmers should be tested in a swimming flume. Strength testing should be done isokinetically,[9] so the force is measured at the speeds required by the sport, and not only statically. Upper body power tests on rowers should involve both arms working simultaneously, and not alternately. The test personnel should be very familiar with the particular sports, in order to give genuinely useful advice to coach and competitor. Field testing may be very useful in monitoring training, to ensure that it is carried out at optimal levels for the required fitness parameters.

To provide incentive for those seeking health-related fitness, there should be a much greater availability of simple but well administered fitness tests, perhaps available in sports centres rather than doctors' surgeries. At many university open days one of the most popular stations is where such tests are on offer to everyone. And one of the most common comments, from competitors and recreational exercisers alike, is the wish for relatively simple testing on a regular basis.

Regarding the uses and the usefulness of testing, this varies with different sports, with differing levels of standard in various sports, and with the various parameters of fitness.

Through three decades of fitness monitoring, the author has always felt that fitness testing can be of greater use in team games and racket sports than in those sports in which performance is measured or timed. Partly this is because in the latter the competitors are in a much better position to assess their own fitness improvement as most of their training will be accurately quantified, and they can perform regular time trials, or trial jumps or throws. The team games and racket sports, together with other non-quantified sports such as martial arts, wrestling, boxing, gymnastics, and stage and ice dance, often involve a greater range of the fitness elements – aerobic and anaerobic endurance, strength, speed, and flexibility – in varying proportions and to different levels. Hence, it is often very useful for their proponents to undergo an all-round appropriate test battery to find out peaks and troughs in their various fitness items, so they can concentrate the training on the weaker areas. Further tests will let them see measures of improvement. Also, following lay-off or injury, the test battery will both spotlight decrements and let the competitors know when they have regained competition levels.

Such laboratory assessment is at its best in aerobic parameters, in terms of $\dot{V}O_2max$ and anaerobic threshold (OBLA); it is reasonably good in the anaerobic parameters of peak power, mean power and rate of fatigue, together with a "recovery index"; if the right equipment is available (i.e. isokinetic dynamometry), assessment is very good regarding muscle force exerted at appropriate contraction velocities; assessment is also very useful regarding body composition, especially if the same tester

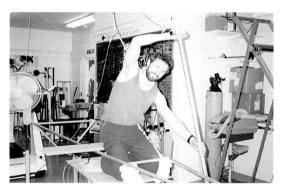

Figure 1.3 A canoeist training on a specific canoe ergometer in the laboratory. The apparatus provides a good indoor simulation and enables the paddler to alter the force or resistance, as well as the frequency of the stroke. He can thus use it as a form of power training

compares a subject against her own previous results. However, laboratory testing tends not to be as effective regarding the measurement of muscle speed or of flexibility. Hence many sports have their own "speed tests", which are various forms of timed sprints or shuttles. Flexibility is much better measured by physiotherapists than physiologists – and again the sports themselves (e.g. gymnastics, dance) often have their own tests.

In sports such as middle and distance running, roller training for Nordic skiing, road cycling, triathlon, swimming, rowing, and slalom and sprint canoeing, field measures of heart rate and blood lactic acid can often be far more useful than corresponding measures in the laboratory, as they can help monitor the training itself and provide valuable feedback for use in adjusting training intensity. In these contexts, the scientist, the coach, and the competitors have to know each other well, and be able to function as a complete unit. Usually the feedback would take the form of comparing heart rate and lactate levels over a standard distance at a set time. The results can, for example, be used to calculate the reduction in time for the training distance. Or the results may be used to ensure, for example, that a steady "aerobic run" genuinely is just that. This would require that the runners maintain a blood lactate level of around 2 mmol/l and not 3 mmol/l or higher, as they often tend to!

In the major competition situation – the Olympic Village or equivalent – the most valuable measures are from the weighing scales and the fat callipers. The former are useful in the detection of a dehydrative loss in weight (e.g. of 1–3% compared to the previous day), and both are useful in helping to detect early effects of the tendency to overeat, through boredom, nervousness, and profusion of food.

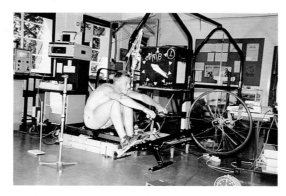

Figure 1.4   Rower training on a rowing ergometer in the laboratory. The athlete is using the laboratory equipment to train on between bouts of filming for ergomechanical analysis

14

Field, home, or practice testing

In the general practice or home setting, there are a number of tests which may be useful, most of which are well explained in the *Eurofit* booklet.[10] Although the Eurofit test battery was designed for school use, the booklet is a most useful, simple, and inexpensive manual. All the equipment items for these tests, plus instructions, may be obtained from laboratory suppliers – such as Simon Skett Esq, Cranlea Ltd, Sandpits Lane, Acacia Road, Bourneville, Birmingham B15. The value of such home or practice tests is as much in their motivational value as anything else. Nevertheless, they may be useful in identifying major areas of weakness, or in establishing baselines against which to measure improvement from training, both normally and on recovery from layoff, injury, or illness.

On the aerobic side, there is first the accurate training diary record of morning pulse count. This may give advance warning of impending illness, or indeed of the overtraining syndrome, with otherwise unexplained rises of 10 bpm from normal baseline levels. There are submaximal cycle ergometer tests with appropriate nomograms; or step tests, to 50–45 cm, with stepping at 20, 25, or 30 steps per minute (metronome settings of 80, 100, or 120) for 5 minutes or until unable to continue, and a 30 second pulse count starting from 1 minute after the end of stepping; the raw score from this being multiplied by six and used to divide 100 times the stepping time (in seconds) to give a figure which usually varies between 50 and 180 – the higher the better. If there is adequate floor space, then the 20 metre shuttle test is probably the best "field" measure of leg-driven aerobic fitness. Cassette instruction and timing tapes are readily available.

There is no satisfactory home/practice measure of anaerobic parameters, although pull-ups, press-ups, the bent-arm hang, and sit-ups, may be used to assess muscular endurance in the respective areas.

A hand-grip dynamometer assesses grip strength, and the vertical jump (especially with the Lewis nomogram[11]) and the standing broad jump give a measure of leg power, as does the medicine ball throw for upper body power.

There are no satisfactory measures of speed, although a timed 10 × 5 metre shuttle run may be useful – as will its equivalents on the squash, badminton, or tennis court, or rugby, football, and hockey pitches, or indoor playing areas.

For flexibility, the "sit and reach" test, on an appropriately calibrated box, gives a measure of hamstring/lower lumbar flexibility.

Body composition may be readily assessed with skinfold callipers, e.g. the Harpenden callipers on the four "Durnin sites" – biceps, triceps, suprailiac, and subscapular. The more expensive electrical impedance techniques are not necessarily more accurate, being particularly susceptible to changes in body water.

15

As a last point, it should always be remembered that physical fitness is but one element in the total preparation for many sports. Lack of appropriate fitness or its loss (especially following a failure to maintain fitness throughout the competition season[12]) *may* be the reason for relative underachievement, but defects in items mentioned above in the introduction, such as tactics, techniques, equipment, psychology, nutrition, dehydration, or subclinical illness or injury, may be equally responsible – as may the sheer quality of the opposition!

References

1 Koutedakis Y. Seasonal variations in fitness parameters in competitive athletes. *Sports Med* 1995;**19**(6):373–392.
2 Saltin B. The physiological and biochemical basis of aerobic and anaerobic capacities in man: effect of training and range of adaptation. In: Russo P, Gass G, eds. *Proceedings of the 5th Biennial Conference on Exercise, Nutrition and Performance*. Sydney, Australia: Cumberland College of Health Science, 1985, pp. 41–78.
3 Hazeldine R. *Strength training for sport*. London: The Crowood Press, 1990.
4 Sale DG. Neural adaptation to strength training. In: Komi PV, ed. *Strength and power in sport*. Oxford: Blackwell Scientific, 1992, pp. 249–265.
5 Zernicke RF, Loitz BJ. Exercise-related adaptations in connective tissue. In: Komi PV, ed. *Strength and power in sport*. Oxford: Blackwell Scientific, 1992, pp. 77–95.
6 Radcliffe JC, Farantinos RC. *Plyometrics: explosive power training*. Champaign, IL: Human Kinetics, 1985.
7 Sharp NCC. Physiology and fitness for squash. In: Reilly T and Lees A, eds. *Proceedings of the 2nd World Congress of Science and Racket Sports*. London: E and FN Spon, 1998.
8 Eston R, Reilly T, eds. *Kinanthropometry and exercise physiology laboratory manual*. London: E and FN Spon, 1996.
9 Koutedakis Y, Agrawal A, Sharp NCC. Isokinetic characteristics of knee-flexors and extensors in male dancers, Olympic oarsmen, Olympic bobsleighers and non-athletes. *J Dance Med Sci* 1998;**2**(2):63–67.
10 Tuxworth W, *et al. Eurofit – European tests of physical fitness*. Council of Europe Committee for the Development of Sport, 1988. Obtainable from UK Sports Council, 16 Upper Woburn Place, London WC1H 0QP.
11 Matthews DK, Fox EL. *The physiological basis of physical education and athletics*, 2nd edn. Philadelphia: WW Saunders, 1976, pp. 499–500.
12 Koutedakis Y, Sharp NCC. Seasonal variations of injury and overtraining in elite athletes. *Clin J Sports Med* 1998;**8**(1):18–21.

2 Warm-up and stretching

NANCY LAURENSON

Warm-up and stretching exercises have slowly evolved to become an essential component of most athletes' training programmes. These exercises are widely perceived to prepare for the activity ahead, improve physical performance, and prevent sports-related injuries. Stretching as a basic component is also regarded as a necessity for maintaining and improving range of motion (ROM).[1,2] As these exercises are performed prior to the principal physical activity, they can be viewed as providing a continuum from rest to activity. The benefits have been widely debated,[3-6] although clinical, experimental, and qualitative observations suggest a link between warm-up and improved performance. Certainly, this belief is upheld by most athletes, coaches, physiotherapists, and doctors.

Warm-up

Physiology

As a general rule, warm-up exercises should precede any exercise period and be as sport-specific as possible in order to enhance all body systems in preparation for activity. A warm-up period usually involves activation of large muscle groups with an elevation of body core temperature. Many of the benefits of warm-up derive from the physiological mechanisms based on temperature-dependent principles of skeletal muscle as described by Bergh and Ekblom[7] and Bennett.[8] An elevation in body temperature leads to greater mechanical efficiency of the contracting muscles[9] because of the decreased viscosity of the tissue. As muscle and connective tissue temperature rises, stiffness decreases and extensibility increases.[9-11] With increased muscle temperature, a change in tissue mechanical behaviour also leads to more forceful and rapid muscle contractions.[7]

Safran *et al*[12] also reported that a decrease in musculotendinous stiffness in rabbit musculature, as a consequence of warm-up, increased the length and force required to tear the musculotendinous unit as compared to a similar musculature that was not subjected to warm-up and was thus more stiff. Additionally, Strickler and colleagues[13] found that passively warmed muscle was more extensible than cold muscle. It was alleged that this increased extensibility could afford some protection from strain injury for warmed muscle. Both these and further studies[1,14,15] provide a biomechanical explanation of the mechanisms by which warm-up may reduce the incidence of musculotendinous injury.

Increased body core temperature also influences those factors that are rate process-dependent such as enzymatic reactions as well as the Bohr effect, which facilitates a more complete dissociation of oxygen from haemoglobin while increasing the release of oxygen from myoglobin. It also accelerates the rate of metabolic processes and heightens the sensitivity of nerve receptors thereby decreasing the overall time of nerve impulse transmission. These physiological processes are important for athletes in sports where skill and complex movements demand fast action and proper central nervous system (CNS) interaction to control intricate movements.

As warm-up increases in intensity, it influences the cardiovascular system by increasing cardiac output with a rise in heart rate and stroke volume and prompting a shift in blood flow distribution which results in improved blood flow to the working skeletal muscles. These mechanisms provide for the subsequent delivery of substrates and removal of metabolic waste products.

Methods

There are a variety of warm-up techniques available to increase body temperature and prepare the individual for exercise. Warm-up methods can be placed in the following categories: passive warm-up, general warm-up, and specific warm-up.

Passive warm-up involves the use of an external heat source to warm the body. Common examples of this form include saunas, hot tubs, and steam baths as well as electrical modalities such as heat pads and diathermy. The advantage of passive warm-up is that it allows sufficient warming of the tissue without physical exertion which may be useful for injured athletes prior to stretching a strained muscle or during breaks in competition to keep muscles warm, prevent muscle spasm or reduce pain. It is not the method of choice, however, when preparing for an exercise session or competition, as there is no skill component or mental rehearsal to accompany the warming of body tissue. Additionally, muscles and joints will not have been taken through set patterns or the full range of motion (ROM) which the athlete is about to undertake.

General warm-up tends to be the most widely used pattern of preparation for physical activity. It often takes the form of general light activity involving the major muscle groups to increase overall body temperature. Activities such as easy jogging, general callisthenics, and easy

18

rhythmic actions constitute the bulk of exercises. The advantage of a general warm-up is that the movements can apply to a variety of activities or sports, are easy to prescribe, and are effective in increasing body temperature if properly executed. Some disadvantages are that it may not be specific to some sports like gymnastics, which are highly skill- and technique-oriented; in addition, an athlete may in fact do too little or too much without a more prescribed programme.

Specific warm-up tends to be just that: exercises aimed at a particular individual in a specific sport or activity. Movements tend to be similar to the activity about to take place, but are incorporated at a reduced level. The principal aim is to prepare the individual both physically and mentally, especially prior to performance or competition involving special skills or coordination. This form of warm-up varies greatly amongst individuals and sports, even between members of the same team or those competing against each other in the same event.

There is often a degree of crossover between the three methods, especially between general and specific warm-up. Often athletes will begin with an easy general warm-up followed by a more specific programme tailored to their individual sporting needs.

Intensity and duration

The intensity and duration of any warm-up must be defined according to an athlete's own physical capabilities and will also reflect other factors such as environmental temperature, time of day, training vs competition, and other needs of the athlete. As a person becomes more physically conditioned, the amount of time and effort put into a warm-up will need to intensify because of the adaptive training response.[1] Acclimatisation to heat will also result in a person responding more efficiently to the increase in temperature, thus it will take longer to reach an optimal body core temperature. Therefore, a "recreational" athlete will need a far less intensive warm-up than an elite or more conditioned athlete.

A rise in core temperature of $1-2°C^{16}$ is usually sufficient to achieve the temperature-related benefits of warm-up. The increase in temperature and metabolic rate is noticeable usually by mild sweating and a slight increase in heart rate and breathing frequency. Warm-up, however, should not be so strenuous as to cause fatigue. The duration of any warm-up depends on the following: the individual and the activity, the environmental temperature, the time taken to achieve other goals of the warm-up such as mental and skill rehearsal. A warm-up of 5–10 minutes is often considered suitable for light or recreational activity, especially if the exercises form the basis of a general warm-up. This brief warm-up would alter significantly for a sprinter about to compete in a 200 m sprint where the warm-up, including stretching, might easily take up to an hour.

Injury prevention

It is generally accepted that a warm-up prior to exercise lowers the risk of injuries,[1,17–19] although some authors[20] dispute this claim. The available evidence to date is somewhat limited due, mainly, to the difficulty of conducting well controlled research. The reduction in incidence of injuries that is claimed is associated with an increase in tissue temperature sufficient to bring an increased blood flow to the exercising muscle as well as an increase in extensibility to the tendons, ligaments, and other connective tissue.[9] Both Heiser and colleagues[21] and Ekstrand and colleagues[22] concluded from their studies that inadequate warm-up and muscle tightness were associated with strains to the soft tissue.

Safran et al[12] found that muscle which was previously warmed displayed different mechanical behaviour to cold or unconditioned muscle. They were able to demonstrate by in vitro experiment that a greater force and increase in length were needed to tear isometrically preconditioned (warmed) muscle showing a relative increase in muscle elasticity. They concluded that physiological warming was beneficial in preventing muscular injury by increasing the elasticity of the muscle–tendon unit and length to failure. This conclusion was confirmed by Rosenbaum and Hennig[14] in their study on 50 male athletes where changes following static stretching and a 10 minute run warm-up resulted in improved muscle compliance and force development as well as decreased electromyographic (EMG) activity in the triceps surae muscle. The authors inferred that these changes could be viewed as reducing the risk of injury and enhancing performance.

Warm-down

A warm-down can be defined as a group of exercises performed immediately after an activity which provide an adjustment from exercise to rest.[23] These exercises are just as important as the warm-up, although they are often overlooked, especially following competition or a team game. The primary objective of warm-down following intense exercise is to prevent blood pooling in the lower extremities, therefore impeding the clearance of metabolites from the previously exercising muscles. By continuing to use the lower limbs, venous return is prevented from falling excessively by the action of the skeletal muscle "pump". This pump assists venous return by rhythmically squeezing the veins in the lower limbs, causing them to "empty" towards the right side of the heart. If intense exercise is stopped suddenly with no continued movement, venous return can drop precipitously, compromising cerebral perfusion. This may result in a fainting episode to remedy the shift in circulation.

A further objective of warm-down often combined with stretching is to help reduce delayed onset muscle soreness (DOMS)[24] or pain and to promote muscular relaxation. Whether warm-down or stretching have any beneficial effect on DOMS has been debated and is further discussed in the section on stretching (see below). Although the scientific data is controversial, much anecdotal evidence exists which supports the belief that warm-down and stretching help alleviate muscle soreness and the associated pain.

Finally, if stretching is to accompany the warm-down, it is advisable to perform the stretches immediately following the principal exercises in order to benefit from the higher tissue temperatures.

Psychological influence

The psychological aspects of warm-up have been well documented by Syer and Connolly,[25] although aspects of this area need further research. Warm-up prior to exercise can be used mentally to rehearse and prepare an athlete for an upcoming event or competition. Particular attention can be paid to an individual's emotional state and specific needs during this time. Generally, an individual or a team can attune to those factors which may otherwise affect a performance adversely, such as tension, or despondency, or faulty equipment. Factors which cannot be changed, like the weather, can be dealt with appropriately by individuals learning to change their response to the situation. Warm-up also acts as a constructive outlet for athletes' anxiety and frustration prior to competition.

Different psychological tools used in a warm-down can also be beneficial, i.e. the use of various meditation and relaxation techniques in the final phase of the warm-down period can enhance self-esteem. As the influence of psychology and psychological strategies surrounding sport becomes more accepted, this area is bound to grow in its application and use.

Stretching

Introduction

Stretching, like warm-up, is an important preparatory activity prior to exercise. Stretching exercises are the method(s) by which ROM increases around a joint. Flexibility can be defined as ROM around a joint or a series of joints or articulations; it is influenced by the bone and joint structure, as well as by the connective and soft tissue surrounding the joint. Flexibility should be regarded as joint-specific, although often it is incorrectly referred to in a general sense. Therefore, stretching to improve flexibility must focus on specific movements and on the muscles and joints unique to that movement.

Stretching as a primary component of fitness has been neglected; it is often assumed that an athlete, indeed a coach, "knows" how to stretch. This basic assumption underlies one of the primary problems governing stretching: the techniques are not well taught, possibly because there is a reluctance to acknowledge its importance as a basic component of fitness and there are still many individuals who query its benefits. Additionally, it is not always easy to perform a stretching exercise which must make correct use of body position and technique to derive maximum benefit.

Benefits

The ability to move a joint easily through a ROM should be considered essential for a healthy body. Any individual who is restricted from movement due to disease or injury may suffer in their athletic performance or daily activities. The relative importance of flexibility as a component of physical fitness was first described by Cureton in 1941.[26] In this review, Cureton stated that leisure or recreational activities required a certain degree of flexibility. This view has been upheld and expanded by most experts in the field of physical conditioning and fitness, although until recently much of the data supporting this view was based on empirical rather than experimental evidence.[27] Most coaches and medical practitioners would agree that an appropriate ROM is essential in order to develop a good overall base of fitness and for successful performance. However, divergent views on the importance of flexibility in athletic performance result mainly from the lack of consistent scientific definitions, measurements, and determinants of flexibility.[28]

The potential benefits of incorporating a stretching programme into a training programme, or indeed as part of a general fitness regime can be described as virtually unlimited. This can be illustrated by modelling flexibility as a useful tool in meditation in order to unify both the mind and body; in turn this can be helpful in reducing stress and tension. Yoga, as an example, is a widely practised discipline which incorporates both the psychological and physical aspects, using various stretching positions or postures aligned with mental preparation to achieve a relaxed state.

There are many proponents who claim that stretching prior to and after exercise prevents injury and enhances or aids performance. As supporting evidence, there are few if any individuals or teams who do not engage in a warm-up and stretching session prior to competition because of one or more of these beliefs, despite the lack of much hard scientific data. This discussion will be further developed in the section, injury prevention, in this chapter.

Another important benefit of a stretching programme is the muscular relaxation it promotes. By helping to relax muscles, excessive tension is reduced. Chronic tension such as contracture is well known to shorten muscle which may reduce muscle strength as well as produce muscle tightness. Posture and muscular symmetry are also highly influenced by a stretching programme. Likewise, an individual needs to have good posture to execute well-controlled stretches. This subject is addressed in the section, posture and muscular symmetry, in this chapter.

There is empirical evidence that adequate mobility in the lower back, for example, may aid in reducing back disorders. Certainly, a well functioning lumbar spine needs an acceptable ROM in order to stay problem- or pain-free. Stretching exercises incorporated into a warm-down have also been stated to help reduce muscle soreness, although there is disagreement regarding both the aetiology concerning muscle pain or soreness and whether stretching does reduce or eliminate it.

Wessel and Wan[29] concluded from their study that a stretching protocol, performed either before or after eccentric exercise, does not reduce DOMS. However, they studied sedentary subjects not used to exercise or stretching. It is likely that the one-off static stretching sequence itself (sitting hamstring stretch: 10 repetitions, each held for 60 seconds with a 10 second rest in between) may have caused some muscle damage in this study. Smith et al[30] reported that in subjects unaccustomed to exercise, static stretching in itself can induce DOMS. It is also known that this sitting stretch position for hamstrings is not reliable in controlling pelvic position.[31] A proper hamstring stretch is dependent on pelvic and back position. It is not clear whether Wessel and Wan controlled for pelvic position or technique in the hamstring stretching sequence. Rodenburg et al[32] studied the effect of a combination of a warm-up, stretching exercises, and massage on DOMS. The combination of all three protocols reduced some negative effects of eccentric exercise, but the results were inconsistent, suggesting a need for better controlled experiments yielding a more uniform picture of the influence of stretching and warm-up on DOMS.

Preparation or follow-up to exercise

Following warm-up or warm-down, stretching exercises should be performed as dictated by the athletes' needs, goals of the training programme, environmental factors, and any other extenuating factors such as a recent injury or post-competition muscle tightness. In achieving and maintaining an adequate ROM the ultimate goal dictates that there are no marked adhesions or abnormalities in or around the joint nor any muscular strains or limitations. Williford et al[33] found that large muscles which are actively warmed prior to stretching appear to produce significant gains in ROM when compared to stretch only or to control groups. Additionally, Wiemann and Hahn[34] reported that ROM in the hamstrings was increased and electromyographic (EMG) activity decreased following a short term static and ballistic stretch as well as a 5 minute stationary cycle warm-up. Their results indicated, however, that while warm-up exercises such as stationary cycling reduced muscle resting tension, no decrease in tension was found in short term stretching alone. This suggests that warm-up exercises are important in reducing muscle tightness.

Performance enhancement

The data supporting the importance of appropriate levels of flexibility in enhancing, indeed maximising performance are increasingly positive. A poor ROM may limit an individual's stride length or gait pattern and inhibit muscle power. Godges et al[2] found that a well controlled static stretching programme performed at the hip resulted in significant improvement in gait economy. Gleim and associates,[35] however, did not find such a correlation between muscle tightness and treadmill walking or jogging. Their method of assessing whether an individual was "loose", "normal", or "tight" was based on gross observation and may not have been reliable.

Research by Wilson et al[36] concluded that experienced male power-lifters had gains of 5.4% in performing rebound bench press lifts, compared to a control group following a training regime which included shoulder flexibility exercises. It was postulated that performance enhancement resulting from flexibility training was directly related to a reduction in the series–elastic component stiffness of the muscles and tendons involved.

Injury prevention

Evidence to support the claim that stretching alone prevents injuries is contradictory, owing much to the complication in conducting research that isolates stretching (from warm-up) as a protocol. Additionally, it is difficult, if not unethical, to conduct research which aims to cause injury in a person to determine what prevents it from occurring. The relationship between flexibility and injury has been stated by Gleim and McHugh[28] to be multi-factorial and possibly more complicated than originally supposed. These researchers review in detail the debate on this subject.

Yet, there are many authors who state that adequate ROM or flexibility may increase an athlete's ability to avoid some injuries.[24] Indeed, athletes with suitable flexibility may be able to use their body more effectively. When an injury situation presents itself, the muscles and joints involved may be able to withstand the extreme torque or stress which a less flexible person could not resist. Each sport has its own inherent risks and the requirements to be fit to play. Flexibility should be included: it is essential to have a ROM that slightly exceeds that which is required for the sport in order to compensate for any movements that take a joint beyond that which is usually needed.

Ekstrand et al[17] found a correlation between muscle tightness and strains in a prospective study of senior division male soccer players. A prophylactic programme of warm-up and proprioceptive neuromuscular facilitation (PNF) stretching combined with a warm-down resulted in a 75% reduction in injuries when compared to a control group of players. In a further study, Worrell and colleagues[37] compared isokinetic strength and flexibility measures between hamstring-injured and non-injured athletes matched by motor dominance and sport. Results indicated that the injured extremity was significantly less flexible than the non-injured extremity within the hamstring-injured group, and the hamstring-injured group was less flexible than the non-injured group. Data in this study also support the conclusion that flexibility was the single most important characteristic of the hamstring-injured athlete, not muscle strength or hamstring/quadriceps muscle group ratio, although both were implicated. In a retrospective study, Heiser et al[21] also concluded that a greater emphasis on stretching along with a strength training programme designed to increase hamstring/quadriceps muscle imbalances resulted in a reduction of primary and recurrent injuries in American football players.

Most frequently it is the antagonist muscle as well as its tendinous attachment which is torn due partly to its inability to relax rapidly as well as the large contractile force of the agonist, and any momentum which accompanies the movement. Too often, blame is directed stating that stretching did not in fact prevent an injury. It is imperative that an injury is qualified. It is hard to see how stretching can prevent all injuries, especially acute or contact injuries involving bone or cartilage. Finally, the area is complicated by the unquestionable role that chance plays in an acute injury.

Posture and muscular symmetry

Posture and muscle balance are extremely important when undertaking a flexibility programme. Too often this aspect is overlooked when teaching flexibility exercises, resulting in the stretching programme being less effective in achieving its goals. In order to perform a stretch correctly an individual must adopt the correct posture and starting position. Sullivan and colleagues[31] concluded in their study "Effect of pelvic position and stretching method on hamstring muscle flexibility" that pelvic position was more important than stretching technique in increasing hamstring flexibility. Following this, any stretching technique used should be based on the goals of the individual as well as muscle symmetry or balance.

Tight muscles tend to have an increased tone; this can influence the antagonist, causing it to weaken, precipitating a muscle imbalance with the agonist. This in turn can predispose an athlete to increased injuries such as muscle strain.[19,37,38] Thus the ultimate aim of any stretching programme is to maintain muscle balance. This is achieved by incorporating correct stretching techniques taking account of posture balanced by proper strengthening exercises.

It is recommended that athletes maintain a specific strength ratio between agonist and antagonist: for example, in quadriceps and hamstrings, the strength ratio should be a minimum of 60% hamstring to quadricep strength to avoid injury. Likewise, an athlete with a 10% or greater strength difference between a major muscle and its contralateral side is felt to be at greater risk for muscle–tendon injury to the weaker muscle group.[19]

Limitations to flexibility

There are a number of factors that determine a person's ROM or loss of ROM around a joint. Flexibility can be improved upon at any age, given the appropriate training; however, neither the rate nor potential for improvement will be the same for each individual. Limitations to flexibility can be broadly defined into both general and specific categories. General reasons for ROM limitation include gender, age, and somatotype of an individual.

Women tend to be more flexible than men due partly to anatomical differences, although not all discrepancies can be attributed to this. Specifically, women tend to be broader in the hips, the pelvic region being adapted for childbearing. It has also been suggested that women have a greater potential for flexibility due to their lower centre of gravity and shorter leg length.[23] To some degree, however, social and cultural influences in sport and activity dictate a person's flexibility state. One needs only to look at sports such as male gymnastics or karate and power-lifting to note the extensive ROM seen in these athletes.

The ageing process of muscle follows a collective decline in function that appears to affect flexibility as much as it affects strength. It is highly variable, depending on the individual, the muscle or the joint itself, and the extent to which a person remains active as well as injury- and disease-free.

An attempt to relate somatotype to flexibility has been investigated over the years although the research is inconsistent.[23] What appears to be more important is the specificity governing flexibility; ROM is joint-specific. Therefore, it follows that if an individual is flexible in one joint, it is not automatic that this same ROM applies to any other joint. This concept is based on the premise that different musculatures, soft tissue, and bony structures are uniquely involved in full joint movement. Thus there is no one measurement which will give a reliable overall flexibility rating or characteristic for an individual.

More specific reasons governing limitations to ROM include the type of connective tissue and its properties (such as scar tissue) both in the muscle and around the joint. This is an influential component and in the majority of individuals is the primary limitation to ROM. Other limitations include: the bone and joint structure; tension of the muscle (due to the stretch reflex); lack of strength and/or coordination in the muscle; certain pathologies and injuries such as osteoarthritis and the temperature of the soft tissue (see physiology of warm-up earlier in this chapter).

The viscoelastic nature of muscle, tendons, ligaments, and connective tissue suggest that a stretching regime will result in greater flexibility or ROM at a particular joint.[15] A muscle can lengthen up to 50% of its resting length; as it stretches, the connective tissue with both its viscous and elastic properties also stretches. A loss of ROM to a joint often occurs as a result of strains or sprains to the muscle and other soft tissue. An injury to the soft tissue can induce inhibition to the joint as well as cause excessive scar tissue to form, especially if rehabilitation is poor.

Hypermobility

An extreme ROM or laxity in a joint, often termed hypermobility, may result in increased predisposition to joint injuries such as subluxation or dislocation. An excessive degree of stretch is best avoided, although ROM varies in its natural degree among individuals.

If a person has hypermobile joints, it is of paramount importance to strengthen the surrounding muscles to bring the joint more into balance and control. It is critical that ROM is not augmented, especially at the expense of strengthening. Joints which are hypermobile tend to be more susceptible to injury, especially in contact sports. In gymnastics, for example, individuals do have excessive ROM as this is what the sport requires; however, in those gymnasts who are well trained, this large ROM at a joint is balanced by strong muscles.

Some clinicians state that an excessive increase in flexibility can decrease joint stability; this in turn would predispose the individual to various sprains or strains to the soft tissue. In theory this may sound plausible, yet Requa and Garrick[39] state there is little evidence to support that this is what actually happens. They contend that flexibility training usually occurs as part of an inclusive programme where adequate strength and muscle balance are improved through full ROM; therefore, joints are not any more prone to injury.

Stretching techniques

There are principally three traditional techniques by which to describe stretching in a sporting context: **static**, **ballistic**, and **proprioceptive neuromuscular facilitation** (PNF). Both static and ballistic methods of stretching have been used for many years. All three methods and their variations increase flexibility and therefore can be recommended, each with its own advantages and disadvantages.

Static stretching

Static or slow stretching is possibly the oldest and the most common technique in use. It is produced by taking a joint and its associated antagonistic muscle group(s) to end or near end-of-range and holding the lengthened position as tension slowly decreases. Recommendations for length of hold vary considerably from as short as 3 seconds to 60 seconds and longer. Based on neurophysiological principles 10 seconds appears to be a minimum duration to induce relaxation in the muscle by invoking the inverse myotatic reflex as discussed in applied neurophysiology of stretching, later in this chapter. Repetitions of up to three to four times per muscle group have been suggested, although there is no consensus on whether it is best or even needed to repeat a stretch so many times. Data are inconclusive or lacking regarding whether to hold a stretch for 60 seconds or to hold the same stretch for 20 seconds and repeat three times.

This method tends to be the safest to perform, and is therefore often reasoned to have the least associated injury risk.[40] Lengthening a muscle to its end ROM and holding it there in a static stretch seems unlikely to produce injury to the soft tissue unless the muscle is overstretched or body positioning is incorrect.

Arguments against static stretching claim that the technique, because of its relative ease, may be performed at the expense of other methods such as ballistic and PNF stretching, which incorporate a strengthening component to the stretch.

Ballistic stretching

This form of stretching has had few advocates in recent years.[23,24,39,41] Most authors cite the danger involved in performing this stretch as exceeding the extensibility limit of the tissues as a result of the repetitive bouncing actions. A ballistic stretch usually involves rhythmic type movements that may extend to full range. The term dynamic flexibility is often interchanged with ballistic, and refers to the maximum ROM of a joint during a ballistic movement, or its ease of movement within the obtainable ROM. Gleim and McHugh[28] state that the important measurement in dynamic flexibility is "stiffness", a mechanical term defined as the resistance of a structure to deformation or the opposite of compliance.

The major debate against ballistic stretching involves the following issues: tissue adaptation; muscle soreness from small tears of the tissue, termed microtrauma; and initiation of the stretch reflex. When tissues are stretched too quickly, there is no time for adaptation to occur; permanent lengthening of tissues is dependent on long duration stretch under low force. The swinging motion of ballistic stretching also produces an angular momentum that may exceed the absorbing capacity of the tissue being stretched.[23] Therefore, flexibility may not be optimally developed. In fact, overstretching may occur leading to muscle soreness and injury. Over time, this may lead to build-up of scar tissue which, in due course, can alter the biomechanics of the joint.[39,41] In addition, the stretch reflex is activated when a sudden stretch is applied causing the muscles to contract. If the stretch is continually repeated the increased tension will not allow for muscular relaxation, one of the purposes of stretching.

Ballistic stretch, however, mirrors most types of activities such as kicking, jumping, and throwing; thus there is an argument that it may have an important role in maintaining flexibility in sports like the martial arts, track and field, and dance which involve fast repetitive movements performed to full ROM. If such ballistic actions are not practised, and at speed, then injury may occur in performance during explosive actions. In their study of dancers, Moscov et al[42] found that exercises which improved static flexibility did not equally improve dynamic flexibility, although the authors stated that dynamic flexibility is possibly a more valid indicator of success in ballistic activities like dance. Ballistic stretching, if undertaken, should only take place in a properly controlled environment where the individual is well warmed up, is fully aware of the dangers involved in the stretch, and knows how to execute the movement properly.

PNF stretching

The techniques used in PNF stretching were first devised in the 1950s and employed by physiotherapists for treating patients with various types of neuromuscular paralysis or joint mobility deficits. Their use in a sporting context to improve flexibility is a relatively recent conversion. This form of stretch typically involves a partner, although there are ways to do PNF stretching without one.

There are a number of different PNF techniques currently in use in sport with three techniques – hold–relax (HR), contract–relax (CR) and contract–relax agonist–contract (CRAC) – arguably being the most popular as well as the most effective non-therapeutic stretching methods.[1,43] All involve some combination of alternating contraction and reflex relaxation of both the agonist and antagonist muscle groups, invoking stretch receptors in the muscle as well as the tendon (see applied neurophysiology of stretching, opposite).

In a straight-leg hamstring stretch using a HR technique the muscle is first taken to its lengthened position. The individual pushes against the partner's resistance to produce an isometric contraction in the antagonist muscle (hamstring) as the partner opposes the contraction. This position is held for 10 seconds at which time the hamstring muscles relax while the partner increases passive pressure to further increase ROM. The sequence is then repeated, usually three times. The CR technique is a variation in which the hamstring muscles are isotonically contracted, so that the leg moves toward the floor during the push phase. The CRAC technique is identical to HR, except that following the push phase the agonist muscle (quadriceps) contracts (the individual maintains the leg in a straight position) for up to 10 seconds before the relaxation phase, at which point a passive stretch is applied to the antagonist muscle. There is some debate regarding force of contraction in the push phase of a PNF stretch; currently, most advocates state a submaximal versus a maximal muscular contraction is all that is required to produce optimal results.

Etnyre and Lee[43] compiled a comparative summary of stretching techniques which overwhelmingly found that PNF methods produced a greater ROM than static or ballistic stretching methods, suggesting that these methods are more effective overall.

Moore and Hutton[44] demonstrated in well trained female gymnasts using three different stretch techniques (static, CR, and CRAC), that maximum range of hip flexion was obtained with the CRAC stretch technique. This technique appeared to be the preferred method for achieving maximum gains in flexibility, possibly because the subjects were well motivated, experienced and there was sufficient time to practise the procedure. The authors concluded that if comfort and limited training time were major factors then static stretching was the more desirable technique to employ.

Other methods

Stretching can also be classified by the more therapeutic approach generally used by physiotherapists, termed active and passive. Active stretching now has a more defined basis in the sporting context. Active stretching involves moving an agonist in an isometric or isotonic contraction to its full range; length of hold can vary. This form of stretching is most useful as it applies to movement in general and helps extend not only the ROM of a joint but also develops strength and control in the surrounding muscle. A classic example would be a dancer doing an arabesque which involves standing on one leg while actively extending the hip keeping both knees straight and the pelvis neutral. The degree of ROM achieved would depend on hamstring, hip, and lower spine flexibility as well as standing leg, lumbar spine, and abdominal strength and control.

Passive stretching involves movement where the individual makes no active contribution. Rather, the work is performed by an outside force, such as a spring or traction, or by another person. Often passive stretching is employed because the agonist is injured or weakened, or attempts to inhibit the antagonist fail. Some benefits of passive stretching include partner-based stretching. However, there are some contraindications to passive stretching:

- Passive stretching taken to extremes of ROM may be painful and cause damage to muscle and connective tissue.
- The retention of flexibility may be jeopardised due to the limited motor learning response of the agonist. This in turn may affect muscle balance.

Applied neurophysiology of stretching

The musculotendinous system has an intrinsic protective system comprised of muscle spindles and Golgi tendon organs (GTOs). The primary function of these sensory nerve receptors, which are involved in the stretch reflex, is to prevent overstretching of the passive joint structures and the muscle/ tendon unit.

The primary stretch receptors in skeletal muscle are the muscle spindles which are found encased in connective tissue lying parallel to the contractile units. They are sensitive to changes in length of the muscle as well as the rate or velocity of stretch. When muscle spindles fire, they initiate the stretch reflex which acts to contract the stretched muscle thereby taking tension off the muscle spindle allowing relaxation to occur. The GTOs are responsible for detecting tension in a tendon and are primarily located in the musculotendinous junction. They tend to lie in line with the transmission of force from muscle to insertion at the bone; unlike the muscle spindle, they therefore lie in series with the muscle rather than in parallel. GTOs are stimulated by passive stretch as well as by contraction of the muscle, although they are most sensitive to excessive tension generated by contraction or by elongation of the tendon. When this occurs, an inhibitory impulse is sent to the muscle causing a reflex relaxation which removes the excess tension. This is termed the inverse myotatic reflex or autogenic inhibition. The action of the GTOs is powerful enough to override the

31

excitatory impulse of the muscle spindles and is a protective mechanism which prevents injury, especially shearing from attachments to both tendons and muscle.

When a static stretch is initiated, the muscle spindles fire which causes the muscle to contract reflexly and therefore to resist the stretch. If the stretch of the muscle continues for at least 6 seconds,[1] the GTOs respond by causing a reflex relaxation that further invokes the muscle to stretch through relaxation before the extensibility limits are exceeded. The effectiveness of static as well as PNF stretching is based in part on these neurophysiological principles.

Stretching guidelines

General principles for flexibility training should include the following:

- Begin the stretch session having decided on the type of stretching method, the stretch exercises themselves, and any variations to be used. These decisions will be determined in part by length of time, goals of the stretch session, and any limitations placed upon the individual.
- Emphasise breathing, using deep slow breaths and focusing on the exhalation to bring about greater muscle relaxation. Avoid breath-holding at all times.
- Focus on the muscle being stretched to facilitate a further increase in muscle relaxation and to gain the maximum benefits from the stretch.
- Stretch with warmed muscles as both connective and contractile tissue is more receptive to lengthening; this will give a more effective stretch and eliminate any potential strains due to stretching cold tissue.
- Stretch after an active warm-up, but before engaging in an energetic activity, training session, or performance. Likewise make sure stretching follows a training and/or warm-down period.
- Position the body correctly, watching overall posture. Correct placement of the hip and lumbar spine is especially important.
- Hold stretches for longer duration (10–60 seconds) when performing a static stretch to utilise the full neurophysiological reflex benefits. The stretch can be repeated, often to increase ROM, especially if the muscle is relaxed.
- When performing a ballistic or dynamic stretch ensure the muscles and joints are well warmed up. Start off with mid-range movements at slower speed before continuing on to more difficult end-of-range movements at speed.
- PNF stretching should only be undertaken by those individuals with appropriate training, especially when performing stretches post-injury or as part of a rehabilitation programme.

- Avoid stretching that is painful or severe. Overstretching can cause muscle strains and defeats the objective in the first place. A muscle can be taken to its end-of-range, assuming this is pain-free, but avoid further increases in ROM.
- Stretching on a daily basis would be ideal to maintain ROM; however, at a minimum, stretching exercises should comprise equal importance along with other components of fitness in a training programme. To this end, how often flexibility is performed varies between individuals, depending on the many limiting factors which may be implicated, the goals of the stretching programme, and the sport or activity involved.

Stretching exercises

The ability to improve or maintain flexibility around a joint is easily achieved by incorporating a programme of exercises which are suitable for an individual and consistent with his/her sport, level of performance, overall goals, general characteristics, such as gender or age, and any limitations (e.g. previous injuries or a hypermobile joint). The following set of exercises are a useful list of some of the more practical and effective stretches that can be quite easily used by most athletes of any age. The exercises have been chosen as some of the better if not the most effective stretches for the major muscle groups. A more exhaustive listing of stretches, especially at an advanced level, can be found in Alter's *Science of flexibility*.[23] However, the given exercises are quite adaptable and variations and modifications are easily applied. Try to be creative and assess the overall goals.

Those athletes with any limitations should be made aware of any contraindications and avoid a particular stretch as necessary. Before performing the stretches, an individual must ensure he/she is well warmed up and suitably dressed in exercise clothes approriate for the temperature and activity. Often after a warm-up an individual may throw on a sweatshirt or track suit to maintain body heat during the stretching session. Remember to follow the advice given in the section on stretching guidelines to gain the most from any stretch. It cannot be emphasised enough that posture, beginning position, type of stretch used (static vs PNF), and execution of the stretch or the overall technique are what depict a "good" stretch and ·make it effective.

Terminology

The stretches are described in terms of:

- **Muscle/joint stretched** This characterises the primary muscle(s) to be stretched, although both the joint and secondary muscles will also be

33

affected, especially if variations of the main stretch are employed. It is important to be aware of overstretching the muscle or causing strain to the joint.

- **Beginning position** The initial start to a stretch will help determine the overall effectiveness. Be aware of good posture, especially in the back, pelvis, and shoulders and correct any positional faults before you proceed with the stretch.
- **Execution of stretch** A description of how to perform each stretch will follow. Decisions regarding the type of stretch used must be made prior to the execution. Often, a combination of methods is used, such as actively moving a limb (slowly and controlled) through a full ROM followed by a static stretch with a long hold. Try to relax during the stretch by utilising correct breathing techniques. All stretch exercises should be performed on both limbs or sides to ensure balance.
- **Cautions and points to consider** Each exercise will have its own safety issues to consider in executing the stretch. This section will detail any such items as well as contraindications for special groups.
- **Variations of the theme** This section will highlight the many variations that can be used with a stretch. This may involve a positional change or use of a towel for instance to increase leverage in a stretch. Many of the variations will challenge an individual as they become more proficient in the exercises as well as altering the training regime to alleviate boredom. Often the straight traditional form of a stretch will not be sufficient in terms of extending the muscle or joint to full ROM and a variation will overcome this. Many of the stretches can be enhanced with a partner, especially using PNF techniques. Not all variations can be highlighted, therefore it is important to individualise a programme to suit each individual's specific needs and preferences.

Stretch 1: achilles tendon stretch

Muscle/joint stretched: Gastrocnemius (with knee extended); soleus (with knee flexed).

Beginning position: Start standing facing a wall or other similar support using your arms for stability. Position your right leg back, keeping the knee straight, foot flat and perpendicular to the wall with the heel down. This stretches the gastrocnemius. Repeat the same stretch bending the knee. This targets the soleus. The opposite forward leg is relaxed and slightly bent.

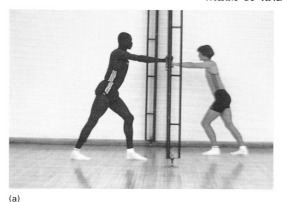

(a)

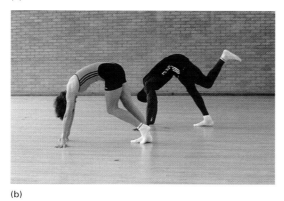

(b)

Figure 2.1   Achilles tendon stretch: (a) standard technique; (b) variation

Execution of stretch: After positioning the feet lean forward bending the elbows and keeping the hips in line with the shoulders. This should increase dorsiflexion of the right ankle.

Cautions and points to consider: Watch heel and hip position. Make sure weight is pushed forward and downward. Remember to switch legs and stretch each calf.

Variations of the theme: This stretch can be performed with the foot in external or internal rotation which stresses the medial and lateral sides of the achilles and calf. A more advanced form of this stretch is to place the hands on the floor in pike position, head and neck in line with the shoulders with the feet in the same position as described above. This also stretches the hamstrings, shoulders, and upper spine especially if you push downward. Another variation involves standing on the back of a stair and dropping the heel downward; this will increase the stretch in the achilles and calf.

35

Stretch 2: running stretch

Muscle/joint stretched: General groin region: hamstring and gluteals of the right forward leg; iliopsoas (hip flexors), rectus femoris of the left extended rear leg.

Beginning position: In a standing position with feet hip width apart in parallel position lunge forward with the right leg, bending the knee at 90° (or wider if flexibility allows). Keep the foot flat and in line with the knee and body. Support your weight with your arms placed to either side of the forward knee.

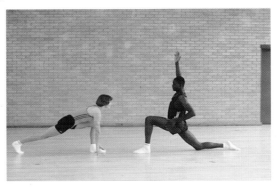

Figure 2.2   Running stretch

Execution of stretch: (i) Press your weight downward through the pelvis allowing the arms to relax and elbows to bend as needed. Initially, keep the extended left leg relatively straight and in line with the body. After holding the stretch for the required duration, (ii) bend the rear extended knee down to the floor and relax the foot. Press forward. Hold the position and balance; extend the upper trunk keeping the abdominals tight and placing the left hip in extension. Your left arm can be extended overhead for balance or both arms placed on your hips or a supporting chair.

Cautions and points to consider: Keep the weight of the right knee over the whole foot and watch for any movement from the centre line. In (ii) watch for any tilting movements of the pelvis. Ensure the left extended knee is kept bent in a wide angle and the hip and trunk are extended in order to stretch iliopsoas. In some individuals placing a towel or mat under the left knee prevents any soreness to the patella.

Variations of the theme: In (i) you can place both arms inside the right knee while rotating the knee slightly outwards to gain more ROM. In (ii)

36

a slight variation in stretch to the hip flexors will occur if the left hip is rotated slightly inward.

Stretch 3: straddle stretch

Muscle/joint stretched: Hip adductors including gracilis; hamstring and spinal extensors.

Beginning position: Sitting, place your legs in an open straddle position with your spine straight and your feet pointed upwards. Keep the pelvis in neutral position.

Execution of stretch: Make sure the hands are "grounded" and placed on the floor and/or on the legs to control the stretch. Try to press forward in an anterior tilt of the pelvis keeping the spine relatively straight. As you press forward try to open your legs wider. Make sure the shoulders are relaxed and the abdominals are contracted. Rotate the shoulders and the trunk so they turn "square" over the right hip and leg. Keeping this position, rest the left hand on the right leg across the knee and the other hand can press into the floor to the side of the right leg to maintain stability. Press forward as before.

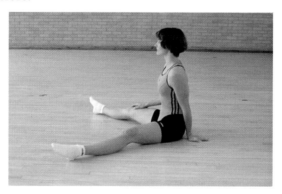

Figure 2.3   Straddle stretch

Cautions and points to consider: For those who find this a difficult stretch, the main aim is just to sit straight and try to tilt the pelvis forward or hollow the back. This will stretch both the adductors and the hamstrings. Watch curving the thoracolumbar junction in an attempt to bring the head down towards the floor. **Do not try to touch the head towards the**

37

floor! The emphasis should be a relatively straight spine, pelvis in anterior tilt, relaxed shoulders, and tight abdominals. Make sure the knees and especially the feet do not roll inward.

Variations of the theme: Using a towel placed around the foot may help control the stretch and keep correct positioning.

Partner stretch: This stretch can be performed with a partner who pushes from the back using their leg as a brace placed up against the athlete's spine while holding on to their shoulders to keep correct pelvic and shoulder positions. This forward press coupled with proper breathing can enhance the stretch. A second partner stretch can be performed with a partner sitting astride in front of the athlete with their feet placed just above the inside of the athlete's knees. The partner links arms with the athlete above the elbow and gently pulls the athlete forward. The athlete must keep the spine straight while tilting the pelvis forward. Again, emphasise correct posture and breathing.

Finally, a degree of lateral side stretch can be made by stretching the arms up and over to either side making sure the extended arm is kept relatively straight and externally rotated and the elbow is positioned alongside the ear.

Stretch 4: groin stretch

Muscle/joint stretched: (i) Hip adductors; gluteal muscles. (ii) Hip adductors.

Beginning position: (i) Start standing with legs wide apart and feet turned out approximately 45°. Squat down with thighs parallel to the floor and knees bent at a 90° angle. (ii) Sit up straight with knees bent and soles of the feet together; grasp the lower leg or ankle and allow the elbows to rest on the knees or legs

Execution of stretch: (i) Gently press the knees open with the elbow, positioning each knee over the foot and stabilising the body. (ii) Slowly lean the trunk forward keeping the pelvis in neutral or anterior tilt and press the knees downward and hold.

Cautions and points to consider: (i) Make sure the foot is not externally rotated too far and that the knee is positioned over the foot. The bent knee must form a 90° angle or wider for the stretch to be effective. This stretch

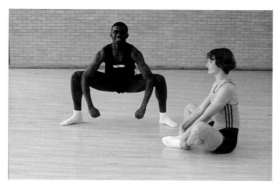

Figure 2.4   Groin stretch: version (i) on left and (ii) on right

may place stress on the medial meniscus; avoid if stretch is painful. (ii) Watch the position of the spine which should be kept straight as you lean forward; do not drop the head.

Variations of the theme: In (ii) alter the position of the feet by pulling in closer to the pelvis for a more advanced stretch or releasing away for a more relaxed or easy stretch. A PNF stretch can also be added: as you press down on the knees with your elbow resist this by pulling upward; an isometric contraction will follow. Hold for 10 seconds then relax. Repeat in a hold–relax PNF stretch.

Stretch 5: lateral side stretch

Muscle/joint stretched: Latissimus dorsi; oblique abdominals; quadratus lumborum; teres major.

Beginning position: (i) Stand with feet hip- or shoulder-width apart and arms loosely at your sides. Relax the knees and shoulders and make sure the abdominals are contracted. (ii) Sit in a comfortable crossed-leg position. Make sure the abdominals are contracted and shoulders are relaxed.

Execution of stretch: In (i) and (ii) reach upward with the right arm and lean towards the left side. Keep the right arm extended and internally rotated and the crook of the elbow by the right ear. In (i) the left arm can relax by the side (more advanced) or be placed on the hip or down the left thigh for support. In (ii) the left arm, externally rotated, provides support with a bent elbow and relaxed shoulder.

39

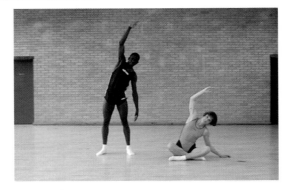

Figure 2.5   Lateral side stretch: version (i) on left and (ii) on right

Cautions and points to consider: (i) and (ii) Ensure that there is no rotational movement about the spine. The hips and shoulders should be kept "in-line" facing forward; the emphasis should be directed not only on lateral flexion, but an upward extension. Keeping the abdominals contracted will help control any outward hip displacement.

Variations of the theme: At an advanced level stretch (i) can also be performed kneeling with the left leg abducted to stretch the hip adductors. A caution: this may impart a valgus force to the knee or overstretch the medial ligaments.

Stretch 6: quad stretch

Muscle/joint stretched: Rectus femoris; vastus intermedius, vastus lateralis, vastus medialis; iliopsoas.

Beginning position: (i) Stand on your left leg holding on to a wall or other support. Bend your right knee and grasp the ankle from behind with the right hand. (ii) Lie prone with knees together. Relax your head on your left arm. Bend your right knee and reach around and grasp your ankle.

Execution of stretch: (i) Pull your leg backward keeping the knees together and the pelvis in neutral position. (ii) Lengthen your leg from the hip then extend the hip and pull the knee backward trying to raise the thigh off the floor.

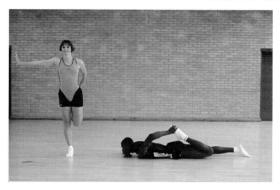

Figure 2.6   Quad stretch: version (i) on left and (ii) on right

Cautions and points to consider: **Avoid allowing the knee to drift outward!** (i) Try to avoid leaning forward or tilting the pelvis, which increases the lumbar curve. Keep your spine straight and as you pull the leg back contract your abdominals and try to lengthen through the knee. (ii) Check for correct position, especially knee and hip placement. Keep the abdominal muscles tight. This position is unsuitable for women in the latter stages of pregnancy.

Variations of the theme: The greater the knee flexion the more intense the stretch in the lower rectus femoris. As hip extension increases there is a greater stretch on the upper rectus femoris. If there is difficulty in grasping the ankle a towel can be wrapped about the ankle for better leverage and pelvic control.

Stretch 7: hamstring stretch

Muscle/joint stretched: Hamstring muscle group.

Beginning position: Correct technique: In (a) lie on your back; relax your shoulders and keep your head on the floor. Clasp your hands behind your right knee and draw the bent leg up to your chest. Keep the left knee slightly bent and the foot flat on the floor (beginner) or the left leg extended, knee straight, and in neutral position (advanced).

Execution of stretch: Straighten the right leg slowly while maintaining the position of the left leg. The knee may straighten fully (more advanced) or be slightly bent (easier), depending on an individual's ROM and how

41

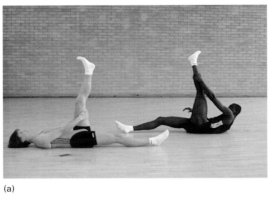

(a)

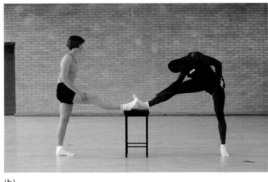

(b)

Figure 2.7   Hamstring stretch: (a) correct (on left) and incorrect (on right) technique; (b) advanced variation, showing correct (on left) and incorrect (on right) technique

"tight" the hamstrings might be. The stretch often starts with a bent right knee, keeping the foot up towards the ceiling, before progressing on to a straighter leg.

Standing variation: A more advanced variation of this stretch (b) involves standing and placing the right leg on a table or other support while facing forward. Keep the hips in line with the shoulders and avoid externally rotating both the standing and stretching leg. Bend forward over the right leg keeping an anterior tilt to the pelvis. The goal is to lean forward emphasising a straight spine and try to bring the abdomen, not the head, down towards the thigh.

Cautions and points to consider: Incorrect technique: stretch (a) is easily done quite poorly! Often an individual tries to straighten their right leg fully, although they do not have the flexibility to do so. This usually causes them to lift their head and buttocks and tense their shoulders. The left leg

42

often drifts off to the side and is not kept in neutral alignment as the pelvis tilts posteriorly. Muscle spasms often occur in the leg due to overstretching.

Variations of the theme: Using a towel increases the leverage and control in stretch (a). Wrap a towel around the foot of the right leg instead of using your clasped hands. This is effective when doing your own PNF stretches. Alter the emphasis of the hamstring muscles being stretched by internally or externally rotating the right hip. Incorporate dynamic leg raises combined with active stretching to increase strength as well as ROM. This stretch is well adapted to using a partner to perform either passive or PNF stretching techniques.

Stretch 8: spinal rotator stretch

Muscle/joint stretched: Spine; hip abductors and external rotators; oblique abdominals.

Beginning position: Begin by lying on your back. (i) Bend the right knee towards your chest and hold it with your left hand. Place your right arm abducted to the side at a 90° angle. (ii) Bend both knees towards your chest. Abduct both arms to 90°.

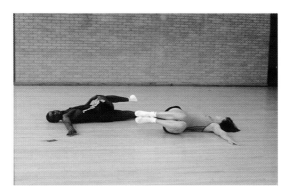

Figure 2.8   Spinal rotator stretch: version (i) on left and (ii) on right

Execution of stretch: (i) Make sure the left leg is extended fully as you rotate your right leg across your chest towards the floor. Press down on the right knee as you tuck your left hip under. Keep the right shoulder pressed to the floor and the arm extended, palm flat. (ii) Rotate both knees to the left, while pressing the right shoulder to the floor.

43

Cautions and points to consider: (i) Be careful not to overstretch by trying to bring the right knee to the floor. Keep the left leg fully extended. (i) and (ii) Watch the position of the right shoulder. Keep the abdominals contracted.

Variations of the theme: By altering the angle of hip flexion you will emphasise the stretch of different muscles in the hip abductors and level of the spine. A more advanced version of this stretch can be performed by straightening the right leg after you cross the chest. Make sure the right leg is bent as you cross the chest and return to neutral to avoid too much stress on the spine.

This stretch combines well with the hamstring stretch (a) (Stretch 7).

Stretch 9: spinal twist

Muscle/joint stretched: Spine; hip abductors.

Beginning position: Begin in a sitting position, legs fully extended. Make sure that the spine is straight.

Execution of stretch: Bend your right knee and cross the right leg over the left placing the right heel as close to the left hip as possible. Support the position with your right arm placed around the back, hand on the floor. Rotate your chest towards the right bringing your left hand or elbow to the lateral aspect of your right leg. The stretch can be increased by pulling

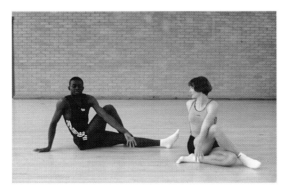

Figure 2.9   Spinal twist: correct technique for standard (on left) and advanced (on right) version

the right knee in closer to your chest and rotating around more. Repeat the sequence on the other side.

Cautions and points to consider: Try to relax the shoulders by depressing them. It is vital that the spine is kept straight. This stretch may be difficult for those with a knee injury. The position is also difficult for pregnant women in the third trimester or those who carry excessive fat around the abdomen.

Variations of the theme: Rotate your trunk to the left side, "opening up" and placing the left hand behind your buttocks for support. Bring the right arm across the right knee. A more advanced version involves bending the left leg under the right. The heel of the right foot is then placed just in front of the bent left knee. Make sure your weight is distributed evenly on the pelvis and you do not lean to the left side.

Stretch 10: gluteal stretch

Muscle/joint stretched: Gluteal muscles; upper hamstring.

Beginning position: Begin by lying on your back. Bend the right knee towards your chest. Bend the left knee to 90° and place the left ankle on top of the right knee and hold the right knee with the right hand on top of the left ankle.

Execution of stretch: Grasp the right shin with your left hand as it weaves between your legs and pull both legs forward as a unit. At the same time

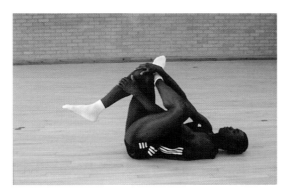

Figure 2.10 Gluteal stretch

45

try to push the left knee open which places a stretch on the left gluteals and abductors.

Cautions and points to consider: This is often a difficult stretch to perform initially. Thus it may require some modifications in hand placement. Be careful not to arch the back in trying either to perform or further the stretch. Watch that you do not hold your breath and concentrate on contracting abdominals. Finally, relax your shoulders on the ground.

Variations of the theme: For a more advanced stretch alter the angle of flexion at the right hip by drawing the leg in a closer angle towards the chest. Press the left knee away from the centre to enhance the stretch.

Stretch 11: back extension

Muscle/joint stretched: Anterior lumbar spine; abdominals.

Beginning position: Lie prone on the floor with your body extended.

Execution of stretch: Place your palms by your chest with your hands facing forward. As you exhale, slowly press your hands down on the floor pushing your arms upward, keeping your hips flat on the floor. Extend as far as comfortable, keeping your elbows bent and your shoulders relaxed and depressed. Hold the stretch and relax to controlled breathing. Maintain your head in a relaxed position in line with the upper thoracic spine.

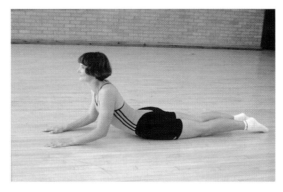

Figure 2.11   Back extension

Cautions and points to consider: At first it is best to extend only as far as resting your elbows on the ground. As ROM increases you may want to extend further, however you must keep your elbows bent and shoulders depressed. This stretch is not advisable for pregnant women due to the lying prone position. Additionally, it only emphasises the lordotic position of the back which the forward weight of the pregnancy places a woman in. Contracting the gluteal muscles may prevent excessive compression on the lower back.

Variations of the theme: A more advanced position places the hands further down toward the hips, giving a greater extension in the lumbar spine and stretch to the abdominals.

Stretch 12: back flexion

Muscle/joint stretched: Lumbar spine; thoracic spine; latissimus dorsi; deltoid.

Beginning position: (i) Begin by lying face down on the floor in a four-point position with the arms extended above the head, hands flat on the floor. (ii) Lie flat on the floor on your back and draw your knees toward your chest using your hands.

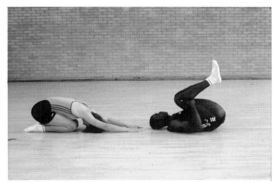

Figure 2.12 Back flexion: version (i) on left and (ii) on right

Execution of stretch: (i) Extend the arms as far as comfortable trying to keep elbows towards the floor, although they will be slightly raised if arms are fully extended. At the same time, the trunk and buttocks are pressed towards the floor and heels respectively to try to accentuate the stretch.

(ii) Take a deep breath and as you exhale press the knees down toward the chest trying to relax the head and shoulders.

Cautions and points to consider: Remember to control your breathing in both stretches. These exercises flex the lumbar spine without adding pressure to the upper spine and are useful for those suffering from lower back stiffness and pain.

Variations of the theme: In (i) and (ii) the stretches can be performed with the knees drawn apart in a V shape which places a different emphasis on the lumbar spine. This variation is also suitable for pregnant women who find the traditional position impossible in the last trimester. A further variation in (ii) involves opening the knees to either side of the chest and pressing the hands down on the soles of the feet which point to the ceiling; as you exhale press down even further on the heels. Try to bring the thighs down parallel to the floor.

Partner stretch: A partner can aid any of the above stretches by gently pressing on the lower back in (i) or the top of the knees in (ii) to increase ROM.

Stretch 13: combined abdominal and trunk stretch

Muscle/joint stretched: Iliopsoas; abdomen; lumbar spine; shoulder.

Beginning position: Start by sitting on the floor with the right leg straight in front of you, the left leg internally rotated at the hip and flexed at the knee to form a hurdler's stretch. Ensure that you are sitting with your hips square.

Execution of stretch: Flex the right knee bringing the foot towards your body. Place your right hand behind the right hip and start to push the hips forward as the trunk externally rotates to the right. Allow the hips to lead the movement as you extend the left arm upward and externally rotate. The head should relax as you focus backwards. Body weight should be taken through both knees and the right arm as the body forms a strong triangular base.

Cautions and points to consider: This stretch looks more complicated than it is! It is a very good stretch of the abdominals and trunk region, a difficult area to stretch. Make sure the hips are fully extended when executing the

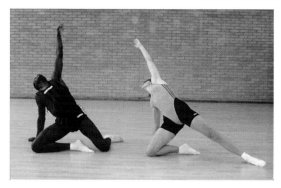

Figure 2.13   Combined abdominal and trunk stretch: correct technique for standard (on left) and advanced (on right) version

movement, and that the focus is backward to gain the full benefits of the stretch.

Variations of the theme: Altering the position of the right arm or drawing your legs in a more open position will alter the emphasis as well as the degree of rotation of the stretch to the spine and trunk. This stretch (advanced) can also be performed with the left leg abducted in a one-leg side straddle; as you extend the leg keep it straight in neutral position, pointing the toes.

Stretch 14: shoulder stretch

Muscle/joint stretched: Triceps; deltoid and pectorals.

Beginning position: (i) While standing relaxed, raise the right arm and position the hand behind the head and as far down the back as possible. (ii) Start standing and clasp the hands together behind your back.

Execution of stretch: (i) Move the left elbow behind the back with the hand reaching upward as far as possible. Ideally the fingers of both hands grasp. (ii) Keep both elbows extended and try to raise both arms upward while maintaining an upright position.

Cautions and points to consider: Watch that you don't allow your lower back to move into excess lordosis. In (ii) make sure the shoulders are relaxed and depressed while performing the stretch. It is quite normal for one arm to have more ROM than the other in both stretches.

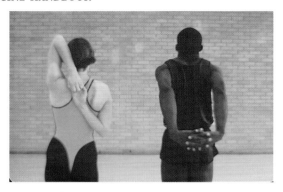

Figure 2.14   Shoulder stretch: version (i) on left and (ii) on right

Variations of the theme: (i) If you have trouble clasping your hands grab a towel and hold it between your hands; with time slowly move your fingertips closer together.

Stretch 15: triceps, deltoid, and posterior capsule

Muscle/joint stretched: (i) Triceps; (ii) deltoid; posterior capsule; triceps; infraspinatus; teres minor.

Beginning position: Begin by either standing or sitting upright in a chair.

Execution of stretch: (i) Raise your right arm and press your hand down your back between the shoulder blades. Place your left hand on your right

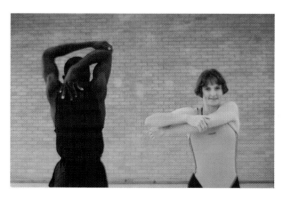

Figure 2.15   Triceps, deltoid, and posterior capsule: correct technique for (i) on left and (ii) on right

elbow for added leverage. Using your left hand push your right arm backwards and down the back keeping your head straight. (ii) Grasp above the right elbow with your left hand and pull the right arm across your chest.

Cautions and points to consider: Be careful not to hyperextend the lumbar spine when performing (i).

Variations of the theme: Stretch (i) can also be performed with both arms at once. With your hands, grasp the opposite elbow and raise both arms as high and far back as comfortable. The emphasis on stretch (ii) can be altered by raising or lowering the elbow.

References

1 Shellock FG, Prentice WW. Warming-up and stretching for improved physical performance and prevention of sports related injuries. *Sports Med* 1985;**2**: 267–78.
2 Godges JJ, MacRae H, Longdon C, Tipberg C, MacRae P. The effects of two stretching procedures on hip range of motion and gait economy. *J Orthop Sport Phys Ther* 1989;**10**(9):350–7.
3 Asmussen E, Boje O. Body temperature and capacity of work. *Acta Physiol Scand* 1945;**10**:1–2.
4 Genovely H, Atamford BA. Effects of prolonged warm up exercise above and below anaerobic threshold on maximal performance. *Eur J Appl Physiol* 1982; **48**:323–30.
5 Ingier I, Stromme SB. Effects of active, passive or no warm-up on the physiological response to heavy exercise. *Eur J Appl Physiol* 1979;**40**:273–82.
6 Karpovich PV, Hale C. Effect of warm-up on physical performance. *JAMA* 1956;**162**:1117–19.
7 Bergh U, Ekblom B. Physical performance and peak aerobic power at different body temperatures. *J Appl Physiol* 1979;**46**:885–9.
8 Bennett AF. Thermal dependence of muscle function. *Am J Physiol* 1984;**247**: R217–R229.
9 Sapega AA, Quedenfeld TC, Moyer RA, Butler RA. Biophysical factors in range-of-motion exercise. *Physician Sportsmed* 1981;**9**(12):57–65.
10 Lehman JF, Masock AS, Warren CG, Koblanski JN. Effect of therapeutic temperature on tendon extensibility. *Arch Phys Med Rehab* 1970;**8**:481–7.
11 Wilson GJ, Wood GA, Elliot BC. The relationship between stiffness of the musculature and static flexibility: an alternative explanation for the occurrence of muscular injury. *Int J Sports Med* 1991;**12**(4):403–7.
12 Safran MR, Garrett WE, Jr, Seaber AV, Glisson RR, Ribbeck BM. The role of warm-up in muscular injury prevention. *Am J Sports Med* 1988;**16**(2):123–9.
13 Strickler T, Malone T, Garrett W. The effects of passive warming on muscle injury. *Am J Sports Med* 1990;**18**(2):141–5.
14 Rosenbaum D, Hennig EM. The influence of stretching and warm-up exercises on Achilles tendon reflex activity. *J Sport Sci* 1995;**13**:481–90.

15 Taylor DC, Dalton JD, Seaber AV, Garrett WE, Jr. Viscoelastic properties of muscle tendon units: the biomechanical effects of stretching. *Am J Sports Med* 1990;**18**:300–9.
16 Gillette TM, Holland GJ, Vincent WJ, Loy SF. Relationship of body core temperature and warm-up to knee range of motion. *J Orthop Sports Phys Ther* 1991;**13**(3):126–31.
17 Ekstrand J, Gillquist J, Lilzedahl S-S. Prevention of soccer injuries. Supervision by doctor and physiotherapist. *Am J Sports Med* 1983;**11**:116–20.
18 Hess GP, Capiello WL, Poole RM, Hunter SC. Prevention and treatment of overuse tendon injuries. *Sports Med* 1987;**8**:371–84.
19 Safran MR, Seaber AV, Garrett WE, Jr. Warm-up and muscular injury prevention. An update. *Sports Med* 1989;**8**(4):239–49.
20 vanMechelen W, Hlobil H, Kemper HCG, Voorn WJ, de Jongh HR. Prevention of running injuries by warm-up, cool-down, and stretching exercises. *Am J Sports Med* 1993;**21**(5):711–19.
21 Heiser TM, Weber J, Suillivan G, Clare P, Jacobs RR. Prophylaxis and management of hamstring muscle injuries in intercollegiate football players. *Am J Sports Med* 1984;**12**(5):368–70.
22 Ekstrand J, Gillquist J. The frequency of muscle tightness and injury in soccer players. *Am J Sports Med* 1982;**10**:75–8.
23 Alter M. *Science of flexibility*, 2nd edn. Champaign, IL: Human Kinetics, 1996.
24 Arnheim DD, Prentice WE. *Principles of athletic training*, 8th edn. St Louis: Mosby, 1993.
25 Syer J and Connolly C. *Sporting body sporting mind: an athlete's guide to mental training*. New York: Simon and Schuster, 1990.
26 Cureton TK. Flexibility as an aspect of physical fitness. *Res Exercise Sport* 1941; **12**(Suppl):381–94.
27 Beaulieu JE. *Stretching for all sports*. Pasadena, CA: Athletic Press, 1980.
28 Gleim GW, McHugh MP. Flexibility and its effects on sports injury and performance. *Sports Med* 1997;**24**(5):289–99.
29 Wessel J and Wan A. Effect of stretching on the intensity of delayed-onset muscle soreness. *Clin J Sports Med* 1994;**4**:83–7.
30 Smith LL, Brunetz MH, Chenier TC, *et al.* The effects of static and ballistic stretching on delayed onset muscle soreness and creatine kinase. *Res Q Exercise Sport* 1993;**64**(1):103–7.
31 Sullivan MK, Dejulia JJ, Worrell TW. Effect of pelvic position and stretching method on hamstring muscle flexibility. *Med Sci Sports Exercise* 1992;**24**(12):1383–9.
32 Rodenburg JB, Steenbeek D, Schiereck P, Bär PR. Warm-up, stretching and massage diminish harmful effects of eccentric exercise. *Int J Sports Med* 1994;**15**(7):414–19.
33 Williford HN, East JB, Smith FH, Burry LA. Evaluation of warm-up for improvement in flexibility. *Am J Sports Med* 1986;**14**(4):316–19.
34 Wiemann K and Hahn K. Influences of strength, stretching and circulatory exercises on flexibility parameters of the human hamstrings. *Int J Sports Med* 1997;**18**:340–6.
35 Gleim GW, Stachenfeld NS, Nicholas JA. The influence of flexibility on the economy of walking and jogging. *J Orthop Res* 1990;**8**:814–23.
36 Wilson GJ, Elliot BC, Wood GA. Stretch shorten cycle performance enhancement through flexibility training. *Med Sci Sports Exercise* 1992;**24**:116–23.

37 Worrell TW, Perrin DH, Gansneder BM, Gieck JH. Comparison of isokinetic strength and flexibility measures between hamstring injured and noninjured athletes. *J Orthop Sports Phys Ther* 1991;**13**(3):118–25.
38 Knapik JJ, Bauman CL, Jones BH, Harris J McA, Vaughan L. Preseason strength and flexibility imbalances associated with athletic injuries in female collegiate athletes. *Am J Sports Med* 1991;**19**(1):76–81.
39 Requa R, Garrick J. Sports epidemiology and injury prevention. In: Johnson RJ, Lombardo J, eds. *Current reviews of sports medicine.* Philadelphia: Current Medicine, 1994.
40 Smith CA. The warm-up procedure: to stretch or not to stretch? A brief review. *J Orthop Sports Phys Ther* 1994;**19**(1):12–17.
41 Norris CM. *Flexibility principles and practice.* London: A&C Black, 1994.
42 Moscov J, Lacourse MG, Garhammer J, Whiting H. Predictors of dynamic hip flexibility in female ballet dancers. *Impulse* 1994;**2**:184–95.
43 Etnyre BR, Lee EJ. Comments on proprioceptive neuromuscular facilitation stretching techniques. *Res Q Exercise Sport* 1987;**58**(2):184–8.
44 Moore MA, Hutton RS. Electromyographic investigation of muscle stretching techniques. *Med Sci Sports Exercise* 1980;**12**(5):322–9.

3 Medicines in sport

RICHARD BUDGETT AND ROSLYN CARBON

Sportspeople have the right to professional medical care, which includes the right to appropriate medication for any medical condition from which they may suffer. Unfortunately, because of previous drug abuse by some athletes certain classes of drugs are prohibited (proscribed) by sporting governing bodies. The use of prohibited drugs may be detected by urine testing conducted either at competition or during training. This chapter outlines suitable prescribing within current doping control regulations.

A given class of drugs may be banned for two main reasons:

1. They are believed to confer a competitive advantage and hence contravene the ethics of fair play.
2. Use of the drug without medical indication causes undue risk of side effects and endangers health.

Different sports and even the same sport in different countries may have different rules governing the use of medications. For the purposes of this chapter the current regulations of the Medical Commission of the International Olympic Committee (IOC) will be followed unless otherwise stated. It is important to note that such rules are continuously subject to review and may change with little notice. Any queries relating to the use of medication by an athlete should be directed to the governing body medical officer of his/her sport or more general enquiries can be made to the UK Sports Council, Ethics and Anti-Doping Directorate (0171 380 8000).

Proscribed drugs

The classes of drugs prohibited during sporting competition are as summarised in Tables 3.1 and 3.2.

Anabolic agents

These include testosterone and the synthetic anabolic/androgenic steroids as well as the beta-adrenergic drug clenbuterol used in asthma. They are abused for their positive effect on protein synthesis and hence (presumed) increase in muscle bulk and strength. Anabolic steroids have considerable androgenic side effects and can cause hepatocellular damage and fluid retention.

Diuretics

This class of drugs can be used to increase renal excretion of other banned substances and hence used to manipulate urine testing. They cause dehydration and are banned for use in "making weight" (i.e. getting down to a defined weight limit) in weight category sports.

Stimulants

All sympathomimetics, amphetamines, and cocaine are banned. For ephedrine, cathine, and methylephedrine the definition of a positive is 5 μg/ml of urine. For phenylpropanolamine and pseudoephedrine the definition of a positive is 10 μg/ml. If more than one substance is present, the quantities are added and if the sum exceeds 10 μg/ml the sample is considered positive. Caffeine ingestion is limited to that which results in a urine level below 12 μg/ml. This equates to approximately five cups of strong coffee but is subject to individual variation and the level of hydration.

> ● Beware of stimulants such as ephedrine, pseudoephedrine, and phenylpropanolamine in many over-the-counter preparations

Bromantan, which was abused by a number of Eastern Block athletes in Atlanta, has now been included as a stimulant and masking agent.

Topical use of vasoconstricting sympathomimetic drugs is allowed in the case of phenylephrine contained in nasal or ophthalmological preparations.

Table 3.1 Class of drugs banned **during** competition

Stimulants, e.g. amphetamine, bromantan, caffeine (>12 μg/ml), cocaine, ephedrine

Anabolic agents*, e.g. methandienone, nandrolone, stanozolol, testosterone, clenbuterol, DHEA

Diuretics*, e.g. acetazolamide, frusemide, hydrochlorothiazide, triamterene, mannitol, androstenedione

Peptide and glycoprotein hormones*, e.g. growth hormone, corticotrophin, chorionic gonadotrophin, erythropoietin

Narcotics, e.g. diamorphine (heroin), morphine, methadone, pethidine

Masking agents*

* Also banned out of competition.

Table 3.2   Other drugs subject to restrictions

Corticosteroids   Route of administration restricted to topical, inhalation*, local or intra-articular injection*

Beta-blockers   Restricted in certain sports. Refer to regulations of national or international sports federation

Local anaesthetics   Route of administration restricted to local or intra-articular injection*

Marijuana ⎫   Restricted in certain sports. Refer to regulations of national or
Alcohol ⎭   international sports federation

---

* Written notification of administration should be given to the relevant medical authority, except for dental application of local anaesthetics.

Adrenaline may be used with local anaesthetic to stem bleeding and clearly its systemic use must not be withheld in the case of a medical emergency such as anaphylaxis or cardiac arrest.

Narcotics

Morphine and its derivatives are banned as analgesia during sporting competitions. Codeine, dextropropoxyphene, dihydrocodeine, dextromethorphan, diphenoxylate, and pholcodeine are now allowed.

Peptide and glycoprotein hormones and their analogues

Several naturally occurring hormones and their releasing factors are now commercially available. Growth hormone and chorionic gonadotrophin have anabolic effects while erythropoietin increases red cell mass and hence oxygen carrying capacity of the blood. They all have significant side effects and should not be used without a defined medical indication.

Masking drugs

Methods to mask or interfere with urine testing are also banned. Uricosuric drugs such as probenecid that promote excretion of other banned substances are proscribed. Bromantan is now included.

Other regulated drugs

Some classes of drugs are subject to certain restrictions which may vary from one sport to another.

Beta-blockers, which lower heart rate and ablate tremor, are banned in the technique sports such as pistol shooting. Alcohol, marijuana, and sedative antihistamines are banned in the modern pentathlon.

The use of corticosteroids presents a rather bewildering array of regulations. All topical use, both as creams in dermatological conditions and inhalations for asthma and rhinitis, is allowed. Corticosteroid injections for management of musculoskeletal problems are allowed for intra-articular, bursa or tendon sheath pathology. However, intramuscular injection for systemic purposes and both oral and rectal corticosteroids are banned.

Local anaesthetic injections are generally allowed in most sports but must be used with appropriate caution. However, procaine is not allowed. Medical officers must never put the athlete's health at risk by masking pain to allow too early a return to competition.

Prescribing within the doping regulations

It is important to remember that the concept behind the doping regulations of "unfair advantage" is situation-specific and hence the rules for competition testing are more stringent than those for random out-of-competition testing. Hence all of the above regulations apply at the time of competition, but during training only the anabolic agents (including peptide hormones), diuretics, and masking agents are proscribed and tested for.

At all times the health of the athlete must be considered first and medical treatment should not be denied unnecessarily. Hence it is legitimate for an athlete to be allowed treatment with ephedrine-containing medicine for an upper respiratory tract infection out of competition.

If an athlete has a legitimate need for a proscribed medication, application can be made through the sport's governing body medical officer to the IOC or relevant international medical board for special dispensation.

The following is appropriate medical care of athletes within the doping guidelines for given conditions.

Injury and pain management

Treatment of injury in athletes usually centres on physical therapy, including the basics of rest, ice, compression, and elevation in acute episodes. Very often the acute inflammatory phase of an injury can be controlled by non-steroidal anti-inflammatories used either orally, topically, intramuscularly or as a suppository. All non-steroidals are allowed although it is inappropriate to use them for prolonged periods or in very high dosage simply to mask pain.

Corticosteroid and/or local anaesthetic injections are part of an allowable treatment regimen but written notification of dosage and route of administration must be sent to the chief medical officer of any major competition. A similar letter of declaration from the treating doctor is required out of competition for the athlete to present should they be dope tested.

All simple analgesics such as aspirin and paracetamol as well as codeine are allowed. It is pertinent to remember that some countries ban the carriage of codeine through customs and this may incur significant penalties, including imprisonment. Morphine derivatives, including pethidine, are prohibited during competition. Caffeine is included in many over-the-counter analgesic products and athletes must be aware that the legal limit of 12 µg/ml of urine can easily be exceeded with such preparations and must not take them during competition. It is really only safe for athletes to self-administer single name generic drugs, such as paracetamol, rather than proprietary compounds unchecked by medical personnel.

Serious injury or pain must always be treated on its merits and if clinically appropriate narcotics should not be witheld. In this instance the athlete would then be withdrawn from any competition. However, injectable or rectal non-steroidal anti-inflammatories (such as diclofenac) are often as effective for severe pain.

Cardiovascular conditions

It is quite likely, especially amongst veteran populations, that some competitive athletes will be hypertensive. Diuretics and, in some sports, beta-blockers are banned but they are also poor choices for athletes. Diuretics will increase the risk of dehydration while beta-blockers decrease cardiac output and hence aerobic capacity. Exercise itself has been shown to decrease blood pressure in the moderately hypertensive and hence the need for medication may actually be reduced in some athletes. Antihypertensives such as calcium channel blockers and angiotensin converting enzyme inhibitors **are allowed** and do not have detrimental effects on exercise performance.

Other categories of cardiac drugs, such as the anti-arrhythmics, digoxin, and nitrates, are all allowed.

Food additives

Many athletes consume high levels of vitamins and minerals to supplement their diet. Herbal remedies and amino acid supplements are also commonly used. None of these preparations are banned in their own right. However, care must always be exercised by athletes when they consume a compound of unknown constituents as there have been several celebrated cases of elite athletes testing positive for stimulants contained in such products.

Recently creatine, contained naturally in meat, has been marketed to be consumed at up to 20 times the normal daily intake. At levels of 5 g taken four times per day it has been shown to decrease fatigue induced by repetitive sprint training. While this may then define creatine as an ergogenic aid, it is not currently banned because it is classed as a food. The long term health implications of consuming creatine in supraphysiological doses have not yet been determined.

Treatment of specific conditions

Asthma

Asthma in athletes must be properly controlled for the sake of their health. It is a potentially fatal condition, and doping control regulations must not and should not interfere with optimal treatment and control.

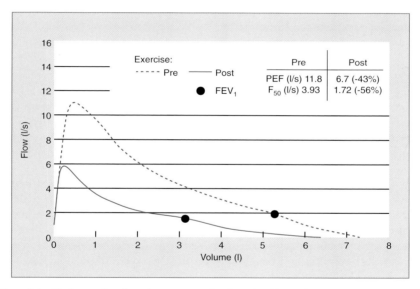

Figure 3.1   Expiratory flow loops in an untreated asthmatic athlete before and after exercise; FEV₁ is significantly lower post exercise. PEF=peak expiratory flow; F₅₀=flow at 50% of FVC (forced vital capacity); FEV₁=forced expiratory volume in one second. (Reproduced with permission of Dr Mark Harries, British Olympic Medical Centre)

In healthy athletes ventilatory capacity does not limit performance. However, in athletes with asthma, which is often exercise-induced, ventilation can become the limiting factor. The flow loops in Figure 3.1 show the greatly reduced air flow with asthma which leads to oxygen delivery to the lungs becoming the limiting factor in aerobic performance.

Beta-2 agonists

All beta-2 agonists are banned during competition because they are stimulants. There are three exceptions which are allowed by inhalation only:

- Salbutamol (Ventolin)
- Terbutaline (Bricanyl)
- Salmeterol (Serevent).

All other inhalers are banned, and *none* (including salbutamol and terbutaline) are allowed orally. This should not cause a problem for most athletes, and it is worth remembering that stimulants are not banned out of competition. Clenbuterol is an exception in that it is considered to be an anabolic agent as well as a stimulant, and so is banned out of competition. It is only used in veterinary practice in this country. Interestingly all the beta-2 agonists have a weak anabolic effect but, apart from clenbuterol, would need to be taken in doses that would produce unwanted side effects such as tremor and tachycardia.

Corticosteroids

All corticosteroids, such as beclomethasone (Becotide) and budenoside (Pulmicort), are allowed by inhalation but none is allowed orally. This causes no practical difficulties in the control of asthma in most athletes as inhaled corticosteroids are very effective, especially if used through a spacer device.

However, there are some athletes who require a short course of high dose oral corticosteroids (such as prednisolone 40 mg per day for 5 days) to treat a very severe deterioration in their asthma. This is allowed out of competition, but **oral prednisolone is banned in the week leading up to a competition**, because all drugs taken in the week before a doping test should be declared. Therefore an athlete whose asthma is so bad that they require oral prednisolone should withdraw from any competition in the week following completion of the course, or risk a positive dope test, although it is unlikely they will be fit to compete. In certain exceptional cases permission may be sought *before* competition from the appropriate regulatory authority.

Other drugs

Sodium cromoglycate (Intal) and the anticholinergic drugs such as ipratropium bromide (Atrovent) are allowed. Thus the commonly used emergency treatment of ipratropium and salbutamol via a nebuliser is allowed even during competition.

Theophylline (e.g. Slo-Phyllin) and aminophylline (e.g. Phyllocontin Continus) are also allowed, but are not often used in athletes due to their side effects. Beware of proprietary theophylline preparations which may contain other substances which are banned such as ephedrine (e.g. Dodo tablets and Franol tablets).

Notification

The IOC and most governing bodies have introduced mandatory reporting of any athlete requiring salbutamol, terbutaline, salmeterol, or corticosteroids by inhalation during competition. This notification should be to the medical officer or medical committee of the governing body. Thus any doctor treating an elite athlete for asthma should give them a note to send on to the medical officer or committee. At national or international competitions, notification of all the members of a team on inhalers should be given to the relevant medical authority at the competition by the team doctor, or the team manager if there is no doctor.

Notification was introduced to try to reduce the excessive use of inhalers, particularly beta-2 agonists, which in some sports had reached 80%.

Hay fever and allergies

All antihistamines such as terfenadine (Triludan) and cetirizine (Zirtek) are allowed.

As in the treatment of asthma, the corticosteroids such as betamethasone (Beconase) and budesonide (Rhinocort) are allowed by nasal inhalation but, contrary to the practice for respiratory corticosteroid inhalers, notification to the governing body or competition medical officer is not required. Furthermore, ophthalmic and nasal application of stimulants such as xylometazoline are permitted but not the use of ephedrine-containing medicines.

Another pitfall in the treatment of hay fever is with the ephedrine and pseudoephedrine contained in some nasal sprays which can be bought without a prescription (e.g. Otrivine). They may also cause rebound congestion. Furthermore the use of systemic steroids via intramuscular injection (e.g. Kenalog) is banned.

Due to these limitations it may be worth considering desensitisation in athletes whose allergy is not well controlled.

Treatment of acute anaphylaxis should never be withheld if treatment with adrenaline or hydrocortisone intravenously or intramuscularly is clinically indicated.

Eczema

All topical corticosteroids such as hydrocortisone, clobetasone, and betamethasone are allowed. If athletes wash frequently with soap this can worsen eczema, so they should use emollients and minimise the use of soap. This should lessen the amount of topical steroid required.

Upper respiratory tract infections

Leading up to and during competition great care must be taken not to prescribe topical or systemic nasal decongestants containing stimulants (e.g. pseudoephedrine).

Symptomatic relief can be obtained using paracetamol, aspirin or ibuprofen. Gargling with chlorhexidine, povidone-iodine or soluble aspirin and the use of local anaesthetic lozenges and spray can help symptoms of sore throat.

Codeine, pholcodeine, and dextromethorphan are now all allowed by the IOC and can be used as cough suppressants.

Topical corticosteroids such as triamcinolone (Adcortyl in Orabase) or hydrocortisone (Corlan), as well as mouthwashes and local analgesics can be used in oral and perioral ulceration such as aphthous ulcers.

All antibiotics are allowed. However, probenecid, which can be used to reduce the excretion of penicillin, is banned both in and out of competition because it may interfere with the excretion of banned drugs.

Diarrhoea and vomiting

Diarrhoea is a common problem in athletes and can be treated with appropriate rehydration solutions and antidiarrhoeals such as Lomotil (diphenoxylate and atropine), loperamide, and codeine, but not morphine (in Kaolin and Morphine mixture).

For the symptomatic relief of vomiting, antihistamines, phenothiazines, domperidone, and metoclopramide are allowed. However metoclopramide is more likely to cause extrapyramidal side effects, including oculogyric crisis, in young adults. The sedative antihistamines (e.g. chlorpheniramine) are not allowed in the modern pentathlon, and would interfere with performance in most sports, so are generally not recommended.

Since all antibiotics are allowed, they can be used for the prevention and treatment of traveller's diarrhoea (e.g. ciprofloxacin, trimethoprim).

Gastrointestinal disease

Antacids, ulcer healing drugs (e.g. H_2-antagonists), and laxatives are all allowed.

Irritable bowel is a common problem in athletes, especially with the stress of training, competition, travel, and dietary changes. If dietary manipulation and appropriate counselling do not help, then antispasmodics (e.g. hyoscine, propantheline, mebeverine) or peppermint oil are allowed and can be useful.

The only problem is with corticosteroids. As mentioned previously, all topical preparations are allowed (e.g. betamethasone ointment perianally) but not oral or rectal prednisolone during competition. Thus inflammatory bowel disease (ulcerative colitis and Crohn's disease) can be difficult to manage. The aminosalicylates (e.g. mesalazine and sulphasalazine) are allowed in competition, but competitors may require prednisolone for many months or years to control the disease, or intermittently to control unpredictable acute attacks.

Fortunately, it is possible to obtain permission to use corticosteroids from the appropriate authority *prior* to competition. In the case of the Olympic Games this is the IOC Medical Commission; for world championships, the international governing body; and for national championships, the national governing body. The application should come from the national medical officer or committee through the appropriate governing body. Thus any doctor treating an athlete who may need oral or rectal prednisolone must notify the national medical advisor to that sport. A well documented case has to be presented for permission to be given.

Central nervous system

Antipsychotics, antidepressants, antiepileptic and antiparkinsonian drugs are all allowed. Hypnotics (sleeping pills) and anxiolytics can be useful after and during long journeys across time zones. They are also often used for anxiety-induced insomnia before competition, but a drug such as temazepam or zopiclone should not be given to competitors unless they have tried it before and so know the effect it will have on them. They will probably perform better after a night of poor sleep than with drug-induced drowsiness. The only sport to ban all sedative CNS drugs is the modern pentathlon.

Melatonin is used by some athletes in an attempt to speed recovery from jet lag and to promote sleep. It is not banned, but great caution is advised in its use. Melatonin is not licensed or available in the UK and has unpredictable effects, including prolonged drowsiness in some individuals. If taken at the wrong time it may even slow adjustment to new time zones. It should only be taken with the advice of experts as part of a full strategy to overcome jet lag as quickly as possible.

Stimulant appetite suppressants such as dexamphetamine, pemoline, and fenfluramine are banned.

Hormones

There is no limitation in the treatment of thyroid disease except that beta-blockers are banned in some sports such as shooting, diving, modern pentathlon, and bobsleigh, but this should not interfere with the treatment of a thyrotoxic crisis.

During the Nagano Olympic Games the IOC banned the use of insulin in non-diabetics, but the management of insulin-dependent diabetic athletes is of course unaffected by this rule.

All progestogens and oestrogens are allowed, so there is no problem with contraception, including emergency contraception (PC 4), which is effective for 72 hours after unprotected intercourse. Two packets of the pill can also be taken without a break to avoid menses during competition. Progestogens such as dydrogesterone and norethisterone can be used in the treatment of dysmenorrhoea and dysfunctional uterine bleeding.

Obviously anabolic agents are banned. ACTH (tetracosactrin) is banned but rarely used in medicine and not available in the UK because of its unpredictable response.

Gonadotrophins such as human chorionic gonadotrophin (HCG) used in subfertility have anabolic properties in male athletes and so are banned in and out of competition, which could produce a problem if a female athlete needs IVF and has not responded to clomiphene.

Growth hormone is also banned, however a child requiring growth hormone must not be denied treatment, and it should be possible to obtain permission from the appropriate authority if the indications are sound. Erythropoietin used to treat the anaemia of chronic renal failure is banned because it raises haemoglobin with an effect similar to blood doping.

Travel medicine

All vaccinations and antimalarials are allowed. Antibiotics, such as ciprofloxacin and rehydration solutions may be needed for traveller's diarrhoea and are allowed.

"Social drugs"

Alcohol and marijuana (which can be detected in the urine for several weeks) are subject to restrictions in certain sports, especially where intoxication may be dangerous (e.g. bobsleigh and skiing). At the Nagano Winter Olympic Games in 1998 testing for marijuana was extended to other sports. The IOC President, Juan Antonio Samaranch, issued a statement that "The Olympic Movement would shortly ban 'soft' drugs such as marijuana. An athlete, above all an Olympic athlete, has to be an example to youth. We will try to extend this ban to all international federations." Nicotine is not controlled.

The drugs which cause the most problems are the stimulants. Amphetamines and cocaine are increasingly used by young people and, as well as all the other dangers, an elite competitor faces suspension if any is present in a urine sample.

Drug testing

In the UK drug testing of athletes is carried out by the Sports Council Doping Control Unit. Normally this is under the auspices of the national or international governing body. If a national governing body does not have adequate regulations and a satisfactory testing programme their Sports Council grant is at risk. Thus the majority of sports run their doping control programme through the Sports Council.

At the Olympic Games testing is carried out by the IOC medical commission under the rules of the IOC. These testing procedures are the standard which all sports follow so the athlete can expect the same procedure wherever the testing is carried out.

Out-of-competition testing will only be carried out on previous internationals and those registered for national team selection. In-competition testing is carried out at national and international competitions on any competitor. Thus most club level competitors will never be tested, although as a member of their sport they are bound by the rules of their governing body, which generally includes doping control.

Details of the testing procedures can be obtained from the UK Sports Council, Ethics and Anti-Doping Directorate, 10 Melton Street, London NW1 2EB, but in summary they are:

1. Notification of the athlete by an independent sampling officer (ISO). Normally they will be given up to an hour to report for testing, and chaperoned during that time.
2. Reporting for testing. Sealed non-alcoholic drinks should be available. A representative can accompany the athlete (e.g. a coach or doctor).
3. Selection of a collecting vessel.
4. Providing the sample. Sufficient clothing has to be removed so that the ISO can directly observe the competitor passing urine (generally 100 ml). Only the competitor should handle the sample.
5. Selection of sample containers by the competitor.
6. Breaking the security seals by the competitor.
7. Division of the sample between the A and B sample bottles by the competitor.

8. Sealing of the samples by the competitor.
9. Recording the information, including any medications taken in the previous week.
10. Certification of the information. The competitor (and their representative if present) and the ISO should check the form and sign it if satisfied. The competitor is then given a copy and is free to go.
11. The samples are transferred to an accredited laboratory by a secure chain of custody with only seal and sample numbers and a list of medication, but no means of identifying the competitor.
12. The analytical result is reported to the relevant governing body.

The doctor to a team should be familiar with these procedures and when possible accompany the competitor to testing. This will help to minimise

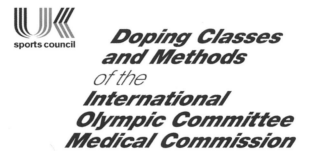

United Kingdom Sports Council
Ethics & Anti-Doping
Walkden House
10 Melton Street
London NW1 2EB

Tel: (44) 0171 380 8030

WARNING

Medications prescribed by your doctor may contain prohibited substances. Some vitamin, herbal and nutritional substances may contain prohibited substances, such as Guarana, Ma Huang, Chinese Ephedra.

The substances listed on this card are only examples of substances permitted or prohibited by the IOC. Not all sports adopt the IOC Medical Code. If in doubt check with your governing body or with the UKSC Drug Information Line.

USE OF THESE PRODUCTS IS AT YOUR OWN RISK.

31 January 1998

(a)

Figure 3.2

66

any possible trauma by relieving the athlete of the responsibility of making sure that the procedures are correctly followed. The doctor can ensure that all drugs are declared. This is not mandatory but advisable.

It is sensible for a team doctor to take a careful drug history from all competitors well before competition. If a banned substance is being taken inadvertently then the competitor must be counselled and educated. If a banned medication is revealed only at the time of drug testing then it must be declared and the circumstances fully documented with any mitigating circumstances. The subsequent positive test will necessitate a hearing by a panel from the appropriate governing body, and a full declaration will help mitigate against any disciplinary procedure.

The following are examples of classes and methods prohibited in sport:

Classes	Stimulants eg. amphetamine, bromantan, caffeine (above 12mcg/ml), carphedon, cocaine, ephedrine, certain beta 2 agonists. Narcotics eg. diamorphine (heroin), morphine, methadone, pethidine. Anabolic Agents eg. methandienone, nandrolone, stanozolol, testosterone, clenbuterol, DHEA, androstenedione. Diuretics eg. acetazolamide, frusemide, hydrochlorothiazide, triamterene, mannitol. Peptide & Glycoprotein Hormones & Analogues eg. growth hormone, corticotrophin, chorionic gonadotrophin, erythropoietin, and all respective releasing factors and their analogues.
Methods	Blood Doping Pharmacological, Chemical & Physical Manipulation eg. substances and methods that alter the integrity and validity of the urine; eg. probenecid, catheterisation, urine substitution.
Classes of drugs subject to certain restrictions	Alcohol & Marijuana Restricted in certain sports. Refer to regulations of national or international sports federations. Local Anaesthetics Route of administration restricted to local or intra-articular injection*. Corticosteroids Route of administration restricted to topical, inhalation*, local or intra-articular injection*. Beta-blockers Restricted in certain sports. Refer to regulations of national or international sports federations.

* Written notification of administration should be given to relevant medical authority, eg. governing body medical officer, except for dental application of local anaesthetics.

Treatment Guidelines
Examples of permitted & prohibited substances

	ALLOWED	*BANNED*
ASTHMA	sodium cromoglycate, theophylline, salbutamol*, terbutaline*, salmeterol*, beclomethasone*, fluticasone*, (*by inhalation only & written notification of administration should be given to relevant medical authority).	products containing sympathomimetics eg. ephedrine, isoprenaline, fenoterol, rimiterol, orciprenaline.
COLD/ COUGH	all antibiotics, steam & menthol inhalations, permitted antihistamines, terfenadine, astemizole, pholcodine, guaiphenesin, dextromethorphan, paracetamol.	products containing sympathomimetics eg. ephedrine, pseudoephedrine, phenylpropanolamine.
DIARRHOEA	diphenoxylate, loperamide, products containing electrolytes (eg. Dioralyte, Rehidrat).	products containing opioids eg. morphine.
HAYFEVER	antihistamines, nasal sprays containing a corticosteroid or xylometazoline, eyedrops containing sodium cromoglycate.	products containing ephedrine, pseudoephedrine.
PAIN	aspirin, codeine, dihydrocodeine, ibuprofen, paracetamol, all non-steroidal anti-inflammatories, dextropropoxyphene.	products containing opioids, caffeine.
VOMITING	domperidone, metoclopramide.	

(b)

Figure 3.2 (continued) Aide-mémoire *card issued by the UK Sports Council. The card folds to credit card size*

67

Summary

The list of banned drugs has evolved over the past few decades and will continue to change. In all cases the health and safety of the athlete should be the overriding priority, and in the vast majority of cases it is possible to give optimal treatment using permitted drugs administered via a permitted route. The Sports Council provides a useful reminder card which is a valuable *aide-mémoire* for athlete and medical officer alike, and is shown in Figure 3.2. This information is also available on the page before the section on Gastrointestinal Drugs in the *British National Formulary*.

Addendum: Summary of IOC regulations for drugs which need physician written notification (June 1998)

Substances	Prohibited	Authorised with notification	Authorised without notification
Selected beta-agonists*	Oral Systemic injections	Inhalatory	
Corticosteroids	Oral Systemic injections Rectal	Inhalatory Local injections Intra-articular injections	Topical (anal, aural, dermatological, nasal, ophthalmological)
Local anaesthetics†	Systemic injections		Dental Local injections‡ Intra-articular injections‡

* Salbutamol, salmeterol, terbutaline: all other beta-agonists are prohibited.
† Except cocaine, which is prohibited.
‡ In agreement with some International Sports Federations, notification may be necessary in some sports.

---

4   Anabolic steroids and ergogenic aids: their use and abuse

PIRKKO KORKIA

Introduction

Throughout history athletes have sought to improve their performance through dietary and other practices such as the use of stimulants, analgesics, herbs, and hallucinogens. Success in sport has always been associated with fame, privilege, and financial rewards; as Tony Sharpe, a Canadian sprinter and colleague of Ben Johnson has said "The glory is too sweet, the dollars are too much".[1] The margin between winning and losing is often minute and the use of banned performance enhancing agents can be just too tempting. The perceived power of one of the most notorious of such agents, anabolic steroids, is typified in a statement by Dr Astaphan, Ben Johnson's medical supervisor, who said that the axiom among athletes is if they do not take it, they will not make it.

Ergogenic aids comprise any procedure or agent that enhances energy production, energy control, or energy efficiency during sports performance. They are often classified as physical, mechanical, biomechanical, nutritional, psychological, and pharmacological substances or treatments. When an athlete considers whether or not to use an ergogenic aid, three main factors must be considered: the safety, efficacy, and legality of the substance or procedure.

Athletes are known to employ a variety of drugs to improve performance, including human growth hormone (HGH), thyroid hormone, insulin, human chorionic gonadotrophin (HCG), clenbuterol, and gamma hydroxy butyrate (GHB) to mention a few. This chapter will consider the use of anabolic steroids in some detail while an update will be provided on blood doping, stimulants, caffeine, creatine, bicarbonates, diuretics, and the contraceptive pill.

What are anabolic steroids?

In 1939, Boje suggested that sex hormones might prove useful for sportspeople in improving their performance and five years later data published from animal and human studies provided support for his speculations. Testimonials from body-builders, who were prominent in the late 1940s and 1950s, suggest that various forms of testosterone were by then already in use[2] and the awesome success of Soviet weight-lifting teams in the 1950s lead to the realisation of the potential of these drugs. Their use quickly spread from strength and power sports to American football and other team games, endurance sports, and finally to the "look good" factions outside sport. They are mainly used in attempts to increase lean body mass, decrease fat mass, allow greater volumes of training at greater intensities, and to increase motivation and decrease feeling of fatigue.

Man-made derivatives of testosterone, anabolic steroids, produce two distinct actions, comprising **anabolic** (tissue building) and **androgenic** (male producing) effects and, despite efforts to dissociate the two, all anabolic steroids have some androgenic effect and are thus recognised as anabolic–androgenic steroids (AS). The virilising effects of AS, which are especially evident in children and women, make the androgenic effects of AS undesirable. Testosterone influences the development and function of practically every organ in the body and it appears that the target tissue is more important in determining the behaviour of the drug, rather than the drug itself; for example muscles hypertrophy, while sebaceous glands increase their rate of secretion. The drug has been modified to slow down its degradation and it is mainly used in injected (oil-based and water-based) and oral form.

Anabolic steroids have a number of important medical uses, some of these are listed in Table 4.1.

Table 4.1   Medical uses of anabolic steroids

- Replacement therapy for men with deficiency or absence of endogenous testosterone
- Anaemia caused by deficient red blood cell production
- Control of metastatic inoperable breast cancer
- Advanced osteoporosis
- Male contraceptive
- Stimulate appetite and induce a sense of wellbeing in terminal patients
- Treatment of male menopause

The American Medical Association is uncertain about the beneficial value of AS as adjunct therapy for conditions such as:
- Protein deficiency
- Patients convalescing from severe infections, surgery, burns, trauma, and cytotoxic drug therapy

Controversies on the action and effects of anabolic steroids

The postulated mechanisms of their action include the stimulation of protein synthesis, resulting in increased muscle mass,[3] antagonism of catabolic effects of glucocorticoids which are released in response to training permitting more intensive training,[4] and central nervous system effects, which increase motivation and energy, and decrease fatigue.[5] Many of these effects, however, are yet to be clearly established and studies investigating the effects of AS on aerobic capacity and endurance, body composition, and strength performance have been contradictory. Results, even from the same laboratories, have led to inconsistent conclusions.[6,7] Reasons for the lack of agreement on the efficacy of AS are related to factors such as small sample size, lack of dietary control, variable training status of subjects, differences in type and dose of drug used, length of use, and placebo effect.[2] The following paragraphs will provide some flavour of the controversy which exists regarding the main classes of the effects of AS on performance.

Aerobic capacity and endurance

Due to the red blood cell producing effects of AS, it has been postulated that their administration may increase oxygen binding capacity and therefore maximum oxygen uptake ($\dot{V}o_2$max), but research evidence for this is contradictory and the validity of $\dot{V}o_2$max as an indicator of endurance performance or an index sensitive enough to detect changes has been questioned. Anecdotal and interview reports with high level track and field athletes have suggested that they may allow more frequent high intensity training, and if this is true, AS would benefit almost any top level athlete from the long distance to middle distance runners whose training loads cannot be increased without this leading to overtraining syndrome and injury. This is the main attraction that AS offer for endurance athletes.

Body composition

AS are used to increase lean body mass while decreasing fat mass. The wide variability in research studies has led to inconsistent results, although a large number of reports do indicate that lean body mass increases in response to weight-lifting, even in those with no prior experience. It is generally accepted that provided the athlete's diet is adequate, AS can contribute to increases in body weight, often in the lean mass compartment. Increased protein synthesis is achieved through the action of steroid-receptor complexes when the athlete is stressed. This explains the idea

71

promoted by AS users that as long as you train hard (new muscle tissue contains new receptor complexes), eat, and take AS, you will grow.[8]

Strength performance

About half of scientific studies reviewed by Lombardo[9] report improvements in strength and it is generally accepted that AS together with high intensity exercise and appropriate diet can improve muscular strength in some individuals. Individuals respond to AS in a highly variable manner, which also complicates the interpretation of research outcomes, particularly in studies involving few subjects.

Track and field records, particularly in women's throwing events, set between the early 1980s and 1990s have shown a decline. In 1984, 23 men put the shot over 21 metres whereas in 1991 only one man managed over 21. Women's javelin has seen a decline from 80 metres to just over 60, and a similar declining trend has been evident in times for the 1500 metre run. It is widely believed that the decline is a result of less systematic drug use by athletes, partly due to more intense targeting by the dope testing authorities. Dr Robert Voy, who was the chief medical officer for the US Olympic Committee, states that "In men, steroids offer an unfair advantage, but in women, that advantage is probably magnified ten times".[10]

Perceived benefits

Interviews with and anecdotal evidence given by AS users consistently agree with powerful positive effects[11] (Figure 4.1) and in competitive body-building their use is often considered as an essential part of training.

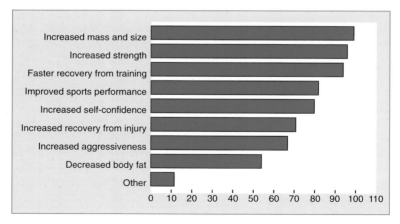

Figure 4.1 Perceived benefits of anabolic steroids reported by 110 users ("always", "very often", and "often" responses combined). For full details of the study, see Korkia and Stimson[11]

72

Although anecdotal and interview information must be interpreted with great care, it should not be ignored.

Sports authorities themselves have been accused of abetting and encouraging drug use. For example, in the past the Australian Institute of Sport has been dubbed the "Australian Institute of Steroids" because of scandals linking the management and coaching staff with alleged systematic use of the drugs. In the early 1980s the Italian athletics federation was found to be involved in "steroid programmes organised and paid for by Nebiolo's FIDAL".[1] Also, Ben Johnson's doping is alleged to have been an open secret within sport but withheld from the public to preserve a clean image and to ensure shattering of world records. The medical profession has been implicated in the fine-tuning of their use, while sporting officials may have protected the users.

Who uses anabolic steroids and how widely are they used?

Hard evidence for drug use in sport is scarce. The Dubin Report (Canada, 1990) investigated the issue for 11 months and heard 122 witnesses. It concluded that AS in particular were being used by athletes in almost every sport, most exclusively in weight-lifting and track and field. During this investigation, Dr Astaphan, Ben Johnson's doctor, testified that his help was sought by 32 athletes from 12 countries, including Britain. These included volleyball players, cyclists, skiers, and track and field athletes. The Black Report (Australia, 1989) estimated that 89% of men were alleged to use them at all levels of competition and 80% of women at national and international levels. In Britain, it has been difficult to obtain reliable information about the prevalence of AS in sport. Although the governing bodies of sport and those responsible for doping control in the UK maintain that drug use is minimal and that the "cheats" are being caught, rumours among participants about the use of AS and growth hormone are rife. These anecdotal reports are not based on any hard evidence, but lack of documentation should not be taken as very informative because, if AS use were more widespread than commonly acknowledged, in spite of testing programmes, it would not be in the interest of either elite competitors or governing bodies for this to be revealed.

Although the use of AS in sport has been a hot media issue, testimonials and research suggest that it is more common among competitive body-builders and those who aim to improve their musculature or appearance.[11,12] The author of one of the most popular "underground" steroid handbooks has stated that the popularity of AS is directly linked to the popularity of body-building.[13]

Table 4.2 Commonly used anabolic steroids in the UK

Anadrol (oxymetholone)
Anapolon (oxymetholone)
Anavar (oxandrolone)
Andriol (testosterone undecanoate)
Androtardyl (testosterone enanthate)
Androxon (testosterone undecanoate)
Dianabol (methandrostenolone)
Deca-Durabolin (nandrolone decanoate)
Equipose (boldenone)*
Finajet (trenbolone)*
Goldline (testosterone)
Halotestin (fluoxymesterone)
Heptylate (testosterone)
Nilevar (norethandrolone)
Omnadren (Polish Sustanon)
Parabolan (trenbolone)
Premastril (dromostanolone)
Primobolin (metholone)
Oxytasona (portuguese Anapolon)
Sustanon (propionate, phenylpropionate, isocaporate and decanoate)

---

* Veterinary preparations.

Comprehensive lists and descriptions of AS and their effectiveness as reported by users can be found in Phillips[13] and Wright.[14] Table 4.2 contains a list of commonly used AS.[11] It is important to realise that some drugs are preferred at different stages of the "cycle" depending on what the user aims to achieve, for instance, "cutting", "size", "strength", "bulking", "maintenance", or "muscle hardness". A body-builder preparing him/herself for a contest would choose preparations according to their effectiveness (or the individual's sensitivity to a particular drug) in producing the desired outcome. The combinations tend to be a result of trial and error rather than scientific study. The drugs are taken in cycles, which for men often vary from 6 to 12 weeks on AS followed by 10 to 12 weeks off AS. Women's cycles tend to be shorter, often half of those reported by men. Within a cycle a large number of different AS may be used but not necessarily all at the same time. Users believe that some preparations work synergistically and this is one of the reasons for "stacking" or taking two or more different AS at the same time. Anabolic steroid "underground handbooks" normally detail theories behind different cycling regimes. Their main aim, according to these handbooks, is to promote the effectiveness (receptor site saturation prevents further improvement) of the drug while minimising their side effects, especially in the long term. These regimes are a result of trial and error, explaining the diversity. Table 4.3 shows selected examples of cycle theories reported by users. Although AS users tend to take them in cycles, many will use them continuously, irregularly and further, some take "maintenance" dosages while off AS. Talking to AS users, it is clear that they long to get back on them because of the

Table 4.3 Cycle theories

- **Diamond pattern** Start with minimal dose of one or more AS, increase dose for several weeks and then decrease for several weeks to ensure that body's own testosterone production works before AS use ceases
- **Inverted pyramid** Start with a maximum dose and then decrease it gradually. Popular with athletes who are likely to be tested
- **Three-week blitz** Use one drug at a time for 3 weeks, changing the preparation over a 15 week period

---

decrease or lack of increase in muscle size associated with cessation of use. To avoid a pronounced decline, HCG is taken for a few weeks before coming off AS.

"Natural" body-building organisations also exist and their members compete drug-free. Studies reporting on the prevalence of AS use in British gymnasia have estimated that up to 46% of clients may have used them[11] and their use appears to be common in gyms around the country. Over 4% of technical college students had taken them in a Scottish survey[15] and data from schools and gyms elsewhere have been very similar.[16] Users are commonly from diverse groups, ranging from teenagers to those near retirement age, of both sexes, and from a wide variety of occupations, including manual workers and top professionals.[11]

Why are drugs outlawed in sport?

First and foremost, drug use is seen as cheating and success is a result of external factors rather than talent. They are therefore seen to provide an unfair advantage. There is also concern about the potential for physiological and psychological harm, and some feel that drug use may encourage others to follow suit to maintain parity. On closer examination, however, each point is seen to contain some inconsistencies.

Patterns of use: anabolic steroids, anabolic agents, and other drugs

The type and dose of AS taken tends to depend on a number of factors. Sportspeople who are likely to be tested either after competition or out of competition tend to take oral forms because their clearance time is short (3–5 days), whereas body-builders who do not face drug testing are unrestricted in their choice. Numerous studies have shown that AS are taken mainly by injection and orally, with fewer women using injections.

75

Dosages

It is also common for AS to be taken at up to 100 times or more the recommended therapeutic dosages. As an example, Table 4.4 shows drugs

Table 4.4 Dosages used by a rugby player and a body-builder (mg per week)

Rugby player	Body-builder
Dianabol 420 mg – 10 weeks	Dianabol 35–175 mg – 2 weeks
Anavar 140 mg – 6 weeks	Sustanon (testo) 500 mg – 6 weeks
Anadrol 700 mg – 6 weeks	Deca-Durabolin 400 mg – 6 weeks
Deca-Durabolin 400 mg – 5 weeks	Oxytasona 350–1050 mg – 6 weeks
Tamoxifen 70 mg – 10 weeks	Tamoxifen 210 mg – 8 weeks
HCG 2000 IU – 6 weeks	HCG 2000 IU – 2 weeks
The cycle lasted for 16 weeks	The cycle lasted for 10 weeks

and dosages reported by a rugby player and a body-builder in interviews.[11] It is not uncommon for users to be unaware of the dosages they take because many quantify them as "shots" or "tablets". Many AS come in different strengths and the lack of knowledge regarding dosages may lead to over- or underdosaging. Millar[17] has also demonstrated that AS can be given in far lower doses than currently used by strength athletes with real gains and no major side effects.

Polypharmacy

Polypharmacy is common among AS users. A variety of drugs are used to enhance the effects of AS or to prevent unwanted side effects. A list of other growth agents commonly used in conjunction with AS is given in Table 4.5. Drugs designated as pre-contest drugs for body-building are detailed in Table 4.6. Although not all drugs listed will be used, it is common to use one under most classes presented. Many of these are taken as well by "non-competitive" users. Within the body-building factions use of amphetamines, ephedrine, cannabis, cocaine, and Ecstasy, as well as alcohol, can be expected. This begs the question whether injecting AS users in particular may be drawn into such a drug culture.

Human growth hormone

The use of human growth hormone (HGH) is estimated to be high both in body-building and sport, despite its expense. One of the principal reasons for sportspeople taking HGH is the lack of reliable detection methods. Some users believe that HGH increases muscle size and strength without the side effects caused by AS but anecdotal reports of their effectiveness have remained controversial. Studies have shown increases in size but not

Table 4.5   Growth agents commonly used in conjunction with anabolic steroids

- **Clenbuterol**   an asthma drug designed to promote smooth muscle relaxation. Has a partitioning effect promoting muscle growth and fat metabolism
- **Human growth hormone (HGH)**   a polypeptide secreted by the pituitary gland and now available in synthetic form. It is anabolic and anticatabolic. Views on effectiveness are controversial. Some believe that muscle tissue generated by GH tends to be "weak" with less contractile proteins than in normal muscle tissue. On the other hand, it is known to strengthen connective tissue throughout the body. Cannot be detected in dope testing
- **Insulin growth factor-1 (IGF-1)**   an insulin precursor taken to accelerate protein synthesis. IGF-2 is also used but has not been found effective by many. Can cause fast and extreme hypoglycaemia
- **Human chorionic gonadotrophin (HCG)**   restores spermatogenesis as it acts like LH; it also stimulates secretion of testosterone thus preventing muscle wasting during an off cycle. Athletes use it after switching off from AS before a competition. Some use it to stimulate fat mobilisation. It appears to minimise some of the depressive physical and mental after effects following cessation of an AS cycle
- **L-Dopa**   prescribed for Parkinson's disease, it is sometimes used to elevate endogenous growth hormone levels. Adverse reactions include paranoid and psychotic episodes

Table 4.6   Pre-contest drugs

- **Diuretics**   spironolactone, frusemide to promote muscle definition ("rippled" look)
- **Insulins**   short and long acting insulins to promote glucose uptake by tissues
- **Thyroid hormones** T_3 and T_4 products, Triacana to accelerate fat metabolism
- **Spreading agents**   Thiomucase (injection, oral, or ointment forms) to "spot" reduce fat (it dehydrates fat cells)
- **Anti-oestrogens**   Nolvadex (tamoxifen citrate) to prevent gynaecomastia in men and female fat distribution in women
- **Hypnotics**   triazolam (Halicom) to promote sleep
- **Opiates**   Nubain (Nalbuplin) to alleviate training-related pain in muscles and joints
- **Anti-catabolic agents**   aminoglutethimide (Cytodren)
- **Local steroids**   Esiclene irritates the injected site, thereby enhancing muscle definition

Note that the reasons given by athletes for using particular drugs do not necessarily conform with their therapeutic purpose.

Reports of the use of the following drugs are also common: antibiotics to combat acne; corticosteroids to treat inflammation; erythropoietin which some believe will give their veins a "fuller" look, also to improve workouts through improved oxygen delivery.

strength; indeed the muscles of agromegalic patients (who suffer from overproduction of HGH) have been shown to be myopathic.

Use of masking agents

Various "masking" agents have been taken in attempts to cover up the use of AS and testosterone and include preparations such as Defend (to block the metabolites of AS), epitestosterone (to lower testosterone/epitestosterone ratio), HCG (to alter testosterone/luteinising hormone ratio) and probenecid (to reduce the excretion of certain AS into urine). Probenecid is now banned and epitestosterone levels exceeding 150 ng/ml are taken as evidence of its exogenous use. Some have also tried to dilute urine by ingesting large amounts of fluids and taking diuretics but the detection methods now are extremely sophisticated and minute amounts of prohibited substances can be detected.

Athletes know that they are likely to be tested at competitions and they only need to come off any drugs days or weeks before, depending on the preparation used, to test clean. As Sir Arthur Gold has said "only the ill-advised and careless get caught".

Availability of anabolic steroids

Anabolic steroids appear to be easily available through gyms and mail order; forms can be obtained through some of the body-building magazines. Friends are also an important link, and in sport, coaches have been implicated. In the past, selling AS has been a relatively safe and lucrative business and the growing demand for AS and their limited supply through pharmaceutical companies has been filled by a flourishing counterfeit market; there are instances when dealers have inserted original labels on fake products. The contents, quality, cleanliness, and safety of such products have been questioned; indeed these have led to cases of poisoning and infection.[13]

Sources of information

Friendship networks play a key role in getting into training and taking AS and this tends to be the main source of information for most users, followed by underground handbooks and dealers. It is worrying that those who sell the drugs provide much of the information about drug combinations, "effective" dosages, cycle lengths, and possible side effects. In the absence of reliable medical and scientific information, AS use is largely based on the trial and error results of other users and drug availability from the dealer. Particularly worrying is the unsuitable advice given by men to women users.

In response to the growing number of AS users, a number of needle exchanges and drug agencies have started up clinics and special services for AS users. Currently there are a number of "well steroid user clinics" in Britain. Appendix 1 contains a list of agencies currently offering information and advice to AS users.

Dangers of self-administration of anabolic steroids

Purported adverse effects of AS use have attracted considerable media attention and have been used in campaigns hoping to deter people from the use of performance enhancing drugs. Such drastic and life-threatening side effects have not been substantiated by the medical literature, however, and the incidence of death or life-threatening diseases associated with AS use among sportspeople has been low.[9] Although it may well be that the occurrence of drastic events really is rare, it is also possible that effects do not get reported because of the stigma attached to AS use. Clearly there is a need for reliable information on the side effects associated with long term use. Unfortunately existing studies are short term, extending from a few weeks to no more than a year in most cases. Moreover, these studies tend to involve only therapeutic doses of AS and much of the data are derived from cases where AS were given as part of the treatment of severely ill patients. There is an acute lack of long term prospective studies of high dosage AS use. Attempts to convince AS users of serious adverse effects in the absence of reliable information have had the effect of alienating them from the medical profession.[17]

Although valuable information can be derived from case studies, the resulting perceived associations between AS and any particular condition cannot have the same status as associations derived from controlled studies. The adverse effects of AS that have been postulated are often considered under five general headings: cardiovascular, cosmetic, hepatic, reproductive, and psychiatric. Numerous reviews have been published on the topic.[18,19]

Cardiovascular effects

Adverse effects on plasma lipid profile have been reported in a number of studies[20,21] and this tends to be associated with the use of 17-α-alkylated steroids, oral or parenteral, but not with parenteral administration of androgen esters, even in high doses.[21,22] No consistent change has been reported for total cholesterol. In practice most AS users take the oral forms which will produce a high density lipoprotein cholesterol (HDL-C) lowering effect, therefore increasing the chance of developing coronary heart disease (CHD) in the long term. A similar effect is likely with the widespread use of oestrogen blockers.[22] It is also worth noting that weight-lifting alone will result in increased levels of HDL-C and decreased levels of low density lipoprotein cholesterol (LDL-C), an effect which is offset by the use of AS. HDL-C fractions start increasing after cessation of AS use and tend to normalise within 6–10 weeks.[20] The long term effects of these changes in terms of the development of CHD, atherosclerosis, and cerebrovascular disease are unknown. Increased platelet sensitivity to collagen in subjects over 22 years of age has been found and it is postulated that this may explain some of the thrombotic disease observed in AS users. Elevation of blood pressure is often cited but not well documented and it has been suggested that this may be dose-related. Increased blood pressure is commonly attributed to increased fluid retention. Morphological changes in the myocardium have been reported in animals treated with AS. The

79

effects of AS in 13 users and 12 non-users did not differ in terms of chamber size, dimensions, and systolic and diastolic functions between the groups, but left ventricular hypertrophy has been observed in other studies. Generally, there are few reports of cardiomyopathy, cases of cardiovascular accidents, and myocardial infarction in athletes and weight-lifters.[9] The possibility of thrombotic complications has been highlighted due to increased platelet sensitivity to collagen in weight-lifters using AS. Hyperinsulinism and altered glucose tolerance have also been implicated. These effects are commonly linked with the development of cardiovascular diseases. The use of clenbuterol causes lowering of plasma potassium levels and the combined use of diuretics may further compound this, leading to cardiac conduction abnormalities. Clenbuterol itself is known to cause arrhythmias, myocardial infarctions, and strokes.

Cosmetic effects

These are most pronounced in women and boys, including coarsening of voice, growth of facial and body hair, male pattern baldness, acne, and gynaecomastia (enlarged breasts) in men (Table 4.7). Sevenfold increases

Table 4.7   Common signs of anabolic steroid use

- **Skin**   acne; needle marks in large muscle groups; body hair in women; bruising with minor injuries
- **Face**   deepened voice and facial hair in women; acromegaly; broadened jaws (GH use); redness of the face and neck (use of Retinol A cream); puffiness caused by fluid retention
- **Chest**   gynaecomastia in men and atrophied breasts in women
- **Genital**   testicular atrophy in men and clitoral enlargement in women; infertility
- **Musculoskeletal**   marked muscle hypertrophy; disproportionate development of the neck, shoulders, and chest
- **Other**   insomnia; lack of concentration; mood swings; depression; obsessiveness with gym and extreme body conciousness

in oestradiol (due to aromatisation of testosterone and its associated esters) have been documented in male power athletes taking long term, high dosage AS combinations.[20] Clitoral enlargement is often viewed as a positive effect by women, leading to greater sexual satisfaction, unless enlargement is gross. Although cosmetic effects will not pose a health threat, they may be unacceptable to many women and the appearance-conscious. These effects also tend to be irreversible.

Hepatic effects

The liver is a target tissue for androgens and the main site for their clearance. Due to higher androgen levels, men develop hepatocellular carcinoma more frequently than women. Benign hepatomas and malignant tumours have been reported in patients treated with AS, and tumour regression was observed with the removal of therapy in the latter. It appears that rather than initiating tumours, AS may promote tumour formation by enhancing the effects of carcinogens. Three recent case reports of liver tumours in athletes, associated with AS use, have been documented. It is hypothesised that 17-α-alkylation does not produce more tumours than androgen esters, but increases the likelihood of discovery because of a greater possibility of a rupture due to enhanced fibrinolytic activity. Peliosis hepatis is characterised by blood-filled cysts in the liver and has been associated with androgen therapy in severely ill patients. In healthy patients, such as transsexuals treated with androgens, very few cases have been reported and most have involved 17-α-alkylated androgens.[23] One case of peliosis has also been reported in a woman who was treated with tamoxifen, which is commonly taken by AS users, suggesting an androgen/oestrogenic component. No cases of peliosis hepatis have been reported in athletes. Liver function abnormalities have been frequently observed but mainly when 17-α-alkylated forms were used. Strauss et al[24] reported elevated AST and ALT concentrations in male body-builders and power-lifters regardless of their history of AS use. Muscular exertion can also elevate levels of SGOT and CPK and therefore liver-specific enzymes should be studied, including LDH isoenzyme LDH_5 and ALK-P.

Table 4.8 A selection of 17-α-alkylated androgens

Fluoxymesterone (Halotestin, Ultandren)
Norethandrolone (Nilevar)
Oxymetholone (Anadrol, Androyd)
Metholone (Primobolin)
Methyltestosterone (Android)
Stanozolol (Winstrol)
Methandrostenolone (Dianabol)

The type of drug used, mainly the 17-α-alkylated forms (see Table 4.8), is often instrumental in the development of effects especially related to the liver. It would therefore be incorrect to attribute significant adverse effects to androgens as a general class. It is also important to bear in mind that adverse effects tend to be reversed with cessation of AS use.

Reproductive effects

A dose-dependent depression of luteinising hormone (LH) and follicle stimulating hormone (FSH) release is observed in men as a result of exogenous androgen use. This will lead to a much reduced or negligible sperm count, abnormal sperm morphology, and testicular atrophy.[25] These studies suggest that it takes less than 4 months for normalisation of sperm count but more than 4 months for normalisation of sperm motility and

81

morphology. Recovery will depend on the dose and length of time on AS. In attempts to prevent decreased testicular size and loss of libido, AS users commonly take HCG. There are no reports of permanent infertility in AS users. Menstrual irregularity or cessation of menstruation is common in women users[11] but there are no reports of permanent infertility in women, and a recent conversation with a long term female AS user suggests that menses may return within a few months after cessation of high dose AS use. On the other hand, data from female to male transsexuals show that the long term use of AS at high dosage may lead to the development of polycystic ovaries. This condition is associated with infertility and miscarriages.

Psychiatric effects

Reports of "roid rages" or aggression, mood swings, euphoria, diminished fatigue, changed libido, grandiosity, anxiety, and depression in AS users are widespread. Animal studies have demonstrated a link between testosterone levels, dominance, and aggressive behaviour, and both learning and social factors influence the actual expression of aggression in adulthood. Although an association in 58 16-year-olds between serum testosterone levels and self-reports of physical and verbal aggression in response to provocation and threat have been reported,[26] the extent to which aggressive behaviour produces higher levels of testosterone is not known. Bursts of high intensity exercise are known to elevate plasma levels of testosterone. Androgens have been used in the treatment of mental disorders, especially depression, for over 50 years, often with positive effects and commonly few undesired behavioural effects have been reported. Popular media reports linking "roid rages" to AS use have somewhat sensationalised the issue. Pope and Katz[27] reported in a widely published study that of the 41 AS users interviewed, 5 showed psychotic symptoms, 4 were borderline, 5 reported manic episodes, and 9 developed full affective syndromes during AS use. This work has been used to exemplify problems faced in researching the topic, and the validity of the findings has been seriously questioned. Parrott *et al*[28] studied 21 male AS users who were asked to complete the Buss–Durke Inventory on feelings of aggression, hostility, and guilt while on AS and while off AS. A second questionnaire enquired about aggression in more detail. They reported that feelings of aggression, aggression against objects, verbal aggression, and aggression during training were significantly heightened when high dose AS were taken. Also it was claimed that suspiciousness and irritability were increased during periods on AS. Lefavi *et al*[29] compared 13 current AS users to 18 former users and 14 non-users. The current users scored significantly higher than the other groups on anger-arousal, hyperactivity, aggressiveness, irritability, and euphoria. It is not known, though, whether such anger and irritability necessarily leads to acts of physical violence or whether it is inherent in the self-selected sample of current users. Indeed, Perry *et al*[30] assessed personality disorders in weight-lifters who were either users or non-users and community controls, and they found that the weight-lifters displayed an increased rate of personality pathology and antisocial traits regardless of AS use. Others have found chronic AS users to be more paranoid, schizoid, antisocial, narcissistic, and passive-aggressive than non-users. One prospective double-blind, fixed order, placebo-controlled crossover trial found that varying dose administration of methyltestosterone over a 3 day period resulted in significant, though subtle increases in positive mood, negative mood, and cognitive impairment during the high dose (250 mg/day) condition.[31] In general, it is agreed that irritability is increased in many users and that a few who are premorbid may end up exhibiting irrational or violent behaviour. It is worth noting that cases have been reported where severe depression and suicidal ideas developed after injections of Haldol Decanoate (a neuroleptic), sold on the black market as an AS. The interactions of heavy training, polypharmacy – particularly the use of other drugs of abuse – personality dimensions, expectations, and sensitivity to certain AS makes it immensely difficult to draw any cause–effect relationship between AS use and behaviour. Illicitly sold preparations pose another serious consideration. It is suggested that AS use may cause dependence and that the two most powerful predictors are *"dissatisfaction with body image"* and *"depressed mood"*.[32] The mechanisms for the proposed dependence are unknown, but three mechanisms have been implicated. The positive reinforcement mechanisms involve a brain reward system similar to opioid use. Large and impressive musculature may improve self-esteem, increase social standing, and further a career in sport, for example. Negative reinforcement mechanisms might involve avoidance of depression and other withdrawal symptoms and, importantly, the loss of muscle mass. The latter will be linked with possible loss of social rewards. Avoidance of feeling not big enough has also been implicated.[32]

The aggression or energy and vigour sportspeople derive from AS use is said to facilitate their training through more intensive effort exerted.

Other health-related effects

In the young, AS use may lead to premature closure of epiphyses and therefore stunted growth, although little documented evidence for this exists. Altered thyroid function has been observed. Musculoskeletal injuries are often cited, but no direct link has been demonstrated with AS. Deaths in AS-using body-builders who contracted AIDS through needle-sharing have been reported. Sharing of injecting equipment has been reported in only a few published British studies, although this is contradicted by anecdotal evidence from needle exchanges, which have been in contact with a worrying number of cases. A case of prostate cancer has been linked with AS use, and the possibility of an androgen effect parallel to the risk of breast cancer from the oral contraceptive pill has been drawn. Interviews with AS users have suggested that some users suffer from colds when they are coming off AS.[11] Six HIV-positive homosexual men felt healthier; in particular, they were able to maintain their weight after they started to take AS.[11]

Although clinical trials with therapeutic doses of AS and short term studies of self-administration of AS have not shown substantial and systematic adverse effects it would be premature to conclude that there are few dangers. Large doses, polypharmacy, and the consumption of preparations obtained from the black market may cause unpredictable consequences which may only be realised in the future.

Screening

Table 4.9 shows some commonly suggested blood and urine tests, and the reader is referred to Brower[32] for further details regarding laboratory tests recommended for the screening of AS users.

Table 4.9 Suggested laboratory tests

Plasma lipids TG, HDL/LDL-cholesterol ratio
Endocrine LH and FSH levels, TSH, T_3, T_4, TBG levels
Liver function ALK-P, LDH
Cardiac function baseline ECG for evidence of LVH, echocardiogram if evidence of LVH found
Other electrolytes, urea, serum glucose, haematocrit, RBC, and immunoglobulins

Summary details of the testing procedure used by the UK Sports Council, Ethics and Anti-Doping Directorate are given in Appendix 2.

Other ergogenic aids: an update

Blood doping

Endurance athletes have used numerous and adventurous ways to improve their performance. Classic studies by Ekblom *et al* and Buick *et al* in the early 1970s suggested that total haemoglobin levels and therefore the blood oxygen carrying capacity could be increased by intravenous infusion of blood. This has a similar effect to training at altitude, which leads to increased haemoglobin levels due to lowered ambient oxygen pressure. The aim has been to increase maximal oxygen consumption.

Blood doping involves the withdrawal of two units of blood and separation of the red blood cells (RBC) which are then frozen. When the athlete's RBC count has returned to normal, which may take up to 10 weeks, the thawed cells are reinfused. This practice is illegal but there are no reliable detection methods.

The production of RBC is partly governed by a naturally occurring glycoprotein, erythropoietin (EPO). In 1985, the gene that codes for EPO was cloned and, shortly thereafter, manufactured. In 1987 recombinant EPO (rEPO) became available and is thought to have become widely used by endurance athletes. Studies by Ekblom and Berglund in the early 1990s[33] have shown improvements in maximal aerobic power with rEPO administration. Some athletes have likened the use of rEPO to being connected to a turbo.

The use of rEPO poses serious health threats and a large number of athletes, including orienteers, cyclists, and runners, are suspected to have died as a consequence of its use. Problems tend to arise with increasing viscosity of the blood. This is compounded when dehydration sets in. At haematocrits above 55% the blood viscosity increases exponentially, which then increases the risk of thrombosis and stroke, and other blood vessel occlusions. Currently, there are no reliable methods for detecting rEPO use and, although quite possible, manufacturers are reluctant to add a marker which could be detected in dope testing.

Stimulants

As a class, stimulants include psychomotor and central nervous system stimulants (e.g. cocaine, amphetamines, and caffeine) and sympatho-mimetic amines (e.g. ephedrine, pseudoephedrine, phenylephrine, and phenylpropanolamine). They are used by sportspeople to reduce fatigue, to increase concentration, to decrease sensitivity to pain, to improve endurance, and to increase competitiveness. For example, amphetamines were used during the Second World War by soldiers to ward off fatigue.

The Barcelona Olympics became notorious for athletes getting caught using the stimulant clenbuterol, a beta$_2$-agonist, which is taken to increase muscle mass and to decrease fat mass. It has been found to be a potent partitioning agent in animals but there are no studies of its efficacy in humans. Large numbers of body-builders have found it effective, although there is some controversy over this.

Caffeine and ephedrine are sometimes taken together to increase fat metabolism and resting metabolic rate. Amphetamines have a similar effect. These drugs are readily detectable in urine samples and the athlete needs to check that any decongestants or herbal remedies they plan to take will not contain ephedrine. Some protein powders (for example Triacana) available from health food shops also contain ephedrine but these tend to warn athletes likely to be tested to withdraw from use 5 days beforehand.

A number of recent studies have suggested that, for example, amphetamines can improve performance in terms of speed, power, endurance, concentration, and fine motor coordination. The risks to be considered include elevation of blood pressure and heart rate, thus stressing the cardiovascular system. They can trigger cardiac arrhythmias. Because amphetamines delay the *sensation* of fatigue, athletes may exercise beyond their limits to the point of circulatory failure, leading to death. They may also become addictive because of the euphorigenic and energising effect. Nervousness, anxiety, insomnia, and aggressive behaviour have also been cited. Between 1988 and 1994, 121 athletes in the UK tested positive for using stimulants.

Caffeine

Caffeine is a central nervous system stimulant and its effects are similar to those mentioned above. In the late 1970s Costill published two reports on improved endurance performance in cycling and running. His article in *Runners World* stating that a 2:30 marathon could be improved by 10 minutes got the masses taking caffeine before endurance events. It also earned the IOC ban (which had been lifted in 1972). Studies on its efficacy have been controversial but it seems that moderate to high doses (5–10 mg/kgBW) are required to improve endurance and habituation may affect the result. Improved endurance times are probably caused by increased fat metabolism which conserves limited glycogen stores within the working muscles. In practice, two cups of strong coffee have been recommended 45–60 minutes before an endurance race combined with caffeine ingestion throughout the event using 5 mg/kgBW. Consumption of a realistic amount of caffeine (150–200 mg = 2–3 cups) has improved 1500 metre running and 1500 metre swimming times. The authors speculated that increased rate of carbohydrate metabolism (breakdown) or improved rate of potassium handling during muscle contraction may be responsible.

Weight-lifters and throwers appear to use caffeine to enhance both power and strength and they take it in the form of strong coffee. Beneficial effects of this have not been substantiated by well controlled studies. Short term (<5 min) high intensity (>100% $\dot{V}o_2$max) exercise (STHIX) and repeated bouts of STHIX under laboratory conditions have also been shown to benefit from caffeine administration. The proposed mechanisms include the stimulation of the CNS, enhancement of neuromuscular transmission and facilitation of muscle fibre contractility due to a variety of cellular effects of caffeine. Dosages taken before enhanced STHIX trials involved between 250 mg and 500 mg, or 5–6 mg/kgBW caffeine. Side effects include

86

Table 4.10 Caffeine content of selected products

1 cup of brewed coffee: 50–150 mg
1 cup of strong tea: 10–50 mg
1 can of a soft drink: 50 mg
25 g milk chocolate cocoa: 6 mg
25 g baking chocolate cocoa: 35 mg
Standard dose of some aspirin products 30–128 mg
Caffeine reaches peak concentration in the blood at between 30 and 120 minutes
* IOC ban: 500–600 mg caffeine = 5–6 cups of strong coffee.

diuresis, increased anxiety, and possible gastric upsets. Table 4.10 illustrates the caffeine content of selected food products and the cut-off point for the IOC ban. Remember that the caffeine content of tea depends not only on its content in the tea, but also the infusion time.

Creatine

Creatine (Cr) is naturally found in meat and fish and it is synthesised in the liver, kidney, and pancreas. During a 6 second sprint, for example, 50% of the energy required is from creatine phosphate (CP) and the decline in power output over the 6 seconds mirrors the decline in CP content within the working muscles. Optimal supplementation appears to involve 20 g of Cr per day for 5 days (increases total muscle Cr content by more than 20%) and enables the athlete to maintain their speed/performance close to maximum.[34] Improvements have been recorded in 300 metre and 3000 metre running and in women hockey players who completed ten 30 second sprints with 30 second recovery. The actual mechanism is still under debate, but increased pre-exercise Cr stores lasting longer, increased buffering capacity, and acceleration of CP resynthesis during recovery have been cited. It seems that the greatest increases in Cr concentrations occur in vegetarians and those who have done light exercise during supplementation. A full kilogram of fresh meat is needed to derive 1 g of chemically created Cr.

Because this method is so new, no information is available regarding side effects. Kidney problems have been postulated with prolonged high dose use. It is known that Cr supplementation increases fluid retention and has been detrimental in a 6 km running race, yet magazines are full of adverts (for example for KR10 and Acceler-8) promoting its use among endurance athletes, such as triathletes. Recent evidence suggests that 20 g Cr per day for 5 days may increase calf muscle strength and endurance. It may work for the endurance athletes, as running velocities have been increased during 1000 m intervals. These were followed by improved recovery, thus possibly improving the quality of training so benefiting the endurance athlete. Creatine supplementation has not been banned in sport and its use appears to be very popular. Muscle stores of Cr decline slowly over 6–8 weeks following a 20 g/day for 5 days regime, while maintenance doses of 2 g daily have been found to be effective.

Bicarbonates

Muscle fatigue in sprinting events lasting longer than 10 seconds is partly due to lowered pH levels and tolerance to high intensity exercise may be limited by the body's ability to counteract decreased muscle and blood pH via its buffering system. The majority of H^+ dissociated from metabolic acids produced during exercise are buffered by the bicarbonate ion system. Bicarbonate ingestion (baking soda) has led to improved performance in rowing, cycling, running, and swimming. Factors associated with improved performance include trained subjects, a single maximal bout of exercise lasting from 1 to 7 minutes, or repeated high intensity bouts of exercise (400–3000 metre running or 100–400 metre swimming). The recommended dose is 300 mg/kgBW with 1 litre of water, to be taken 90–120 minutes before the race. Side effects include gastrointestinal discomfort in the short term. Prolonged use is associated with apathy, irritability, muscle spasms, and cardiac arrhythmias.

Diuretics

Diuretics are used most commonly in sports with weight categories, such as boxing, gymnastics, martial arts, and wrestling. They rid the body of excess fluid and have been used in attempts to mask the use of banned substances. There are no other advantages for taking diuretics apart from weight loss, and in fact they may impair performance in events which require moderate to high levels of endurance because of losses in extracellular fluid, including plasma. This also leads to lesser ability to thermoregulate effectively. Loss of body fluids may also result in electrolyte imbalances, mainly sodium and potassium, which may cause muscle cramping and fatigue and, if pronounced, may cause arrhythmias and cardiac conduction problems. Between 1988 and 1994 only two athletes in the UK tested positive for diuretics.

Oral contraceptive pill

The birth control pill contains manufactured oestrogen and progesterone and is considered ergogenic because it controls the athlete's menstrual cycle. Some women feel that their performance is adversely affected because of premenstrual syndrome or painful periods. Some elite women athletes are convinced that they can perform better during the follicular phase (early phase) of the menstrual cycle and in such cases manipulation of the cycle may be attempted to ensure that the competition coincides with the "right time of the month". Side effects of the contraceptive pill may include: nausea, weight gain, fatigue, hypertension, liver tumours, blood clots, and strokes. Side effects, especially weight gain and fluid retention, have been minimised with new low dose triphasic preparations.

Summary

Judge Dubin's report revealed the vast scope of doping in sport, not only in Canada but all over the world. It appears that the IOC and other major sporting authorities have in reality done little to combat this. Potentially harmful drugs, such as AS, GH, and EPO, are being used by sportspeople. Some of these can be detected by the dope tests, while others cannot. In particular, AS use outside competitive sport has increased exponentially in the past 10 years and AS users can now be found in most cities. While widespread use is now acknowledged, there remains a lack of substantive information on the long term effects of this. It is important to realise that polypharmacy, use of protein supplements, vitamin and mineral preparations, together with extremely hard training regimes, makes it difficult to assess the efficacy of AS. Likewise, the causes of side effects (psychological and physiological) associated with the use of AS and the other drugs described, is further confounded with concomitant use of the "traditional" drugs of abuse.

References

1 Simson VYV, Jennings A. *The lords of the rings*. New York: Simon & Schuster, 1992.
2 Yesalis CE, Wright JE, Lombardo JA. Anabolic-androgenic steroids: a synthesis of existing data and recommendations for future research. *Clin Sportsmed* 1989; 1:109–34.
3 Forbes GB. The effect of anabolic steroids on lean body mass: the dose–response curve. *Metabolism* 1985;34:571–3.
4 Boone JB, Lambert CP, Flynn MG, Michaud TJ, Rodriguez-Zayas JA, Andres FF. Resistance exercise effects on plasma cortisol, testosterone and creatine kinase activity in anabolic-androgenic steroid users. *Int J Sports Med* 1990;11: 293–7.
5 Itil T. Neurophysiological effects of hormones in humans: computer EEG profiles of sex and hypothalamic hormones. In Schar EJ, ed. *Hormones, behaviour and psychopathology*. New York: Raven Press, 1976.
6 Hervey GR, Hutchinson I, Knibbs AV, *et al.* Anabolic effects of methandienone in men undergoing athletic training. *Lancet* 1976;2:699–702.

7 Hervey GR, Knibbs AV, Burkinshaw L, *et al*. Effects of methandienone on the performance and body composition of men undergoing athletic training. *Clin Sci* 1981;**60**:457–61.

8 Duchaine D. *Underground steroid handbook II*. USA: Daniel Duchaine, 1989.

9 Lombardo J. The efficacy and mechanisms of action of anabolic steroids. In Yesalis CE, ed. *Anabolic steroids in sport and exercise*. Champaign, IL: Human Kinetics Publishers, 1993.

10 Duda M. Female athletes: targets for drug abuse. *Phys Sports Med* 1986;**14**: 142–6.

11 Korkia PK, Stimson GV. *Anabolic steroid use in Great Britain: exploratory investigation*. The Centre for Research on Drugs and Health Behaviour. A report for the Department of Health, the Welsh Office and the Chief Scientist Office, Scottish Home and Health Department, 1993.

12 US Department of Justice Drug Enforcement Administration. *Report of the International Conference on the Abuse and Trafficking of Anabolic Steroids*. Washington, DC: US Drug Enforcement Administration, 1994.

13 Phillips WN. *Anabolic reference guide*. Golden, USA: Mile High Publishing, 1991.

14 Wright JEW. *Anabolic steroids and sport*, vol. II. North Little Rock: Sports Science Consultants, 1982.

15 Williamson DJ. Misuse of anabolic drugs (Letter). *Br Med J* 1993;**306**:6869–71.

16 Buckley W, Yesalis C, Friedl K, Anderson W, Streit A, Wright J. Estimated prevalence of anabolic steroid use among male high school seniors. *J Am Med Assoc* 1988;**260**:3441–5.

17 Millar AP. Licit steroid use – hope for the future. *Br J Sports Med* 1994;**28**: 79–83.

18 Haupt H, Rovere G. Anabolic steroids: a review of the literature. *Am J Sports Med* 1984;**12**:469–84.

19 Yesalis C, Ed. *Anabolic steroids in sport and exercise*. Champaign, IL: Human Kinetics Publishers, 1993.

20 Alen M, Rahkila P, Marniemi J. Serum lipids in power athletes self-administering testosterone and anabolic steroids. *Int J Sports Med* 1985;**6**:139–44.

21 Thompson PD, Cullinane EM, Sady SP *et al*. Contrasting effects of testosterone and stanozolol on serum lipoprotein levels. *J Am Med Assoc* 1989;**261**:1165–8.

22 Friedl KE, Hannan CJ, Jones RE, Plymate SR. Comparison of the effects of high dose testosterone and 19-nortestosterone to a replacement dose of testosterone on strength and body composition in normal men. *J Steroid Biochem Mol Biol* 1990;**40**:607–12.

23 Lowdell CP, Murray-Lyon IM. Reversal of liver damage due to long term methyltestosterone and safety of non-17α-alkylated androgens. *Br Med J* 1985; **291**:637.

24 Strauss RH, Wright JE, Finerman GA, Catlin DH. Side effects of anabolic steroids in weight-trained men. *Phys Sports Med* 1983;**11**:87–96.

25 Matsumoto AM. Effect of chronic testosterone administration in normal men: safety and efficacy of high dosage testosterone and parallel dose-dependent suppression of luteinizing hormone, follicle stimulating hormone and sperm production. *J Clin Endocrinol Metabol* 1990;**70**:282–7.

26 Olweus DO, Mattsson A, Schalling D, Low H. Testosterone, aggression, physical and personality dimensions in normal adolescent males. *Psychosom Med* 1980;**50**:261–72.

27 Pope H, Katz D. Affective and psychotic symptoms associated with anabolic steroid use. *Am J Psych* 1988;**145**:487–90.

28 Parrot AC, Choi PYL, Davies, M. Anabolic steroid use by amateur athletes: effects upon psychological mood states. *J Sports Med Phys Fitness* 1994;**34**: 292–8.
29 Lefavi R, Reeve T, Newland M. Relationships between anabolic steroid use and selective psychological parameters in male bodybuilders. *J Sport Behaviour* 1990;**13**:157–66.
30 Perry P, Andersen K, Yates W. Illicit anabolic steroid use in athletes. *Am J Sports Med* 1990;**26**:422–8.
31 Su T-P, Pagliaro M, Schmidt PJ, Pickar D, Wolkowitz O, Rubinow DR. Neuropsychiatric effects of anabolic steroids in male normal volunteers. *J Am Med Assoc* 1993;**31**:1232–4.
32 Brower KJ. Assessment and treatment of anabolic steroid withdrawal. In Yesalis CE, ed. *Anabolic steroids in sport and exercise.* Champaign, IL: Human Kinetics Publishers, 1993.
33 Ekblom B, Berglund B. Effect of erythropoietin administration on maximal aerobic power. *Scand J Med Sci Sports* 1991;**1**:88–93.
34 Greenhaff PL, Casey A, Short AH, Harris RC, Soderland K, Hultman E. Influence of oral creatinine supplementation on muscle torque during repeated bouts of maximal voluntary exercise in man. *Clin Sci* 1993;**84**:565–71.

Appendix 1 Sources of information and advice

Institute for the Study of Drug Dependence (ISDD)
Waterbridge House, 32–36 Loman Street, London SE1 0EE
Tel: 0171 9281211

The library holds a comprehensive range of articles, some on anabolic steroids. Leaflets are also for sale.

National Sports Medicine Institute Library
c/o Medical College of St Bartholomew's Hospital, Charterhouse Square, London EC1M 6BQ
Tel: 0171 2510583

Quarterly bulletin on Ergogenic Aids in Sport and a library service.

The UK Sports Council, Ethics and Anti-Doping Directorate
Walkden House, 10 Melton Street, London NW1 2EB
Tel: 0171 3808000

Information on performance enhancing drugs.

The English Sports Council Information Centre
16 Upper Woburn Place, London WC1H 0QP
Tel: 0171 2731500

Library service by appointment.

District Health Authorities may be contacted to find out about local "well steroid user clinics".

For details of testing procedures see Chapter 3, p 65.

5 Medical care for female athletes

ROSLYN CARBON

As increasing numbers of women of all ages and expertise become involved in regular sports participation, it is likely that many will present for management of sports injuries and health problems. The management of the vast majority of such cases presents no difference between the sexes. Injury patterns are more sport-specific than sex-specific and immediate care and rehabilitation programmes are dictated by the severity of the injury and the aspirations of the participant rather than by gender. The health management of the highly trained female does however present some specific aspects related to menstrual function, dietary requirements, skeletal integrity, and pregnancy.

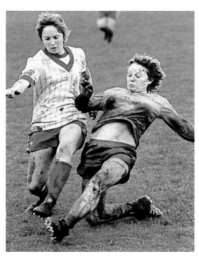

Figure 5.1   Injury patterns are more sport-specific than sex-specific (Reproduced from McLatchie G, Harries M, Williams C, King JB. ABC of sports medicine. London: BMJ Publishing Group, p. 73.)

Too much has been written of the "dangers" of sport for women. The vast majority of active women enjoy improved health, remain fertile and

93

find fulfilment in their sport. Exercise has positive effects on menstrual function, bone mineral density, cardiac risk factors and function, as well as on general wellbeing and psychological health. High level sport poses health and injury risks for both sexes and this requires expert medical care for both prevention and cure.

Nutrition for sportswomen

Iron intake and anaemia

All athletes need a well balanced diet that meets the energy needs of their training programme as well as providing the necessary vitamins and minerals for health. Some sportswomen may have particular nutritional needs in respect of extra iron intake relative to menstrual blood loss, and adequate calcium intake to ensure optimum bone density.

Menstruating women generally require twice the daily iron intake of men – about 15 mg per day. Endurance athletes of both sexes frequently have haemoglobin and iron levels below reference range and this is, in part, due to the haemodilution in response to aerobic training itself. However, some athletes will have true iron deficiency either from low intake or absorption of iron, or from a postulated haemolysis from the repeated microtrauma of training. Hence women endurance athletes, in particular, should ensure adequate iron levels or risk possible fatigue and poor performance. Serum ferritin is probably the best indicator of iron stores and a level below 30 ng/ml should be treated. Meat is the best source of iron and should be eaten daily, although vegetarians can manage to maintain iron stores with a careful diet. Total daily nutrition should exceed 2000 kcal (8300 kJ) and include fortified cereals and bread, green vegetables, and fruit. It is useful to remember that vitamin C (in orange juice) improves iron absorption, while phytic acid (in fibrous cereals) and tannic acid (in tea and coffee) bind iron in the gut and hence limit absorption.

In practice, overt iron deficiency often requires supplementation under medical control. Many athletes find the gastrointestinal disruption of oral iron too debilitating and, if anaemia persists, intramuscular iron in small doses may be necessary.

Calcium and bone mass

All women need adequate calcium intake and regular weight-bearing exercise to ensure optimal bone density. Current guidelines suggest a recommended daily intake (RDI) of 800 mg per day for young (menstruating) women and 1500 mg per day for postmenopausal women who have a lower absorption of calcium.

Physical activity results in increased bone density, especially in those parts of the skeleton exercised, such as the lower limbs in running and the spine in rowing. However, in amenorrhoeic athletes bone mass may be reduced due to a negative calcium balance in response to low oestrogen levels and poor nutrition (see below). Hence calcium intake should be equivalent to that recommended for postmenopausal women. In practice this may be difficult to achieve from diet alone. Athletes must be encouraged not to avoid dairy products, the main source of dietary calcium. Low fat cheese, milk, and yoghurt are excellent nutritional choices for sportswomen. Half a litre of low fat milk and 300 g of low fat plain yoghurt will meet the daily calcium needs of the amenorrhoeic athlete. High protein, tea, and coffee ingestion have a negative effect on calcium status because of increased renal excretion.

Amenorrhoeic athletes on a limited diet will almost certainly need calcium supplementation and consideration should be given to hormone replacement therapy to protect the skeleton from future osteoporosis.

Eating disorder and sport

Anorexia nervosa and bulimia are severe psychological disturbances that often require long term psychiatric care and, especially in the case of anorexia, carry significant morbidity and mortality. Anorexia is characterised by fasting, weight loss, and amenorrhoea while bulimia involves food binges and purging, often with fairly normal body weight.

There is an increasing prevalence of these conditions in Western adolescent populations, with a sex ratio approaching 9:1 toward girls.

Most sports require a low body fat to optimise performance; some have weight categories, and others such as gymnastics and ballet encourage a very thin appearance for aesthetic reasons. Women, however, naturally carry about twice the body fat of men because the physiology of ovarian hormones favours fat deposition. Higher levels of testosterone in men favour an increased lean mass of muscle and bone. Consequently many female athletes constantly strive to maintain a low body fat while at the same time needing to ensure adequate nutrition for their sport and appetite.

There is probably no greater incidence of true eating disorder in athletes compared with the general population, but the stresses of sports participation lead to a high level of abnormal eating practices in athletes. Furthermore, some true anorexics may exercise as part of their obsession with thinness.

Medical personnel, as well as coaches, need to be alert to signs of disordered eating such as gross weight loss or food avoidance. Nutritional advice should be given to athletes without undue pressure for unrealistic and unnecessary weight control. As in any form of medical examination, sensitivity must be used when measuring body weight and fat mass. Body

95

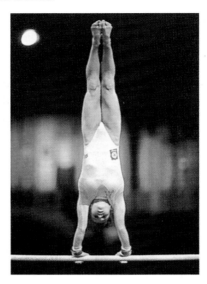

Figure 5.2 Many female athletes will strive to maintain low body fat while needing to ensure adequate nutrition for their sport (Reproduced from McLatchie G, Harries M, Williams C, King JB. ABC of sports medicine. London: BMJ Publishing Group, p. 43.)

fat should be seen as just one variable of health and training assessment rather than a "performance target" in itself.

Should there be evidence of a true eating disorder in an athlete this must be addressed quickly and management sought from a specialist (psychiatrist) in the field.

Reproductive physiology and exercise

The menstrual cycle and sport

In general, exercising women report fewer premenstrual symptoms, including dysmenorrhoea. This is related to the general "dampening down" of the reproductive hormones as a result of regular exercise. The hormonal response to exercise itself also probably improves mood and lessens the perception of symptomatology – akin to the concept of "runner's high".

However, some athletes, especially younger girls, will continue to suffer from heavy bleeding or pain that may interfere with training or competition. Treatment can include simple analgesics such as paracetamol or the short acting anti-inflammatories, including mefenamic acid. Bleeding can be controlled using progestogens such as norethisterone 5–15 mg per day. Alternatively, regular use of the oral contraceptive can limit both pain and menstrual loss.

Management of significant premenstrual symptoms in athletes is similar to the general population. Progestogens or other "remedies" such as vitamin B complex or "evening primrose oil" can be used during the last week of the cycle. Care must be taken not to prescribe banned drugs such as diuretics to competitive athletes.

Menses can be avoided at competition times by continuation of the oral contraceptive beyond the usual 3 week course, but breakthrough bleeding and increased "premenstrual" symptoms may be a problem. Alternatively, an earlier course of "the pill" may be cut short followed by less than the usual 7 days off medication before commencing a 3 week course to create a withdrawal bleed before competition. The athlete should be warned that contraceptive efficacy may be disrupted.

Exercise-related amenorrhoea

The diminution of reproductive hormonal levels induced by exercise can lead to alteration of menstrual function. In a percentage of highly trained athletes this will culminate in loss of menstrual cycling – amenorrhoea – during times of heavy training. However, complete absence of menses is rarely, if ever, only as a result of high levels of exercise. Amenorrhoeic athletes are usually younger, have commonly lost weight and body fat, have nutrition inadequate for their training load, and are suffering psychological stress in response to their lifestyle. The combination of these factors alters the central neurotransmitters in the hypothalamus, and hence pituitary gonadotrophins are diminished and ovarian function ceases. The central mechanism is thought to be related to feedback mechanisms from hormone levels which are altered by regular exercise and other stresses. Possible hormones implicated include the reproductive steroids themselves, the catecholamines, and the "stress" hormones of cortisol and ACTH, and/or the beta endorphins.

In reality, the changes of menstrual function are not simply an on–off mechanism. Rather, some athletes will have more frequent menses due to "luteal inadequacy" from a poorly functioning corpus luteum, others will have menses more than 35 days apart (oligomenorrhoea), and some will lapse into total amenorrhoea.

Delayed menarche is also common in athletic girls, although this is also related to self-selection in that girls who mature late often excel in sport.

Such menstrual disturbances are reversible when the stresses responsible for them are removed. This is often seen when the athlete stops training because of injury or a holiday, or she gains a few kilograms in weight. Hence this "hypothalamic" type of amenorrhoea can be viewed as a "functional" adaptation rather than an "organic" disease, but it may incur significant sequelae.

Secondary effects of menstrual disturbance

Fertility

While an athlete is often unaware of any problems associated with the absence of her menses, the secondary effects of depressed ovarian function may, in time, have negative health sequelae.

Obviously, if an athlete is anovulatory she will be infertile. However, most women in heavy training are not seeking pregnancy and reproductive function will almost always resume with improved nutrition, higher body weight, and lower training load.

In a very small minority, infertility remains a problem and this should be treated in keeping with the persistent hormonal insufficiency. Clomiphene may be used if endogenous oestrogen levels are high enough or, rarely, parenteral gonadotrophin may be required.

Bone mineral density

It is now well recognised that persistent hypo-oestrogenic states such as prolongued exercise-related amenorrhoea can result in loss of spinal bone mineral density (see above). This is because of changes in calcium balance and altered bone turnover in response to hormonal disturbance. Many studies have shown that amenorrhoeic athletes, on average, have lower spinal bone mass when compared with menstruating controls. Vertebral bone is largely trabecular in conformation and this type of bone, which has a rapid turnover rate, is the most susceptible to hormonal inadequacy.

Physical activity is, however, a potent stimulator of bone deposition. Hence normally menstruating athletes will be expected to have above average bone mass. Furthermore, the cortical bone mass of long bones, which is increased in athletes, is largely unaffected by menstrual disturbance.

Amenorrhoeic athletes should not be labelled as having "osteoporosis" in terms of the condition of elderly women in whom minimal trauma is likely to cause acute fractures of the spine, wrist, and neck of the femur. Such fractures do not occur in young athletes. It is more accurate and relevant to term their bone mass as "osteopenic", as young women, unlike the postmenopausal woman, may have the capacity to increase bone mass in the future. It is also likely that bone quality, or collagen matrix, is superior in the young. Research indicates, however, that peak bone mass may be jeopardised in prolongued amenorrhoea. Of significance to long term management is the probability that women who continue to exercise are more likely to maintain bone mass into old age.

Injury incidence

Less obvious than infertility and lower bone mass measurements is the observation that amenorrhoeic athletes have a greater injury incidence.

Interpretation of injury statistics is difficult because there are often confounding factors that cannot be controlled such as training load and poor training techniques. However, several reports indicate that total trauma incidence, including acute as well as chronic overuse injuries, is greater in amenorrhoeics.

Stress fractures have been shown in several studies to occur with increased frequency in amenorrhoeic compared with normally menstruating athletes. It is not known whether this is because athletes who train harder, and become amenorrhoeic, also get stress fractures, or because the coincident alteration in bone metabolism leads to stress fractures.

Diagnosis and management of athletic amenorrhoea

Amenorrhoea is a symptom and not a diagnosis and, as it may herald malignancy or significant endocrine disturbance, an "organic" diagnosis must always be excluded. Because of the known sequelae, athletes must not be encouraged to seek amenorrhoea by overzealous coaches who may see it as evidence of total commitment to training.

Table 5.1 outlines the differential diagnosis to be considered in the young amenorrhoeic athlete. Because spontaneous ovulation may occur during menstrual disturbance, pregnancy should always be considered and investigated early. As indicated above, high levels of physical activity may present as part of the pathology of true anorexia nervosa.

Table 5.1 Differential diagnosis for "athletic" amenorrhoea

Pregnancy
Anorexia nervosa
Primary ovarian failure
Polycystic ovarian disease
Pituitary tumour – hyperprolactinaemia
Virilisation syndromes – e.g. congenital adrenal hyperplasia
Thyroid disease
Genetic disorders ⎫
Anatomical abnormalities ⎭ primary amenorrhoea

Amenorrhoea of 6 months' duration or a delayed menarche beyond 16 years warrant medical assessment.

A thorough history should be taken, noting any change in training and competition, body weight, and dietary patterns which coincide with the onset of menstrual disturbance. Systemic enquiry should focus on symptoms associated with those features of organic pathology within the differential diagnosis.

Physical examination should be entirely normal in hypothalamic, exercise-related amenorrhoea, except the athlete may have low body fat and/or weight.

Signs of eating disorder include emaciation, lanugo hair, and low body temperature and pulse rate in anorexia nervosa; and parotid swelling and occasionally stained teeth with facial telangiectasis from vomiting in bulimia.

Signs of virilisation or hirsutism may be evident in polycystic ovarian disease or certain tumours and endocrine disorders, as well as in anabolic steroid abuse.

Perineal examination is important in the primary amenorrhoeic to exclude anatomical abnormality but ultrasound examination of the pelvis is more accurate and probably preferable to clinical pelvic examination in the young athlete. Genetic abnormalities may present as primary amenorrhoea and chromosomal analysis should be performed early.

If the clinician is satisfied that the onset of amenorrhoea can be explained by weight loss, training, and stress levels, a minimum of investigation can be performed. A serum prolactin can exclude a pituitary tumour. An oestradiol level should be low normal, consistent with the early follicular phase. Very low levels should raise concern about bone health and be followed by gonadotrophin estimation to exclude primary ovarian failure.

Management of exercise-related amenorrhoea.

The underlying causes of exercise-related amenorrhoea need to be discussed with the athlete, along with a clear explanation of the possible short and long term sequelae. An attempt should be made to encourage the athlete to decrease her training load, perhaps trading "quality" for "quantity", reduce the stresses in her lifestyle, and improve her nutrition and gain weight. The clinican should stress the benefits of improved health on physical performance. Amenorrhoea should be seen as one part of overstressing or overtraining that may eventually lead to poor performance.

If the athlete is unwilling to comply with this advice, or is unable to because of current demands of a sporting season, it is reasonable to offer medical treatment to protect bone health. This may take the form of progestogens alone; 15 mg of medroxyprogesterone daily will result in withdrawal bleeds if endogenous oestrogen levels are high enough. Replacement hormonal therapy in postmenopausal doses may be used and this will present minimal further suppression to the reproductive axis. Low dose oral contraceptives may be used, preferably if the athlete has previously had an established menstrual pattern.

However, there is increasing evidence that bone mass improvement is greater with the return of normal menses compared with oestrogen/progesterone administration. The former must always be the aim of medical management.

Pregnancy and the active woman

Many competitive sportswomen succeed in their careers into motherhood. Similarly, many recreational athletes look forward to continuing physical activity during pregnancy and beyond.

While there are several theoretical risks posed by maternal exercise, the haemodynamic and physical adaptations conferred by nature protect the fetus from all but the extremes of conditions. There are now many reports of women undergoing arduous training and completing marathons in early pregnancy while unaware of their condition. These women have gone on to produce healthy babies.

There are, of course, medical complications involving either the fetus, the mother, or both, whereby physical activity may pose a greater risk. Some cardiac lesions may preclude any activity, while diabetic women need close monitoring under specialist care. In cases of threatened abortion women are usually advised to rest completely, although there is little evidence to suggest this will affect the outcome.

Pregnant women have higher iron requirements and this will be particularly so in the physically active. Although a mild "physiologic anaemia" is expected due to haemodynamic volume expansion, serum ferritin should remain above 30 ng/ml. All women seeking conception should take folate supplements (400 μg/day) to minimise the risk of neural tube defect.

Some particular activities are dangerous in pregnancy. These include scuba diving and parachuting, where sudden pressure changes may jeopardise the fetal circulation. Water skiers should wear a wet suit to avoid forceful vaginal douching. Sports with a high level of trauma should probably be avoided, but attempts to give accurate guidelines regarding all levels and types of sport during pregnancy are medicolegally fraught. However, if mother and baby are both well, and this is confirmed by past history and frequent antenatal checks, regular exercise should be encouraged of a type and level with which the woman feels comfortable.

Trauma

Until the second trimester the uterus is safe within the confines of the bony pelvis and thereafter the fetus is protected by the layers of maternal tissue and amniotic fluid. The fetus has been likened to an egg in a jar completely filled with water; the jar must break for the egg to be damaged. In general quite significant trauma, such as a fall from a horse, is necessary to traumatise the fetus. However, no one should be encouraged to continue contact or collision sports into the second trimester, for medicolegal reasons if nothing else. In advancing pregnancy the maternal centre of gravity shifts

101

forward while ligaments loosen through the effect of the hormone relaxin and many women will become less adept at weightbearing activities. This increases the risks of maternal sprains and strains. However, if a woman has particular expertise in a sport she may choose to continue for as long as she feels able, depending on the sport's governing body rules.

Hyperthermia

Animal studies and retrospective data in women have indicated that maternal hyperthermia is a risk factor for neural tube defects in the baby. The prolonged fever (>39°C for 3 days) cited in these reports, however, does not equate with the mild temperature changes experienced during most exercise. Despite fears raised, there are no reports of fetal compromise as a result of hyperthermia induced by exercise. Pregnant women dissipate heat through haemodynamic adaptations including volume expansion and an increased skin blood flow. Sensible guidelines would include exercising during the cool period of the day and ensuring adequate hydration. Sauna bathing and the use of hot jacuzzis must be avoided.

Placental perfusion

Animal studies have demonstrated that uterine circulation is compromised by maternal exercise because of increased blood flow to exercising muscles. However, large numbers of studies of women undergoing jogging and cycling programmes have failed to show any long term problems with fetal growth and development. This is probably because of preferential shunting of uterine blood flow to the placental site during exercise, coupled with the greater oxygen affinity of fetal compared with adult haemoglobin. Furthermore, compromise of uterine blood flow is less evident if the mother is aerobically trained before pregnancy.

Women in late pregnancy should not perform Valsalva manoeuvres during exertion, or exercise while supine, so as not to compromise venous return and cardiac output.

Care of the pregnant athlete includes exclusion of risk factors and encouragement to adopt a healthy lifestyle while continuing exercise at a level that is appropriate to the mother's own fitness level. Attention to good nutrition with the increased requirements of iron, calcium, and folate is vital.

Many women return to sport soon after delivery. Swimming should be avoided until the cervix closes and postpartum loss ceases, although short term use of intravaginal tampons is unlikely to pose a risk of infection after the first week. Early attention must be paid to recovery of the pelvic musculature, with "pelvic floor" exercises and abdominal strengthening using the pelvic tilt position.

Like all women, athletes should be encouraged to breastfeed. They will have high dietary energy requirements and need to consume enough fluids to ensure their milk supply. For comfort, it is always best to breastfeed before exercise and wear a fitted maternity bra.

Contraception for the athlete

Choice of contraception may pose some difficulties for the competitive athlete. Some women, competitive or not, prefer not to use the oral contraceptive (OCP) as it presents something "foreign" to the body. For them the best option is probably simple barrier techniques using condoms and spermicides. Intrauterine devices may be appropriate for women who have previously had children.

Progesterone-only "mini-pills" may be an option, as they do not interfere with ovulation but rather increase cervical mucous viscosity and hence decrease sperm motility. However many women find breakthrough bleeding and menstrual irregularity a problem, and this can be particularly so in the athlete. Reliable contraception requires precise daily dosage and this may prove difficult with training and travel.

As discussed earlier, combination OCPs may offer advantages for the oligo- or amenorrhoeic athlete in whom there is concern for skeletal bone mass.

There has been some research which indicates that maximal aerobic capacity ($\dot{V}o_2$max) may be decreased with use of the combined OCP. However, neither anaerobic capacity nor aerobic endurance at 90% of $\dot{O}_2$max were affected. It is unknown what, if any, effect there is on elite performance. Certainly many athletes have recorded peak performances while using the OCP.

Athletes may express fear regarding weight gain and fluid retention while using the OCP. However, weight change in OCP users is not significantly different from the rest of the population when large numbers of women are studied.

Premenopausal women have lower rates of cardiac disease than men because of the cardioprotective effects of their reproductive hormones. Lipid profiles are improved by oestrogen administration and made worse by progestogens; the combination of both in low dose has little overall effect. Similarly, thrombotic effects are minimised, with progestogens reducing and oestrogens increasing clotting factor activity.

Athletes, of course, have minimal risk factors for cardiovascular disease as they are likely to be non-smokers, have improved lipid profiles, and greater cardiovascular fitness. Hence there is probably little likelihood of adverse health risks posed by use of the OCP by athletes.

Combined OCPs provide reliable contraception, decrease dysmenor-rhoea, and result in light withdrawal bleeds the timing of which can be controlled. On balance they may be the best choice for an athlete.

It is imperative that athletes realise that oligomenorrhoea or even established amenorrhoea do not necessarily ensure anovulation and reliable contraception must always be sought. Condoms, of course, confer protection from sexually transmitted disease and should be encouraged, especially for the travelling athlete.

Conclusion

Those wishing to provide medical care for athletes must have an understanding of the physiologic adaptations that result from training and

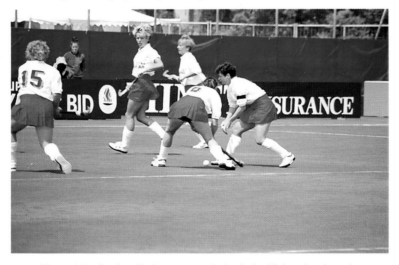

Figure 5.3   Good medical care can optimise the health benefits of exercise

competition as well as having empathy for the competitor's needs and aspirations. Good medical care can optimise the health benefits of exercise while contributing to a greater chance of success in the sporting arena.

6 Sports nutrition

RON MAUGHAN, LOUISE BURKE, AND
MICHAEL GLEESON

Introduction

Motivation, training, and genetic predisposition are considered by many
athletes and coaches to be the cornerstones of successful athletic
performance. However, without proper nutrition, the full potential of the
athlete will not be realised since performance will not be at its peak, training
levels may not be sustained, recovery from injury will be slower, and the
athlete may become more susceptible to injury and infection. The
importance of adequate and appropriate nutrition to athletic performance
is now well recognised and for the sportsman or woman, whether taking
exercise for recreation or competing at the highest level, nutrition ranks
alongside training and injuries as a subject of abiding interest. Despite this,
there remains much misunderstanding of the nutritional principles which
underpin both health and fitness.

The recreational sportsperson is generally concerned with the health
benefits, both physical and psychological, of exercise, including weight
control. At the highest level of competition in sport, nutritional intervention
may make the difference between winning and losing. Although it is clear
that the ability to train and compete will be impaired if the diet is inadequate,
the concept of dietary inadequacy may be quite different for the elite
athlete compared with the sedentary individual or the recreational exerciser.
Performance may be improved by some forms of dietary manipulation,
but the optimum diet will differ between sports and will vary between
individuals. Only general guidelines can therefore be issued, even though
individuals want the prescription of a programme of eating that will make
them a champion. Good nutrition will not make the average individual
into a world class performer, but inappropriate eating habits may prevent
even the best athletes from realising their potential.

Two distinct aspects of the athlete's diet must be considered; the first is
the diet in training which must be consumed on a daily basis for a large
part of the year, and the second is the diet before and during competition.
The athlete's diet should not prevent the performance of consistent hard
training. In most sports, peak performance must be achieved on only a few

105

occasions each year. In some team games (e.g. football, rugby, basketball) competition is frequent, but maximal effort cannot be produced on every occasion. Nutritional requirements vary with the range of activities encompassed by the term sport and the variation in the characteristics of the individuals taking part. For non-competitive activities, and for the individual who exercises for recreational and health reasons, the daily diet forms part of a lifestyle which may be quite different from that of the competitive athlete. The nutritional implications of exercise participation apply equally.

Nutrition for training

Energy requirements

The primary need during periods of training is for the diet to meet the additional nutrient requirement imposed by the training load (accounting for intensity, duration, and frequency) of exercise. In sports involving prolonged strenuous exercise on a regular basis, participation has a significant effect on energy balance. Metabolic rate during running or cycling at 70–80% of the individual's maximal oxygen uptake ($\dot{V}O_2$max), may be 10–15 times the resting rate, and such levels of activity may be sustained for several hours by trained athletes. Even for events which last only a few seconds, as in sprinting or weight-lifting, the top performers may spend several hours per day in training, resulting in very high levels of energy expenditure and a need for a correspondingly high energy intake. Most of the studies reporting dietary habits of athletes show high levels of energy intake, with little difference between competitors in endurance and strength events. After correction for body weight (BW), there is a tendency for higher energy intakes among the endurance and male athletes.

The principal effect of exercise is to increase the rate of energy expenditure during the exercise period itself, but the metabolic rate may remain elevated for at least 12 and possibly up to 24 hours afterwards if the exercise is both prolonged and intense.[1] The effect of this sustained elevation of metabolic rate will be to further increase the energy cost of training. Unfortunately, the recreational exerciser, whose aims include weight loss, is unlikely to benefit from this effect because the duration and intensity of exercise will be too short for it to be significant. The elite athlete who trains once or more per day at the limits of the tolerable load will incur an additional energy cost which may be unwelcome. Maintenance of body weight and performance levels requires a high rate of energy expenditure to be matched by an equally high energy intake. This is to be expected, as a chronic deficit in energy intake would lead to a progressive loss of body mass and a reduced capacity to tolerate high training loads: the process is therefore self-limiting to a large degree. However, data for women engaged in sports where a low body weight, and especially a low body fat content, are important, consistently show a lower than expected energy intake;[2] such sports include gymnastics, distance running, and ballet. There is no obvious physiological explanation for this finding, which has led to the suggestion that it is a result of methodological errors in the calculation of energy intake and expenditure, but it does seem odd that these should apply specifically to this group of athletes. It may be that these individuals are consistently underreporting their actual intake, but it must be recognised that they are a unique group by virtue of their training and competition. There are major difficulties in training at high intensity on a regular basis and maintaining body fat content at a level well below that which would be considered normal. Many of these women athletes have a very low body fat content: a total fat content of less than 10% of body weight is not uncommon in female long distance runners. Secondary amenorrhoea is common in these women, but is usually reversed when training stops[3] suggesting that the menstrual cycle disturbances may be more related to the training load than to the low body fat content.

Protein

Athletes engaged in strength and power events have traditionally been concerned with achieving a high dietary protein intake in the belief that this is necessary for muscle hypertrophy. In a survey of American college athletes, 98% believed that a high protein diet would improve performance. Although a diet deficient in protein will lead to loss of muscle tissue, there is no evidence to support the idea that excess dietary protein will drive the system in favour of protein synthesis.[4] Excess protein will simply be used as a substrate for aerobic, oxidative metabolism, either directly or as a precursor of glucose or fat, and the excess nitrogen will be lost in the urine. Exercise, whether it is long distance running, aerobics, or weight training, will cause an increased protein oxidation compared with the resting state. Although the contribution of protein oxidation to energy production during the exercise period may decrease to about 5% of the total energy requirement, compared with about 10–15% at rest, the absolute rate of protein degradation is increased during exercise.[5] This leads to an increase in the minimum daily protein requirement above the 0.8 g/kgBW recommended for the sedentary population by the World Health Organization. The amount of protein required by speed and strength athletes is 1.2–1.7 g/kgBW, and 1.2–1.4 g/kgBW is recommended for endurance athletes.[4] This will be met by the consumption of a normal mixed diet sufficient to meet the increased energy expenditure (Table 6.1). In spite of this, however, many athletes ingest large quantities of protein-containing foods and expensive protein supplements; daily protein intakes of

Table 6.1 Daily protein intake in grams by diet composition (% of energy intake) and total energy intake

Total energy intake (MJ/day)	Protein intake (g) (as % of total energy intake)						
	5%	7.5%	10%	12.5%	15%	17.5%	20%
5	11	16	22	28	33	39	44
7.5	17	25	33	41	50	58	66
10	22	33	44	55	66	77	88
12.5	28	41	55	69	83	96	110
15	33	50	66	83	99	116	132
17.5	39	58	77	97	116	135	154
20	44	66	88	110	132	154	176
22.5	50	74	99	124	149	174	198
25	55	83	110	138	165	193	221

Assumes energy content of protein $= 22.68$ kJ/g. For a resting sedentary individual the RDA for protein is 0.8 g/kgBW. For most athletes it is probably nearer to 1.4 g/kgBW. Hence, for a 65 kg athlete all the combinations highlighted in bold will meet the RDA for protein.

3–4 g/kgBW are not unknown in body-building and other strength training events.[6] Disposal of the excess nitrogen, principally in the form of urea and ammonia, is theoretically a problem if renal function is compromised, but there does not appear to be any evidence that excessive protein intake among athletes is in any way damaging to health.[4] The recommended diet for athletes, especially those in endurance events, may even contain a lower than normal proportion of protein (when expressed as a percentage of total energy intake) on account of the fact that the total energy demand is increased to a greater extent than is the protein requirement.

Carbohydrate

Under normal circumstances the energy requirements of exercise are largely met by oxidation of fat and carbohydrate, with only a very small contribution from protein oxidation. The higher the intensity of exercise, the greater the reliance on carbohydrate as a fuel: at an exercise intensity corresponding to about 50% of an individual's $\dot{V}O_2max$, approximately two-thirds of the total energy requirement is met by fat oxidation, with carbohydrate oxidation supplying about one-third. If the exercise intensity is increased to about 70% of $\dot{V}O_2max$, the total energy expenditure is increased, and carbohydrate becomes the major fuel. If carbohydrate is not available, or is available in only a limited amount, the intensity of the exercise must be reduced to a level where the energy requirement can be met by fat oxidation. If very high intensity exercise is performed with a high rate of anaerobic metabolism, much of the energy will come from conversion of carbohydrate (primarily muscle glycogen) to lactic acid. This places a high demand on the limited muscle glycogen stores when high intensity interval training or repetitive heavy weight training sessions are carried out. Table 6.2 illustrates some calculations of rates of carbohydrate utilisation for different intensities and durations of exercise.

The rate of carbohydrate utilisation is about 2 g/min at work rates of 70–80% $\dot{V}o_2$max: although endurance training will increase the use of fat as a fuel, the endurance athlete has an increased $\dot{V}o_2$max and an increased ability to work at a high fraction of $\dot{V}o_2$max, so the demand for carbohydrate remains high. Hard training of 1–4 hours at intensities of in excess of 60% $\dot{V}o_2$max, can incur the use of over 300 g of carbohydrate, roughly the total muscle glycogen store. The most rapid and greatest glycogen depletion occurs during short term intense intermittent exercise; here one study found that glycogen content fell by about 80% within 21 minutes at 120% $\dot{V}o_2$max and by a similar amount within 8 minutes at 150% $\dot{V}o_2$max.[7] Environmental conditions influence muscle metabolism. At high altitude and in hot humid conditions where blood flow is redistributed to the skin to effect greater heat loss, the relative contribution of anaerobic glycolysis will be increased and muscle glycogen stores will be more rapidly depleted.

The primary nutritional need is for sufficient carbohydrate intake to enable the training load to be sustained. During each strenuous training session, substantial depletion of the glycogen stores in the exercising muscles (Figure 6.1) and in the liver takes place.[7–9] If this carbohydrate reserve is not replenished before the next training session, training intensity and/or duration must be reduced, leading to corresponding reductions in the adaptive response to exercise training. Exercise performance and endurance capacity improves when muscle glycogen stores are enhanced prior to prolonged strenuous exercise.[10–13] A high carbohydrate diet has been shown to promote better recovery and restoration of endurance capacity the day after strenuous exercise.[14]

Recovery of the muscle and liver glycogen stores after exercise is a rather slow process, and will normally require at least 24–48 hours for complete recovery.[15] The rate of glycogen resynthesis after exercise is determined largely by the amount of carbohydrate supplied by the diet,[16] and the amount of carbohydrate consumed is of far greater importance for this process than the type of carbohydrate (simple sugars or oligosaccharides) or the form of carbohydrate (liquid or solids) (for review, see Coyle[17]). If the diet is deficient in carbohydrate, little restoration of muscle glycogen will occur.[10]

Trained muscle uses a relatively greater proportion of fat than untrained muscle. Recently there has been renewed interest in the suggestion that man might adapt by training on a low carbohydrate, high fat diet. However, benefits to the performance of exercise at higher work intensities which are more relevant to the outcome of most sporting activities have not been observed.[18] While further investigation seems warranted, the current dietary guidelines for athletes recommend a high carbohydrate diet during training

109

Table 6.2 Estimated rates of carbohydrate use during different intensities (%V̇o₂ max) and durations (10–240 minutes) of exercise (running or cycling)

Exercise intensity (%V̇o₂max)	RQ and (% E from CHO)	V̇o₂ (l/min)	E expend (kJ/min)	E from CHO (kJ/min)	CHO use (g/min)	CHO use (g) by total duration (min)[a]					
						10	30	60	120	180	240
Rest	0.75 (17)	0.30	6.0	1.0	0.05	0.5	1.5	3	6	9	12
30	0.77 (23)	1.37	27.4	6.3	0.30	3.0	9	18	36	54	72
50	0.80 (33)	2.28	46.3	15.3	0.73	7.3	22	44	88	131	175
60	0.85 (50)	2.73	55.4	27.7	1.33	13.3	40	80	160	239	319
70	0.87 (57)	3.19	65.0	36.8	1.76	17.6	53	106	211	316	422
80	0.90 (67)	3.64	74.6	50.0	2.39	23.9	72	143	287	430	—
90	0.97 (90)	4.10	85.2	76.7	3.67	36.7	110	220	440	—	—
100	1.00 (100)	4.55	95.1	95.1	4.55	45.5	137	273	—	—	—
130	1.00 (100)	5.92[b]	123.7	123.7	8[c]	80.0	240	—	—	—	—

Calculations assume the following: overnight-fasted subject with a body mass of 65 kg and a V̇o₂max of 70 ml/kg/min (4.55 l/min); a constant metabolic respiratory quotient (RQ) throughout exercise; energy (E) content of carbohydrate (CHO) = 20.9 kJ/g.
[a] Assumes a constant rate of CHO use throughout exercise and intermittent performance of high intensity work rates.
[b] Estimated o₂ requirement.
[c] Estimated rate of CHO utilisation given high anaerobic contribution.

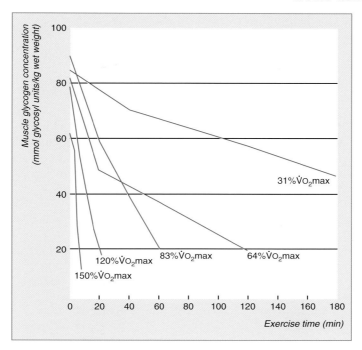

Figure 6.1   Depletion of muscle glycogen from the quadriceps muscle during cycle ergometer exercise of different intensities (%V̇o₂max) and durations. Exercise at 31, 64, and 83% of V̇o₂max was continuous, whereas exercise at the two highest work rates was intermittent with 3 minute (120% V̇o₂max) or 1 minute (150% V̇o₂max) exercise bouts interrupted by 10 minute rest periods. Subjects were male physical education students with a mean V̇o₂ max of 4.46 l/min (61.3 ml/kg/min). Note the speed and extent of glycogen depletion at the higher work rates typical of interval training. (Data from Gollnick et al[7])

periods to support the performance of, and recovery from, each exercise session.

Carbohydrate should provide at least 50% of total energy intake. This is compatible with the additional fuel needs of the athlete. Actual carbohydrate requirements are determined by the training load and body size of the athlete. In situations where training loads are heavy and maximum resynthesis of muscle glycogen is desirable, a daily carbohydrate intake of about 8–10 g/kgBW (i.e. 500–600 g carbohydrate for a 70 kg athlete) may be necessary.[19] This may represent up to 60–70% of total energy intake for some athletes.[20,21] Such high levels of intake are difficult to achieve without choosing compact forms of carbohydrate (e.g. foods high in simple sugars, lower fibre choices of carbohydrate foods, carbohydrate drinks) as well as increasing the frequency of meals and snacks towards a "grazing" eating pattern.

For the athlete training at least once and perhaps even two or three times per day, and who also has to work or study, practical difficulties arise in achieving the necessary energy and carbohydrate intake.[22] Most athletes find it difficult to train soon after food intake, and the appetite is also suppressed for a time after strenuous exercise. The athlete should focus on ensuring a rapid recovery of the glycogen stores between training sessions. This is best achieved when carbohydrate is consumed as soon as possible after the end of training, as the rate of glycogen synthesis is most rapid at this time.[23] At least 50–100 g should be consumed at this time, and a high carbohydrate intake continued thereafter.[16] There is clearly a maximum rate at which muscle glycogen resynthesis can occur, and there appears to be no benefit in increasing the carbohydrate intake to levels in excess of 100 g every 2 hours.[24] Where rapid restoration of muscle glycogen is a critical issue there may be some benefit from ingesting foods that are rapidly digested and absorbed, producing a rapid rise in the blood glucose concentration (i.e. a high glycaemic index).[25] Glucose-containing drinks, potato, rice, and bread belong to this category. Drinks containing glucose or maltodextrins are a practical choice during the post-exercise recovery period, providing a palatable and convenient source of carbohydrate while simultaneously addressing fluid needs. The high carbohydrate and energy requirements of athletes may be difficult to achieve without resorting to a significant intake of snacks and convenience foods. There is, however, no evidence that this pattern of eating is harmful. For the individual who has to fit an exercise programme into a busy day, it is inevitable that changes to eating patterns must be made, but these need not compromise the quality of the diet. When the energy expenditure is very high, drinks and snacks rich in carbohydrate become an essential part of the diet, an increasing proportion of which is consumed between meals, again leading to a "grazing" pattern of eating.[26,27]

Vitamins

There is very little evidence to suggest that the vitamin intake of athletes is inadequate except in those with extremely low or high dietary energy intakes, based on the recommended dietary allowances (RDAs).[28–30] The RDA of any particular micronutrient is defined as the level of intake required to meet the known nutritional needs of more than 95% of healthy persons.[31] Individuals who consume less than the RDA are not necessarily deficient in that nutrient, but the further the actual intake lies below the RDA, the greater the risk of developing a deficiency state that is detrimental to the health of the individual. However, it should be noted that the data used to determine the RDAs often did not include information from athletes, and in most cases the activity levels of the subjects were not reported. Therefore, the RDAs may not be an accurate means of evaluating

Carbohydrate needs for training

Summary: A high carbohydrate diet increases muscle glycogen stores and improves performance of and recovery from prolonged strenuous exercise. An inadequate carbohydrate intake may limit recovery and cause earlier onset of fatigue during exercise. At least half of your daily energy intake should come from carbohydrate (i.e. 50–70% of total energy) and in situations where maximal rates of glycogen synthesis are needed a carbohydrate intake of 8–10 g/kgBW/day is a suggested target.

Practical tips

1 Be prepared to be different – a Western diet is not a high carbohydrate diet.
2 Base meals and snacks around nutritious carbohydrate-rich foods, including wholegrain breads and breakfast cereals, rice, pasta, noodles, and other grain foods, fruits, starchy vegetables (e.g. potatoes, corn), legumes (lentils, beans, soya-based products), and sweetened dairy products (e.g. fruit flavoured yoghurt, milkshakes). Let these foods take up at least half of the room on your plate.
3 Many of the foods commonly believed to be high in carbohydrate are actually high fat foods. Keep to low fat ideas, and promote fuel foods rather than high fat foods.
4 Sugar and sugary foods provide a compact carbohydrate source. They may be particularly useful in a high energy diet, or when carbohydrate is needed before, during, and after exercise.
5 Carbohydrate drinks (e.g. fruit juices, soft drinks, fruit/milk smoothies) are also a compact source for special situations or very high carbohydrate diets. This category includes many of the supplements made specially for athletes – e.g. sports drinks, high carbohydrate powders and liquid meal supplements.
6 When energy and carbohydrate needs are high, increase the number of meals and snacks that you eat, rather than the size of your meals. You may need to be organised to have snacks on hand in a busy day.
7 Choose lower fibre choices of carbohydrate-rich foods when energy needs are high, or when you are eating just before exercise.
8 Eat a high carbohydrate meal or snack containing at least 50 g carbohydrate within 30 minutes after a prolonged session of exercise to speed the recovery of body glycogen stores. Low glycaemic index carbohydrate foods (e.g. oats, lentils, legumes) are less suitable at these meals.
9 Consume carbohydrate during lengthy training and competition sessions when additional fuel is needed.

Based on Burke LM. Practical issues in nutrition for athletes. *J Sports Sci* 1995;**13**:S83–S90.

the nutritional needs of individuals engaged in regular strenuous exercise. Although physical activity may increase the requirement for some vitamins (e.g. vitamin C, vitamin B_2 and possibly vitamin B_6), this increased requirement typically can be met by consuming a balanced high carbohydrate, moderate protein, low fat diet. Vitamin intakes in athletes are correlated with energy intakes up to 20 MJ/day (Figure 6.2a), so

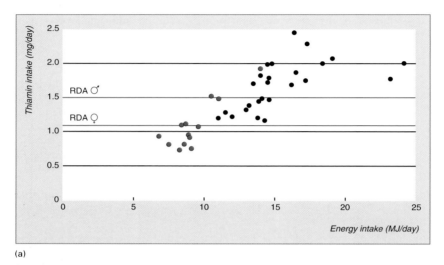

(a)

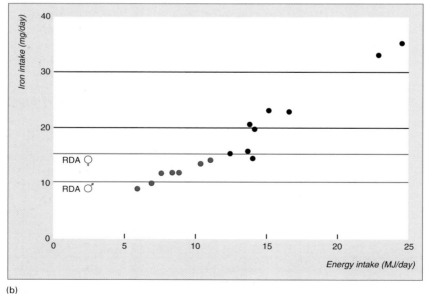

(b)

Figure 6.2

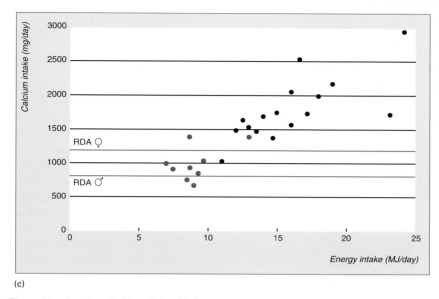

(c)

Figure 6.2 (continued) *The relationship between mean daily intake of dietary energy and thiamin (Vit B₁) (a), iron (b) and calcium (c) in male (closed circles) and female (open circles) athletes. Each point represents a mean value for a group. (Data from Erp-Baart et al[30] and Beek.[32])*

individuals at risk for low vitamin intake are those who consume a low energy and/or unbalanced diet. When the energy intake is very high (>20 MJ/ day), athletes tend to consume a large number of "in-between meals" and high energy sports drinks, often composed mainly of refined carbohydrate, but low in protein and micronutrients, and consequently the nutrient density for vitamins (e.g. Vit B₁, thiamin) drops.[32] Vegetarian athletes will obviously have problems in obtaining sufficient intakes of some vitamins (particularly Vit B₁₂, cyanocobalamin, whose only dietary source is from foods of animal origin) and appropriate education and vitamin supplementation is recommended for these athletes.

Vitamin losses in sweat are negligible[33,34] and there is no indication of increased vitamin excretion in urine and faeces in athletes. In general, vitamin turnover seems to be remarkably unaffected by exercise, but it has been reported that physical training may increase the Vit B₂ (riboflavin) and Vit B₆ requirement which may be a consequence of increased retention of these vitamins in skeletal muscle.[35,36] Adaptations to regular prolonged exercise include an increased biogenesis of mitochondria in skeletal muscles and increased oxidative enzyme activity which might explain the increased retention of vitamins that are co-factors in energy metabolism within the adapting muscle. In summary, the scientific evidence currently available does not support the notion of a generally increased vitamin requirement in athletes. Since the energy intake of most athletes is considerably higher than that of the sedentary population, their intake of vitamins and minerals is also necessarily higher, assuming a well balanced diet. Therefore, additional supplements of vitamins are generally not needed.

Vitamin supplementation

Many papers have been written about the effects of vitamin supplementation on exercise performance. A number of older studies have suggested a potential ergogenic role of vitamins, based on the argument that the RDA may not represent the optimal intake of a vitamin. However, following numerous more recent, better controlled studies, this notion has been discredited.[32,37–40] It is quite well established that marginal vitamin deficiencies can decrease exercise performance, which can be remedied by appropriate supplementation.[41] Severe or prolonged vitamin deficiencies are deleterious to health and would therefore be expected to impair athletic performance. Many athletes still consume large amounts of vitamin and mineral supplements in the (mistaken) belief that this will provide an ergogenic boost. There is no convincing scientific evidence that doses in excess of the RDA improve performance. Consuming very large dosages (mega-doses) of certain vitamins can be harmful. For example, very large doses of Vit C are associated with urinary stone formation and impaired copper absorption, while mega-doses of Vit B_6 can cause sensory neuropathy.

In summary, vitamin supplements are not necessary for athletes eating a diet adequate in respect of quality and quantity. Many athletes are, however, concerned to ensure adequate intakes of vitamins, without the risks of oversupplementation. Athletes and coaches should be educated about dietary practices and safe daily intakes. However, a daily intake of a low dose vitamin preparation, supplying not more than the RDA, will ensure an adequate and safe level of vitamin intake, especially during periods of intensive training or when eating from an irregular and uncertain food supply (e.g. while travelling).

Minerals

The dietary requirement for most minerals is probably increased in athletes compared with sedentary people since prolonged exercise tends to increase losses in sweat and urine. Information based on dietary surveys of athletes and their blood chemistry suggests that iron (Figure 6.2b), calcium (Figure 6.2c), zinc, and magnesium status may be of some concern, especially for young athletes and women of all ages involved in physical activity.[42]

Protein, vitamins, and minerals for training

Summary: Athletes in heavy training have increased protein needs (1–1.5 g/kgBW/day). However, a high energy diet should provide additional protein to meet these targets. A high energy diet chosen from a variety of nutritious foods should also provide adequate amounts of vitamins and minerals to meet any increased requirements. Athletes at risk of suboptimal intakes are those who restrict their food variety (e.g. vegetarians, fad dieters), and those who consume low energy intakes in order to reduce/maintain low body fat/weight levels. Iron and calcium are "at risk" nutrients, especially for female athletes. Professional help should be sought when inadequate eating patterns, menstrual disturbances, or excessive fatigue are present. Clinical management requires proper diagnosis of problems, dietary counselling, and, on occasions, dietary supplements.

Practical tips

1 Enjoy a variety of foods – do not cut out food groups entirely.
2 Mix and match foods at meals: popular diets which advise against food combining are unsound.
3 Include haem iron-rich foods (red meats, shellfish, liver) regularly in your meals – at least 3–5 times per week. These can be added to a high carbohydrate meal (e.g. sauce on pasta).
4 Enhance the absorption of non-haem iron (found in wholegrains, cereal foods, eggs, leafy green vegetables etc.) by including a vitamin C food at the same meal. For example, drink a glass of orange juice with your breakfast cereal).
5 Be aware that some foods (excess bran, strongly brewed tea) interfere with iron absorption from non-haem iron foods. Avoid these items, or separate from meals, if you are at risk of iron deficiency.
6 Iron supplements should be taken only on the advice of a sports dietitian or doctor. They may be useful in the supervised treatment and prevention of iron deficiency, but do not forget other dietary factors.
7 Eat at least three servings of dairy foods a day, where one serving is equal to a glass of milk or a carton of yoghurt. Low fat and reduced fat types are available. Dairy products can be added to a high carbohydrate meal (e.g. milk on breakfast cereal, cheese in a sandwich).
8 Extra calcium is needed if you are growing, having a baby, or breastfeeding. Increase your dairy intake to 4–5 servings a day. Women who are not having regular menstrual cycles also require extra calcium – seek expert advice from a sports medicine doctor.
9 Fish eaten with its bones (e.g. tinned salmon, sardines) is also a useful calcium source, and can also accompany a high carbohydrate meal (e.g. salmon casserole with rice).
10 A sports dietitian can help you to explore and maximise food variety. If you are a vegetarian, or unable to eat dairy products and red meat in these amounts, you will need help to find creative ways or other foods to meet your iron and calcium needs (such as fortified soy products), or to use mineral supplements correctly.

Based on Burke LM. Practical issues in nutrition for athletes. *J Sports Sci* 1995;**13**:S83–S90.

Iron

Iron, as a component of haemoglobin, myoglobin, and cytochromes, is essential for oxidative metabolism. Iron depletion (low iron stores as evidenced by low concentrations of serum ferritin) is commonly reported in both male and female athletes but is not consistently associated with impaired performance. However, if the condition should progress to a state of iron deficiency, then athletic performance is negatively affected.[43] Endurance athletes engaged in heavy training loads commonly have low circulating haemoglobin levels and haematocrit, although total red cell mass may be elevated due to an increased blood volume. This may be considered to be an adaptation to the trained state and is sometimes called "sports anaemia" but has no apparent effect on exercise performance.[44] Plasma volume expansion has been reported to occur within the first few days of a training programme or following increases in the training load in well trained individuals[45] and after single bouts of intense, prolonged or muscle-damaging exercise.[46] This will result in a temporary dilutional anaemia. The incidence of iron deficiency anaemia is rare and is similar among athletes and the general population.[47]

Anaemia   Exercise tolerance will be impaired in the presence of anaemia. Meat provides the most readily available dietary source of iron. Exercise may cause haemolysis of red blood cells, alterations of iron metabolism, increased losses in the urine, and losses due to gastrointestinal bleeding in some susceptible individuals.[48] Hence, regular exercise may increase the dietary requirement for iron. The periodic screening of serum ferritin levels in athletes is recommended as changes in the storage and transport of iron typically precede decreases in functional iron (haemoglobin) levels.

Calcium

A calcium intake of 800–1200 mg/day is recommended to protect against the development of osteoporosis.[49] Calcium intake is one of the factors that influences the development of osteoporosis. The emphasis for the prevention of osteoporosis should be to maximise the body's stores of calcium at an early age and minimise any loss.[50] The performance of regular weight-bearing activity will promote the deposition of calcium in bone.[51] The absence of menstruation (amenorrhoea) or infrequent menstruation (oligomenorrhoea) which are commonly associated with low levels of body fat, low energy intakes, and high levels of physical activity (especially gymnastics, swimming, and long distance running) are also associated with a reduced bone mineral density. In the young female athlete, amenorrhoea may hinder bone growth at a time in development when bone should be forming at its maximum rate. When amenorrhoea is present, increasing the consumption of calcium to 120% of the RDA helps to maintain bone density and allows proper development.[52] Weight-conscious athletes (e.g. gymnasts) may markedly reduce their consumption of dairy products in order to decrease their intake of dietary fat. However, since the main dietary source of calcium is from milk, yoghurt, and cheese, this practice may result in their intake of calcium falling considerably below the RDA. Most low fat dairy products (e.g. skimmed milk, low fat yoghurt) contain similar amounts of calcium as the full fat dairy product, so athletes should be encouraged to include the former in their diet in order to preserve calcium intake.

Zinc and magnesium

Some studies[53,54] have indicated that the intake of zinc among some groups of athletes (wrestlers, female endurance runners, gymnasts) is considerably less than the RDA (15 and 12 mg/day for males and females, respectively). Prolonged exercise may result in significant losses of zinc and magnesium in sweat, and losses of these minerals in urine is also increased as a result of intensive training. Zinc is a cofactor of several enzymes in energy metabolism and is also required for normal immune function and wound healing. Magnesium is an essential cofactor for many enzymes involved in biosynthetic processes and energy metabolism. Hence, supplements of these minerals may be beneficial to those with marginal dietary intakes. However, as with vitamins, one should guard against excessively high dosage of selected minerals due to the potentially toxic effects and mineral interactions.

In summary, most athletes do not require vitamin or mineral supplements, since a well chosen, high energy diet should be more than adequate in terms of quantity and quality to meet any increased requirements resulting from the effects of regular intensive exercise. However, it is possible to identify particular groups of athletes who are at risk of marginal nutrient intake. These are athletes who compete in sports events where a low body weight is essential for success (e.g. gymnasts, dancers) or where they have to compete within a certain body weight category (e.g. boxers, wrestlers, weight-lifters). Participants in these sports are often training frequently and intensively, but consume low energy diets or undergo drastic weight loss regimes in order to maintain or lose body weight prior to competition. The low energy intake (less than 8 MJ per day) in these situations is likely to lead to an inadequate intake of essential micronutrients. This aspect is worthy of special attention, since many of these athletes are very young and still in a period of body growth and development, which could be detrimentally affected by vitamin and mineral deficiencies. Other groups at risk are those who abstain from varied food patterns (i.e. those who consume extremely unbalanced diets with a low micronutrient density) and vegetarian athletes. Nutrition education and micronutrient supplementation are recommended for such sportspeople, but daily supplements of vitamins or minerals should not exceed one to two times the RDA.

Nutrition for competition

The ability to perform prolonged exercise can be substantially modified by dietary intake in the pre-exercise period. This is particularly important for the individual aiming to produce peak performance on a specific day. The pre-exercise period can conveniently be divided into two phases – the few days prior to the exercise task, and the day of exercise itself.

Days before the event

Carbohydrate loading

Dietary manipulation to increase muscle glycogen content in the few days prior to exercise has been extensively recommended for endurance athletes. The suggested procedure was to deplete muscle glycogen by prolonged exercise about one week prior to competition and to prevent resynthesis by consuming a low carbohydrate diet for 2–3 days before changing to a high carbohydrate diet for the last 3 days during which little or no exercise was performed. This procedure can double the muscle glycogen content and is effective in increasing cycling or running performance.[17]

There is now a considerable amount of evidence that it is not necessary to include the low carbohydrate glycogen depletion phase of the diet for endurance athletes. Nor is it necessary to completely deplete muscle glycogen stores before the carbohydrate loading phase. Very prolonged strenuous exercise and especially exercise involving eccentric muscle actions should be avoided in the days before competition since these may cause muscle damage which causes a temporary insulin resistance[55] and a slowing of the rate of muscle glycogen resynthesis.[56] Such exercise will also cause muscle soreness and weakness for several days afterwards. Simply reduce the training load over the last 5 or 6 days before competition whilst increasing the dietary carbohydrate intake. This avoids many of the problems associated with the more extreme forms of the diet. Although an increased pre-competition muscle glycogen content is undoubtedly beneficial, there is a faster rate of muscle glycogen utilisation during exercise when the glycogen content itself is increased, thus nullifying some of the advantage gained.

Consumption of a high carbohydrate diet in the days prior to competition may benefit competitors in games such as rugby, soccer, or hockey, although

Carbohydrate loading for endurance events

Summary: Carbohydrate loading is a technique used by endurance athletes to optimise muscle glycogen levels prior to an event of greater than 90 min duration. The modified strategy is achieved by programming 72 h of exercise taper and a high carbohydrate diet prior to the event. These menu plans provide about 600 g of carbohydrate per day – providing the recommended carbohydrate intake of 8–10 g/kg BW/day for a 60–65 kg athlete. They may need to be adapted for athletes outside this weight range. These menus are proposed for carbohydrate loading days only – while meeting carbohydrate intake goals, they do not meet all the nutrient requirements for everyday eating.

DAY 1: (602 g CHO, 12.2 MJ – CHO = 80% of energy)
Breakfast: 2 cups wheat flake cereal + 250 ml (8 fl oz) skim milk
            1 cup sweetened canned peaches
            250 ml (8 fl oz) sweetened fruit juice
Snack: 2 thick slices toast + scrape marg + 20 g (1 tbsp) honey on each
            250 ml (8 fl oz) sports drink
Lunch: 2 large bread rolls with light salad
            375 ml (12 fl oz) can of soft drink
Snack: Large coffee and roll (unbuttered)
Dinner: 3 cups of boiled rice
            (made into "stir fry" with small amount of lean ham, peas, corn and onion)
            250 ml (8 fl oz) sweetened fruit juice
Snack: 2 crumpets + scrape marg + 20 g (1 tbsp) jam on each
Extra water during day

DAY 2: (605 g CHO, 12.7 MJ – CHO = 77% of energy)
Breakfast: 2 cups oatmeal + 250 ml (8 fl oz) skim milk
            1 banana
            250 ml (8 fl oz) sweetened fruit juice
Snack: 2 muffins + scrape marg + 20 g (1 tbsp) jam on each
Lunch: Stack of three large pancakes + 60 ml (2 oz) maple syrup
            + small scoop ice cream
            250 ml (8 fl oz) sweetened fruit juice
Snack: 50 g (2 oz) jelly beans
Dinner: 3 cups cooked pasta + 1 cup tomato pasta sauce
            2 slices bread
            250 ml (8 fl oz) sports drink
Snack: 1 cup fresh fruit salad
            200 g carton low fat fruit yoghurt
Extra water during day

DAY 3: The athlete may like to switch to a low residue diet to reduce gastrointestinal contents and improve comfort during the event
        For example, use menus for Day 1 or 2, switching to white bread and cereals. From lunch onwards, replace some or all of the solid food with 500 ml (16 oz) snacks of commercial carbo-loader or liquid meal supplements.

Based on Burke LM, Hargreaves M. Eating for peak performance. In: Zuluaga M et al, eds. Sports physiotherapy, Melbourne: Churchill Livingstone, 1995, pp. 707–19.

it is not common practice for these players to pay attention to this aspect of their diet. Saltin and Karlsson[57] showed that players starting a soccer game with low muscle glycogen content, because of inadequate dietary carbohydrate intake in the recovery period after an earlier game, did less running, and much less running at high speed, than those players who ate a high carbohydrate diet and began the game with a normal muscle glycogen content. It is common for players to have one game in midweek as well as one at the weekend, and it is likely that full restoration of the muscle glycogen content will not occur between games unless a conscious effort is made to achieve a high carbohydrate intake.

Although this glycogen-loading procedure is generally restricted to use by athletes engaged in endurance events, there is some evidence that the muscle glycogen content may influence performance of high intensity exercise lasting only a few minutes.[58] A high muscle glycogen content may be particularly important when repeated sprints at near maximum speed have to be made: at major athletics championships, the sprinter who competes in the 100 and 200 m as well as in the relay may be required to run as many as eight or nine races within a rather short space of time. The beneficial effects of a high muscle glycogen content on performance of high intensity exercise may seem surprising in view of the fact that this results in a higher than normal level of blood lactate accumulation,[59] which would normally be associated with reduced performance. However, it is clear that the ability of the muscles to produce energy by anaerobic means is compromised by low substrate levels, leading to a reduced performance capacity.

Day of the event

The importance of pre-event eating depends on the status of the athlete's liver and muscle glycogen stores. An overnight fast may substantially deplete liver glycogen stores; eating on the morning of an event will restore liver glycogen levels. Muscle glycogen stores may not be optimal if the athlete's training or competition schedule has not allowed adequate time (usually at least 24–48 hours) for tapering and refuelling. A high carbohydrate meal, eaten 1–4 hours prior to exercise, will increase carbohydrate availability and may improve exercise endurance.[60] Pre-event meals should also provide fluid to ensure full hydration, and to avoid any foods known by the athlete to cause gastrointestinal discomfort. A meal low in fat, protein, and fibre is generally recommended since these factors may increase the risk of gastrointestinal problems in susceptible individuals. The timing, type, and amount of food chosen for pre-event meals will vary according to the individual athlete and the event.

122

The last hour

It has been common to recommend that intake of carbohydrate, particularly simple sugars, be avoided in the hour prior to strenuous exercise. Such intake may be associated with hyperinsulinaemia, reduced availability of free fatty acids, and a decline in blood glucose levels at the onset of exercise. One study has reported a reduction in exercise endurance, attributed to more rapid utilisation of muscle glycogen, when carbohydrate was consumed 45 minutes prior to exercise.[61] The results of this study have been widely publicised. However, a review of the literature shows that other studies of carbohydrate intake during the hour before the event have not reported negative effects and some have even observed enhanced performance (see Coyle[17]). It appears that increased carbohydrate availability will more than offset the transient changes in exercise metabolism that accompany prior carbohydrate ingestion in most people; however, athletes should experiment with their pre-event eating and identify any negative effects.

During the event

There is scope for nutritional intervention during exercise only when the duration of events is sufficient to allow absorption of drinks or foods ingested and where the rules of the sport permit. The primary aims must be to ingest a source of energy, usually in the form of carbohydrate, and fluid for replacement of water lost as sweat.[62] High rates of sweat secretion occur during hard exercise in order to limit the rise in body temperature. If the exercise is prolonged, this leads to progressive dehydration and loss of electrolytes. Some people may lose up to 2–3 litres of sweat per hour during strenuous activity in a warm environment.[63] Even at low ambient temperatures of about 10 °C, sweat loss can exceed 1 litre per hour. Since the electrolyte composition of sweat is hypotonic relative to plasma, it is the replacement of water rather than electrolytes that is the priority during exercise. Fatigue towards the end of a prolonged event may result as much from the effects of dehydration as from substrate depletion. Exercise performance is impaired when an individual is dehydrated by as little as 2% of body weight, and losses in excess of 5% of body weight can decrease the capacity for work by about 30%.[63] Dehydration impairs mental concentration and skills,[64] and may therefore have even greater effects on the performance of team games and sports involving skill and complex decision making. Sprint athletes are generally less concerned about the effects of dehydration than are the endurance athletes. However, the capacity to perform high intensity exercise, which results in exhaustion within only a few minutes, has been shown to be reduced by as much as 45% by prior prolonged exercise which resulted in a loss of water corresponding to only 2.5% of body weight. Smaller, but substantial, reductions in performance occurred after administration of diuretics or after sweat loss in a sauna; these factors may be especially important to athletes who dehydrate themselves prior to events in order to "make weight". Athletes who travel to hot climates are likely to experience acute dehydration, which will persist for several days and may well be of sufficient magnitude to have a detrimental effect on performance in competition. Dehydration also poses a serious health risk in that it increases the risk of cramps, heat exhaustion, and life-threatening heat stroke.[65]

Oral fluid ingestion during exercise can help restore plasma volume to near pre-exercise levels and prevent the adverse effect of dehydration on muscle strength, endurance, and coordination. Thirst is unreliable as a guide to drinking as a considerable degree of dehydration (certainly sufficient to impair athletic performance) can have occurred before the desire for fluid intake occurs. Athletes should learn to consume adequate fluids during activity so that body weight remains fairly constant before and after exercise. Guidelines for the amounts of fluid to be consumed before, during, and after exercise can only be very general due to the large inter-individual sweating responses, and the varying opportunities to drink during exercise. The American College of Sports Medicine has published new guidelines for fluid replacement during exercise.[66] The summary statement sets general recommendations for fluid intake before and at regular intervals during exercise (see Table 6.3); nevertheless the commentary stongly advises athletes to develop and practise a fluid intake plan to suit their individual needs and circumstances.

The composition of drinks to be taken during exercise should be chosen to suit individual circumstances.[62] Water is suitable for situations where carbohydrate needs can be supplied by the athlete's own body stores and is generally promoted as the most economical choice for events/exercise lasting less than 1 hour. However, the ingestion of carbohydrate is recommended during strenuous exercise of longer duration, or in situations where adequate recovery of fuel stores before the event is impossible (e.g. during tournaments). Carbohydrate consumed during such exercise has been shown to improve exercise endurance and performance (for review, see Coggan and Coyle[67]), and the effects on performance of fluid replacement and carbohydrate provision have been shown to be independent and additive.[68] The primary role of exogenous carbohydrate is to maintain normal blood sugar and enhance carbohydrate oxidation rates when muscle glycogen levels are low.[69] Carbohydrate intake should begin well in advance of the depletion of body fuel stores and associated fatigue; an intake of 30–60 g/h is generally recommended[66] but needs vary according to the individual athlete and their event. The performance enhancing effect of carbohydrate ingestion during prolonged exercise has been recognised but largely ignored for most of the past 70 years.[70] Until recently it was

Table 6.3 American College of Sports Medicine statement on exercise and fluid replacement (1996)

It is the position of the American College of Sports Medicine that adequate fluid replacement helps maintain hydration, and therefore promotes the health, safety, and optimal physical performance of individuals participating in regular physical activity. This position statement is based on a comprehensive review and interpretation of scientific literature concerning the influence of fluid replacement on exercise performance and the risk of thermal injury associated with dehydration and hyperthermia. Based on the available evidence, the American College of Sports Medicine makes the following general recommendations on the amount and composition of fluids that should be ingested in preparation for, during, and after exercise or athletic competition.

1 It is recommended that individuals consume a nutritionally balanced diet and drink adequate fluids during the 24-h period before an event, especially during the period that includes the meal prior to exercise, to promote proper hydration before exercise or competition.
2 It is recommended that individuals drink about 500 ml (about 17 fl oz) of fluid about 2 h before exercise to promote adequate hydration and allow time for excretion of excess ingested water.
3 During exercise, athletes should start drinking early and at regular intervals in an attempt to consume fluids at a rate sufficient to replace all the water lost through sweating (i.e. body weight loss), or consume the maximal amount that can be tolerated.
4 It is recommended that ingested fluids be cooler than ambient temperature (between 15 and 22°C, 59 and 72°F) and flavoured to enhance palatability and promote fluid replacement. Fluid should be readily available and served in containers that allow adequate volumes to be ingested with ease and with minimal interruption of exercise.
5 Addition of proper amounts of carbohydrates and/or electrolytes to a fluid replacement solution is recommended for exercise events of duration greater than 1 h since it does not significantly impair water delivery to the body and may enhance performance. During exercise of less than 1 h, there is little evidence of physiological or physical performance differences between consuming a carbohydrate-electrolyte drink and plain water.
6 During intense exercise lasting longer than 1 h, it is recommended that carbohydrates be ingested at a rate of 30–60 g/h to maintain oxidation of carbohydrate and delay fatigue. This rate of carbohydrate delivery can be achieved without compromising fluid delivery by drinking 600–1200 ml/h of solutions containing 4–8% carbohydrates (g/100 ml). The carbohydrates can be sugars (glucose or sucrose) or starch (e.g. maltodextrins).
7 Inclusion of sodium (0.5–0.7 g/l of water) in the rehydration solution ingested during exercise lasting longer than 1 h is recommended since it may be advantageous in enhancing palatability, promoting fluid retention, and possibly preventing hyponatraemia in certain individuals who drink excessive quantities of fluid. There is little physiological basis for the presence of sodium in an oral rehydration solution for enhancing intestinal water absorption as long as sodium is sufficiently available from the previous meal.

From American College of Sports Medicine.[66]

considered that the inclusion of significant amounts of carbohydrate in exercise fluids might compromise gastric emptying and rehydration goals. However, fluid delivery to the body is not impaired when solutions containing 4–8% (g/100 ml) carbohydrate are ingested during exercise.[66] The renewed interest in carbohydrate intake during exercise is directly associated with the growing commercial market for sports drinks. These drinks, typically 5–7% mixtures of simple sugars and glucose polymers,

Eating and drinking during exercise

Summary: Sweat rates vary according to fitness and acclimatisation levels, intensity of exercise, and environmental conditions. Dehydration causes a reduction in exercise performance with the effects proportional to the degree of fluid deficit. It is important to be well hydrated at the start of exercise and to drink regularly during exercise to replace as much of the sweat loss as possible. Drink to a plan rather than thirst. Carbohydrate intake during prolonged exercise may enhance performance.

Practical tips for intake during exercise

1 Weight changes before and after exercise may give you a guide to sweat losses and your success in replacing these losses during exercise. (A loss of 1 kg is approximately equal to 1 litre of sweat that should be replaced.) Check this from time to time to get an estimate of expected sweat losses in different events and conditions.

2 You cannot train your body to "get used" to dehydration or "toughen up".

3 Previous weight calculations may give you a guide to expected sweat losses. Aim for a drinking plan that replaces most of this while you exercise, keeping nett fluid losses below 1–2 kg. Drink early and frequently at a comfortable rate.

4 Fluid intake opportunities vary with exercise and sports. Aid stations are available in triathlons and marathons but require the athlete to learn to "drink on the run". In many team sports there are formal and informal breaks in play (half-time, substitutions, injury breaks) during which fluid may be consumed.

5 Organise strategies to have suitable fluid needs on hand during exercise, in bottles or vessels that promote fluid availability.

6 Choose fluids that are cool and palatable.

7 Some athletes fear gastrointestinal discomfort from drinking during exercise. Practice, and a programme of small, frequent drinks can usually minimise these problems. Note that dehydration itself may cause gastrointestinal upsets.

8 Carbohydrate intake may enhance performance during events of longer than 1 h, especially if pre-event preparation of muscle and liver glycogen stores has not been ideal. Experiment with a schedule of 30–60 g/h and adapt to your needs. Make sure that intake starts well before you begin to feel fatigued. Your sport may dictate the opportunities to consume carbohydrate drinks and foods.

9 Sports drinks provide an ideal way to meet carbohydrate and fluid needs simultaneously during exercise. An intake of 600–1000 ml/h provides 40–80 g of carbohydrate. You may manipulate the concentration of the drink if carbohydrate needs exceed this fluid ratio, or if you want to use a more dilute solution when replacing very large sweat losses.

10 Solid carbohydrate foods can also be used during exercise to provide additional fuel. This is often seen in sports such as cycling where the risk of gastro-intestinal discomfort is less, and where the athlete needs to carry a compact carbohydrate source. Popular choices include fruit, sandwiches, sports bars, and confectionery.

11 Practise your strategies in training until you are confident of your competition plan.

provide a practical way for an athlete to meet their carbohydrate and fluid needs simultaneously during exercise. Sodium is added to these drinks primarily to enhance palatability and increase fluid intake (see Table 6.3). Athletes undertaking prolonged strenuous exercise are advised to experiment with carbohydrate drinks, or carbohydrate foods where desired, and develop a successful carbohydrate intake plan.

After the event

In the post-exercise period, replacement of fluid and electrolytes can usually be achieved through the normal dietary intake. However, rapid replacement of water and electrolytes in the post-exercise recovery period may be of crucial importance where repeated bouts of exercise have to be performed (say within a few hours) and there is a need to maximise rehydration in the time available. Ingestion of water alone in the post-exercise period results in a rapid fall in the plasma sodium concentration and osmolarity. These changes have the effect of reducing the stimulation to drink (thirst) and increasing the urine output, both of which will delay the rehydration process. Plasma volume is more rapidly and completely restored in the post-exercise period if some sodium chloride (77 mmol/l or 0.45 g/l) is added to the water consumed.[27,71] This sodium concentration is similar to the upper limit of the sodium concentration found in sweat and is close to the sodium content of oral rehydration solutions used in the clinical management of dehydration, but is considerably higher than the sodium concentration typical of commercially available sports drinks (10–25 mmol/l). Optimal rehydration after exercise can only be achieved if the sodium lost in sweat is replaced as well as the water.[72] Hence, if there is a need to ensure adequate replacement before exercise is repeated, extra fluids should be taken and additional salt (sodium chloride) might usefully be added to food (for review see Maughan *et al*[73]). The other major electrolytes lost in sweat, particularly potassium, magnesium, and calcium, are present in abundance in fruit and fruit juices. Mineral supplements containing these are not usually necessary.

In summary, increased fluid intake is necessary to avoid dehydration. It may improve performance during prolonged exercise, especially when sweat loss is high. These fluids may contain some carbohydrate, the concentration of which will be dictated by both the duration of exercise and the environmental conditions. If exercise is of short duration and sweat losses are small, the replacement of salts can be achieved from a normal food intake after exercise.

Nutritional supplements: creatine, alkaline salts, and amino acids

Creatine (see also Chapter 4)

There is no doubt as to the beneficial effects of creatine on high intensity exercise,[74] now widely used by athletes in many different sports. The use of creatine is not currently against the rules of any sport. The normal daily dietary intake of creatine is about 1–2 g: the major sources are meat and fish, so the intake in vegetarians is minimal. Daily creatine turnover is about 2 g, so any shortfall in the dietary intake is met by endogenous synthesis.[75] Harris *et al*[76] showed that ingestion of small amounts of creatine (1 g or less) had a negligible effect on the plasma creatine concentration, whereas feeding higher doses (5 g) resulted in an approximately 15-fold increase. Repeated feeding of creatine (5 g 4 times per day) over a period of 4–5 days resulted in a marked increase of 50% in the total creatine content of the quadriceps femoris muscle. Approximately 20% of the increase in total muscle creatine content was accounted for by creatine phosphate, the short term buffer for ATP resynthesis in muscle.

There appears to be no beneficial effect of creatine supplementation on the peak power output that can be achieved in a range of tests, but the balance of the available evidence suggests that performance is improved in high intensity exercise tasks, especially where repeated exercise bouts are carried out. However, there is no evidence to suggest that creatine supplementation has any beneficial effect on performance of endurance exercise events.

Alkaline salts

Short term high intensity exercise can also be improved by ingestion of alkaline salts prior to exercise to enhance the buffering of the hydrogen ions (acid) produced by anaerobic glycolysis.[58] Some athletes competing in the shorter middle distance events have been known to attempt this. These supplements, often consumed in bulk quantities a few hours prior to competition, include phosphates and sodium bicarbonate. There is some reliable evidence that the latter can improve performance in events where the accumulation of lactate in the muscle is a major cause of fatigue, such as 400–1500 m running. However, in many individuals the consumption of the amount of sodium bicarbonate necessary to alter blood acid-base status sufficiently to influence performance (approximately 20 g) causes gastrointestinal discomfort and diarrhoea. Because of these unpleasant side effects, the practice of bicarbonate loading could temporarily result in inadequate absorption of essential micronutrients and carbohydrate, and so could delay the restoration of muscle glycogen stores after exercise. This could be an important factor to consider for sports events involving competition on successive days.

Amino acids

Consumption of solutions containing branched chain amino acids (leucine, isoleucine, and valine) has been suggested as a method of decreasing the central component of fatigue during prolonged endurance exercise.[77] However, recent well controlled laboratory studies have not found any benefits of branched chain amino acid supplementation.[78,79] Another reason for supplementing athletes' diets with specific amino acids is that some of them may stimulate an increased release of growth hormone. Examples are arginine and ornithine which are believed by many strength athletes to have anabolic effects due to their effect of raising the plasma concentration of growth hormone.[80] However, since intense exercise itself induces a more than 10-fold increase in the plasma growth hormone concentration, which is sustained for at least an hour of recovery,[81] it seems that sprinters and strength athletes will create the effect they are trying to achieve with supplements simply by performing their normal training.

Conclusions

There is no doubt that exercise performance is influenced by the composition of the diet. In spite of this, however, many elite athletes have no clear idea of the nutritional demands of their sport, and often pursue practices which are unhelpful. The main requirements are to ensure that energy intake is appropriate for the level of energy expenditure, after taking account of requirements for growth and of any need to change body mass or fat content. A high carbohydrate intake is necessary to meet the demands of intensive training, and carbohydrate supplementation prior to competition may also be beneficial. If a varied diet is eaten in an adequate amount, it is extremely unlikely that deficiencies of protein or of any of the micronutrients will arise. There may be a need to pay attention to the intake of iron, and possibly also of calcium, especially in female athletes and anyone on an energy-restricted diet. Water intake must be increased to meet the increased losses which occur through sweating, and carbohydrate-electrolyte drinks may be beneficial if consumed during events lasting longer than about 1 hour. Dietary supplements are not recommended, although information is emerging to suggest that creatine supplementation may enhance performance in sprint events.

References

1 Bahr R. Excess postexercise oxygen consumption – magnitude, mechanisms and practical implication. *Acta Physiol Scand* 1992;**144**(Suppl 605):1–70.

2 Stanton R. Dietary extremism and eating disorders in athletes. In Burke LM, Deakin V, eds. *Clinical Sports Nutrition*. Sydney: McGraw-Hill, 1994, pp. 285–306.

3 Drinkwater BL, Nilson K, Ott S, Chestnet CH. Bone mineral density after resumption of menses in amenorrheic athletes. *J Am Med Assoc* 1986;**256**: 380–2.

4 Lemon PWR. Effect of exercise on protein requirements. *J Sports Sci* 1991;**9** (Special Issue):53–70.

5 Dohm GL. Protein as a fuel for endurance exercise. *Exerc Sport Sci Rev* 1986; **14**:143–73.

6 Burke LM, Inge K. Protein requirements for training and "bulking up". In: Burke LM, Deakin V, eds. *Clinical sports nutrition* Sydney: McGraw-Hill, 1994, pp. 124–50.

7 Gollnick PD, Piehl K, Saltin B. Selective glycogen depletion pattern in human muscle fibers after exercise of varying intensity and at varying pedalling rates. *J Physiol* 1974;**241**:45–57.

8 Bergstrom J, Hultman E. A study of the glycogen metabolism during exercise in man. *Scand J Clin Lab Invest* 1967;**19**:218–28.

9 Hultman E, Nilsson LH. Liver glycogen in man. *Adv Exp Biol Med* 1971;**11**: 143–51.

10 Bergstrom J, Hermansen L, Hultman E, Saltin B. Diet, muscle glycogen and physical performance. *Acta Physiol Scand* 1967;**71**: 140–50.

11 Karlsson J, Saltin B. Diet, muscle glycogen and endurance performance. *J Appl Physiol* 1971;**31**:203–6.

12 Widrick JJ, Costill DL, Fink WJ, Hickey MS, McConell GK, Tanaka H. Carbohydrate feedings and exercise performance: effect of initial muscle glycogen concentration. *J Appl Physiol* 1993;**74**:2998–3005.

13 Rauch LHG, Rodger I, Wilson GR, *et al*. The effects of carbohydrate loading on muscle glycogen content and cycling performance. *Int J Sport Nutr.* 1995; **5**:25–36.

14 Fallowfield JL, Williams C. Carbohydrate and recovery from prolonged exercise. *Int J Sport Nutr* 1993;**3**:150–64.

15 Piehl K. Time course of refilling of glycogen stores in human muscle fibres following exercise-induced glycogen depletion. *Acta Physiol Scand* 1974;**90**: 297–302.

16 Ivy JL, Lee MC, Brozinick, JT, Reed MJ. Muscle glycogen storage after different amounts of carbohydrate ingestion. *J Appl Physiol* 1988;**65**:2018–23.

17 Coyle EF. Timing and method of increased carbohydrate intake to cope with heavy training, competition and recovery. *J Sports Sci* 1991;**9**(Special Issue): 29–52.

18 Lambert EV, Speechly DP, Dennis SC, Noakes TD. Enhanced endurance in trained cyclists during moderate intensity exercise following 2 weeks adaptation to a high fat diet. *Eur J Appl Physiol* 1994;**69**:287–93.

19 Costill DL. Carbohydrates for exercise: dietary demands for optimal performance. *Int J Sports Med* 1988;**9**:1–18.

20 Williams C, Devlin JT. *Foods, nutrition and sports performance*. London: E & FN Spon, 1992.

21 American Dietetic Association. Position of the American Dietetic Association and the Canadian Dietetic Association: Nutrition for physical fitness and athletic performance for adults. *J Am Dietetic Assoc.* 1993;**93**:691–6.

22 Clark K. Nutritional guidance to soccer players for training and competition. *J Sports Sci* 1994;**12**(Special Issue):S43–S50.

23 Ivy JL, Katz AL, Cutler CL, Sherman WM, Coyle EF. Muscle glycogen synthesis after exercise: effect of time on carbohydrate ingestion. *J Appl Physiol* 1988;**65**:1480–5.

24 Blom PC, Hostmark AT, Vaage O, Vardal KR, Maehlum S. Effect of different post-exercise sugar diets on the rate of muscle glycogen synthesis. *Med Sci Sports Exerc* 1987;**19**:491–6.

25 Burke LM, Collier GR, Hargreaves M. Muscle glycogen storage following prolonged exercise: effect of the glycaemic index of carbohydrate feedings. *J Appl Physiol* 1993;**75**:1019–23.

26 Brouns F, Saris WHM, Stroecken J, *et al.* Eating, drinking and cycling. A controlled Tour de France simulation study. *Int J Sports Med*, 1989;**10**:S41–S48.

27 Brouns F. *Nutritional needs of athletes.* Chichester: John Wiley, 1993.

28 Beek EJ van der, Barens MF, Listemaker C, van Eck I, Weimar M. De voeding van triatleten. *Geneeskunde en Sport* 1988;**21**:40–7.

29 Saris WHM, Schrijver J, van Erp-Baart AMI, Brouns F. Adequacy of vitamin supply under maximal sustained workloads: the Tour de France. In: Walter P, Brubacher G, Stohelin H, eds. *Elevated dosages of vitamins: benefits and hazards* (*Int J Vit Nutr Res* 1989; suppl 30). Toronto: Hans Huber, pp. 205–12.

30 Erp-Baart AMJ van, Saris WHM, Binkhorst RA, Elvers JWH. Nationwide survey on nutritional habits in elite athletes, part II. Mineral and vitamin intake. *Int J Sports Med* 1989;**10**:S11–S16.

31 Beek EJ van der. Vitamins and endurance training – food for running or faddish claims? *Sports Med* 1985;**2**:175–97.

32 Beek EJ van der. Vitamin supplementation and physical exercise performance. *J Sports Sci* 1991;**9**:77–89.

33 Sargent F, Robinson P, Johnson RE. Water-soluble vitamins in sweat. *J Biol Chem* 1944;**153**:285–94.

34 Consolazio CF. Nutrition and performance. *Prog Food Nutr Sci* 1983;7:1–187.

35 Dreon DM, Butterfield GE. Vitamin B6 utilization in active and inactive young men. *Am J Clin Nutr* 1986;**43**:816–24.

36 Hunter KL, Turkki PR. Effect of exercise on riboflavin status of rats. *J Nutr* 1987;**117**:298–304.

37 Roe DA. Vitamin requirements for increased physical activity. In: Horton ED, Terjung, RL, eds. *Exercise, nutrition, and energy metabolism.* New York: Macmillan, 1989, pp. 172–9.

38 Singh A, Moses FM, Deuster PA. Chronic multivitamin-mineral supplementation does not enhance physical performance. *Med Sci Sports Exerc* 1992;**24**:726–32.

39 Bruce A. The effect of vitamin and mineral supplements and health foods on physical endurance and performance. *Proc Nutr Soc* 1985;**44**:283–95.

40 Weight LM, Myburgh KH, Noakes TD. Vitamin and mineral supplementation: effect on the running performance of trained athletes. *Am J Clin Nutr* 1988; **47**:192–5.

41 Beek EJ van der. Restricted vitamin intake and physical performance of military personnel. In: *Predicting decrements in physical performance due to inadequate nutrition.* Washington, DC: National Academy Press, 1988, pp. 139–69.

42 Clarkson PM. Minerals: exercise performance and supplementation. *J Sports Sci* 1991;**9**(Special Issue):91–116.

43 Sherman AR, Kramer B. In: Hickson JE, Wolinsky I, eds. *Nutrition in Exercise Sport*. Boca Raton: CRC Press, 1989, pp. 291–300.

44 Eichner ER. The anemias of athletes. *Phys Sportsmed* 1986;**14**:122–30.

45 Dressendorfer RH, Wade CE, Amsterdam EA. Development of pseudoanaemia in marathon runners during a 20-day road race. *J Am Med Assoc* 1981;**246**: 1215–18.

46 Gleeson M, Almey J. A rapid and sustained expansion of the plasma volume follows a single bout of muscle soreness-inducing exercise. *J Sports Sci* 1994; **12**:137.

47 Haymes EM. Vitamin and mineral supplementation to athletes. *Int J Sports Nutr* 1991;**1**:146–69.

48 Clement DB, Sawchuck LL. Iron status and sports performance. *Sports Med* 1984;**1**:65.

49 Healthy People 2000. National Health Promotion and Disease Prevention Objectives. Washington, DC, US Department of Health and Human Services, 1990.

50 Halioua L, Anderson JJB. Lifetime calcium intake and physical activity habits: independent and combined effects on the radial bone of healthy premenopausal Caucasian women. *Am J Clin Nutr* 1989;**49**:534–41.

51 Dalsky GP. The role of exercise in the prevention of osteoporosis. *Compar Ther* 1989;**15**:30–7.

52 Myburgh KH, Hutchins J, Fataar AB, Hough SF, Noakes TD. Low bone density is an etiologic factor for stress fracture in athletes. *Ann Intern Med* 1990; **113**:754–9.

53 Erp-Baart AMJ van, van Dokkum W, Saris WHM, Binkhorst RA, Elvers JWH. Magnesium and zinc intake of 25 groups of elite athletes. In: *Food habits of athletes* (thesis of AMJ van Erp-Baart), Katholieke Universiteit, Nijmegen, Netherlands, 1992, pp. 39–48.

54 Fogelholm M. Vitamins, minerals and supplementation in soccer. *J Sports Sci* 1994;**12**:S23–S27.

55 Kirwan JP, Hickner RC, Yarasheski KE. Eccentric exercise induces transient insulin resistance in healthy individuals. *J Appl Physiol* 1992;**72**:2197–202.

56 O'Reilly KP, Warhol MJ, Fielding RA. Eccentric exercise-induced muscle damage impairs muscle glycogen repletion. *J Appl Physiol* 1987;**63**:252–6.

57 Saltin B, Karlsson J. Die Ehrnahrung des Sportlers. In: Hollman W, ed. *Zentrale Themen der Sportmedizin*. Berlin: Springer Verlag, 1972, pp. 245–60.

58 Maughan RJ, Greenhaff PL. High intensity exercise and acid-base balance: the influence of diet and induced metabolic alkalosis on performance. In: Brouns F, ed. *Advances in nutrition and top sport*. Karger: Basel, 1994, pp. 147–65.

59 Kelman GR, Maughan RJ, Williams C. The effect of dietary modifications on blood lactate during exercise. *J Physiol* 1975;**251**:34–35P.

60 Sherman WM, Brodowicz G, Wright DA, Allen WK, Simonsen J, Derbach A. Effects of 4 h pre-exercise carbohydrate feedings on cycling performance. *Med Sci Sports Exerc* 1989;**21**:598–604.

61 Foster C, Costill DL, Fink WJ. Effects of pre-exercise feedings on endurance performance. *Med Sci Sports Exerc* 1979;**11**:1–5.

62 Maughan RJ. Fluid and electrolyte loss and replacement in exercise. In: Harries M, Williams C, Stanish WD and Micheli LJ, eds. *Oxford Textbook of Sports Medicine*. New York: Oxford University Press, 1994, pp. 82–93.

63 Maughan RJ. Fluid and electrolyte loss and replacement in exercise. *J Sports Sci* 1991;**9**(Special Issue):117–42.

64 Gopinathan PM, Pichan G, Sharma VM. Role of dehydration in heat stress-induced variations in mental performance. *Arch Environ Health* 1988;**43**:15–17.

65 Sutton JR, Bar-Or O. Thermal illness in fun running. *Am Heart J* 1980;**100**: 778–81.
66 American College of Sports Medicine. Position stand: exercise and fluid replacement. *Med Sci Sports Exerc* 1996;**28**:i–vii.
67 Coggan AR, Coyle EF. Carbohydrate ingestion during prolonged exercise: effects on metabolism and performance. *Exerc Sport Sci Rev* 1991;**19**:1–40.
68 Below P, Mora-Rodriguez R, Gonzalez-Alonso J and Coyle EF. Fluid and carbohydrate ingestion independently improve performance during 1 h of intense cycling. *Med Sci Sports Exerc* 1994;**27**:200–10.
69 Coyle EF, Coggan AR, Hemmert MK, Ivy JL. Muscle glycogen utilisation during prolonged strenuous exercise when fed carbohydrate. *J Appl Physiol* 1986;**61**:165–72.
70 Hawley JA, Dennis SC, Noakes TD. Carbohydrate, fluid and electrolyte requirements during prolonged exercise. In Kies CV, Driskell JA, eds. *Sports nutrition: minerals and electrolytes* Boca Raton: CRC Press, 1995, pp. 235–65.
71 Nose H, Mack GW, Shi X, Nadel ER. Role of osmolality and plasma volume during rehydration in humans. *J Appl Physiol* 1988;**65**:325–31.
72 Shirreffs SM, Taylor AJ, Leiper JB, Maughan RJ. Post-exercise rehydration in man: effects of volume consumed and sodium content of ingested fluids. *Med Sci Sports Exerc* 1996;**28**:1260–71.
73 Maughan RJ, Leiper JB, Shirreffs SM. Rehydration and recovery after exercise. *Sports Sci Exchange* 1996;**9**(3):1–6.
74 Balsom PD, Soderlund K, Ekblom B. Creatine in humans with special reference to creatine supplementation. *Sports Med* 1994;**18**:268–80.
75 Walker JB. Creatine biosynthesis, regulation and function. *Adv Enzymol* 1979; **50**:117–42.
76 Harris RC, Soderlund K, Hultman E. Elevation of creatine in resting and exercised muscle of normal subjects by creatine supplementation. *Clin Sci* 1992; **83**:367–74.
77 Blomstrand E, Hassmen P, Ekblom, B, Newsholme EA. Administration of branched-chain amino acids during sustained exercise – effects on performance and on plasma concentration of some amino acids. *Eur J Appl Physiol* 1991;**63**: 83–8.
78 Lambert M, Velloza P, Wilson G, Dennis S. The effect of carbohydrate and branched chain supplementation on cycling performance and mental fatigue. *Clin Sci* 1994;**87**(Supplement):53.
79 Hall G van, Raaymakers J, Saris W, Wagenmakers A. Supplementation with branched-chain amino acids (BCAA) and tryptophan has no effect on performance during prolonged exercise. *Clin Sci* 1994;**87**(Supplement):52.
80 Hatfield FC. *Ultimate Sports Nutrition*. Chicago: Contemporary Books Inc, 1987.
81 Nevill ME, Holmyard D, Hall G, Allson P, van Oosterhout A, Burrin JM. Growth hormone responses to treadmill sprinting in sprint and endurance trained male athletes. *J Physiol* 1993;**473**:73P.

7 Caring for a team abroad

TOM CRISP AND ROGER G HACKNEY

Introduction

The job of a team doctor is complicated and demanding, yet enormously satisfying. It is a low profile position with few rewards but demands a dedication to the players. It involves treading the narrow line between familiarity with the team members and having their confidence on the one hand, yet being able to maintain enough distance to make dispassionate decisions about their health and fitness to compete on the other. The confidence of the team management is crucial and team doctors must be able to make decisions on purely medical grounds and resist outside pressures.

Training is essential, especially when dealing with representative and national sides. There are now a number of Diploma and MSc qualifications available that prove the acquisition of a suitable standard of sports medicine expertise. These include courses such as the full time MSc and Diploma courses at the Royal London Hospital and at the Universities of Nottingham and Glasgow, and the British Association of Sport and Medicine programme which will provide basic training. Basic first aid skills are essential, and in addition the practitioner must possess a good understanding of the pathology and epidemiology of injury in a particular sport. In a number of sports medical skills such as advanced life support are now considered essential.

General Practice skills are important since a large part of the role of the team doctor is as the GP to the team, but other areas such as exercise physiology, nutrition, and sports psychology are useful. It is our hope that training schemes will develop to bring the education of a national team doctor up to standards similar to that of any other specialty in medicine. It is not acceptable for a doctor to be present at sporting venues to provide management of a serious injury or illness but be unable to handle such a situation when it does occur. The Football Association (FA) for example, demands at least the possession of a Diploma in Sports Medicine for the appointment of all new team doctors.

Wearing appropriate clothing is important for the doctor, and it is not acceptable to be dressed in smart clothing when it may be necessary to take control of treatment of a neck injury on a wet rugby pitch. Functional clothing signals to the other members of the team that you are ready to participate fully.

A number of specific areas will be discussed in detail, but it is important at this point to stress the need for finite responsibility. On joining a team you need to know whether your responsibilities are to look after the team only, or whether you are also responsible for the spectators (where the size of the crowd does not necessitate a specific doctor); or when abroad, whether you will also be expected to care for an entourage that may include families, referees, officials, and even journalists. The responsibility will differ from team to team, country to country, and even competition to competition. Your first responsibility, however, must always be to the athletes.

Travelling

Travelling is a tiring business. The experienced sports traveller becomes accustomed to the vagaries of timetables, delays, and unhelpful officialdom. The athletes must not allow themselves to become upset by matters beyond their control. Team management should ensure that their charges are protected from hassle as much as possible and sports travellers should be offered advice on dealing with the problems and frustrations of travel.

Jet lag

The body possesses a pacemaker or internal clock that produces circadian rhythms. This pacemaker, if left to run without external stimuli, would run over a period of 25 hours, and is slowed to a 24 hour day by light, and by behavioural factors such as bedtime, meal times, and activity. There are a number of well recognised circadian rhythms which include body temperature, alertness and sleep/wake cycles, kidney function including urine output and potassium secretion, cardiovascular function and resting heart rate, various hormone secretions such as adrenaline, growth hormone, and testosterone, and perhaps most important, athletic performance. Body temperature is probably the most important guide to the phase of the circadian rhythms and performance and sleep/wake patterns are closely related to variations in core temperature.

This is of relevance not only when planning training for specific competition (in order to maximise performance) but also when travelling to different time zones. In a new time zone the body clock will be out of phase, leading to a lack of alertness during the day and a decreased performance. This phenomenon is called jet lag and the symptoms are

135

Advice to be offered to sports travellers

- The team management or the athlete (if travelling alone) must ensure that travel arrangements are as smooth and short as possible. Be wary of venues at a large distance from airports
- To avoid boredom during long journeys take plenty of personal entertainment, e.g. books, playing cards, music, games, etc.
- Food – take some of your own and some evening carbohydrate for prior to sleeping
- Carry anti-travel sickness medication in your hand baggage for aircraft, coach, or boat travel
- In airport lounges, in the event of a delay find a quiet corner, relax, keep hydrated and fed
- Aircraft are pressurised to 5000 feet using dry air which is then humidified, but not up to normal levels. A great deal of body fluid is lost over a long journey. Take extra fluids, but avoid coffee, tea, and alcohol as these act as mild diuretics and lead to further fluid loss. Take a 2 litre bottle of diluted squash in your hand baggage. Sore throat and headache indicate insufficient fluid intake
- When in aircraft, ensure you are comfortable and away from smokers; don't hesitate to ask for a seat upgrade! Tall people should ask for a seat with extra leg room. Take regular walks around the aircraft and avoid stiffness by stretching regularly
- Employ strategies for coping with time change
- Customs often require a long wait. Don't get frustrated
- Visas – international athletes are still stopped from entering a country for competition because they have not obtained the correct entry requirements. Check with your travel agent and ensure documents are in order in good time
- **Always** carry shorts and a pair of training and competition shoes in your hand baggage, and local currency and acceptable credit cards either on your person or in your hand baggage, just in case your luggage goes missing
- **Be self-sufficient**

fatigue, inability to sleep at night, loss of appetite and concentration, bowel upset, headache and general malaise, and of course decreased performance. Studies have shown that muscular strength, psychomotor, and athletic skills are all reduced until jet lag symptoms have abated. The ability to acclimatise to a hot environment is compromised.

The time it takes to adjust to the new time zone will depend on the time difference and the direction (East when time is ahead or West when time is behind that of the time zone left). Travelling East is more difficult to accommodate, though this is less evident in near maximal time zone shifts

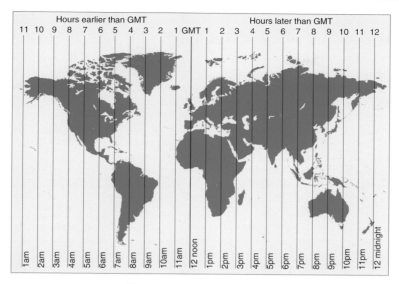

Figure 7.1   Time zone differences

(9–12 hours time difference). To help athletes speed their adjustment, various strategies can be suggested, as detailed in the Box on page 138.

Training and competing abroad

The sportsperson travels for a variety of reasons including squad training, acclimatisation for heat, humidity and/or altitude, and of course competition. Training camps and competitive events are associated with their own particular problems. The extra spare time available and the element of competition inevitable in a training camp may lead to increased risks from overtraining and injuries. The choice of a suitable venue requires a great deal of care and consideration.

Although facilities may be excellent, some venues require the athletes and their medical staff to be very self-sufficient. Extra food, particularly carbohydrate and electrolyte replacement drinks, will need to be part of an individual's baggage. The athletes need a degree of self-discipline (which is sometimes lacking) and a supply of reading material and games to occupy excess spare time.

Major championships

The stresses of competing in a major championship are severe and some athletes have difficulty coping. The unfamiliar pressures include those from

137

Strategies to aid athletes adapt to a new time zone

- Adopt your new time zone as soon as possible (better still if you can do it before departure). You can adapt by up to 2 hours towards the destination time zone before departure, i.e. evening training, instead of morning, before easterly travel
- Go to bed at the appropriate time even if you are not tired, ideally in quiet dark surroundings. Try to avoid daytime naps unless exhausted
- If woken by a full bladder, return to bed and rise at the correct time even if unable to sleep
- Eat meals that are appropriate for the time of day – a small carbohydrate meal before bed and more protein and caffeine in the morning
- Social and especially athletic activities at appropriate times may speed adjustment. Moderate exercise even on the day of arrival will help
- Sedatives and sleeping tablets may help you get to sleep but do not guarantee that you will continue to sleep. They may cause a hangover and should be tried before travel to assess their effects. Alcohol is not a good sedative since it acts as a diuretic and may cause waking during the night
- Allow enough time for acclimatisation before competition
- Remember that even with these strategies it will take approximately 1 day for every two time zones travelling West and 2 days for every three time zones travelling East. For highly specialised skills such as pistol shooting it may take longer than this to adjust

Advice on diet and fluid when competing abroad

- A set of scales and a graph for individuals to fill in to be aware of any changes in weight should be part of the medical room equipment
- Check menus beforehand if possible
- Educate team on possible problem areas
- Encourage athletes to maintain high carbohydrate intake
- Ensure athletes increase fluid intake on the flight and before thirst increases
- Check form and availability of fluid before competition
- Monitor hydration of athletes

the media, and expectations of family and friends. The choice of room mates can be crucial and segregation of teams competing early or late in a championship should be considered.

Medical staff can play an important role in helping athletes settle into the new situation. There is a dearth of organised entertainment and socialising frequently takes place in the restaurants. The medical facilities will often become a social centre which provides medical staff with an

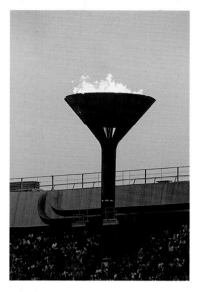

Figure 7.2   Competing in major competitions puts many stresses on the athlete

excellent opportunity to gauge the morale of both the individuals and the team.

The standard of food and drink at major championship events is extremely variable. Adequate intake of food both pre and post competition is vital for optimum performance. Part of the general advice from medical staff should be concerned with eating habits and weight change, with instructions to avoid local ice creams, tap water, or ice in drinks.

Areas of concern when training or competing abroad

- Illness, especially diarrhoea
- Unfamiliar climate or altitude may increase training load and requires compensation
- Altered diet, particularly insufficient carbohydrate
- Increased alcohol consumption
- Stress associated with competing in a major championship
- Food, over/undereating
- Fluid intake
- Sleep/jet lag/boredom

After the competition sportspeople may experience a post-event peak in mood. At such times eating may have a low priority, but athletes must be encouraged to do so. In events where there may be several matches or rounds, carbohydrate consumption must be maintained. Suitable foodstuffs should be available at the medical facilities both at headquarters and at the sport venue, with encouragement to consume early and ample food and fluids.

Acclimatisation

Hot climates

Travelling to a new climate causes problems to athletes, especially if the new environment is hot and/or humid. Physical activity generates a great deal of heat which has to be lost in order to maintain body core temperature within an acceptable range. With exercise, core temperature rises, reaching a level that is more dependent on the intensity of the exercise than the environmental temperature. When body core temperature in exercise rises beyond a given level for an individual, their performance deteriorates. A variety of adaptations occur to reduce the rise in body temperature with exercise in hot climates (see Box).

Adaptations to exercise in the heat

- Earlier production of sweat from larger more sensitive and efficient sweat glands
- Sweat is more dilute, preserving salt
- Greater quantity of sweat, 2 litres per hour or more
- Altered distribution of sweating patterns
- Reduction in the rise of body core temperature
- Plasma volume increases by 10%
- Heart rate decreases
- Adaptation is prevented by jet lag, tiredness, illness
- Hydromeiosis is the effect of reduced sweating when the skin is wet

---

Hot humid environments are more difficult to adapt to, as the humidity reduces the ability of the body to lose heat through evaporation of sweat, and performance will be reduced.

A 1–2% loss of body fluid will result in a deterioration of performance which is significant in terms of competition. Maintenance of body fluid is therefore essential, and various strategies are adopted for this. Fluid intake must increase greatly in hot environments and should be carefully monitored. It may be necessary to weigh athletes before and after training or competition to monitor hydration. The message that "drinking

140

sufficient fluid is essential" requires constant reinforcement. Athletes vary tremendously in their ability to thermoregulate, responses should be closely monitored to prevent those least well adapted from suffering hyperthermia. Heat tolerance will improve over 7–14 days. Acclimatisation can commence prior to travel to a hot environment by the use of extra clothing during training. Over a period of a month the effect will be quite dramatic. The athlete must be warned to expect an initial deterioration in performance.

How to avoid poor performance due to dehydration

- Palatable fluid must be available at all times, but especially before and after competition and training
- Electrolyte replacement fluids should be made to manufacturer's dilutions
- Colour of urine is a good guide to relative hydration. Clear urine indicates a good fluid balance
- Thirst is a poor guide to hydration and is unreliable
- Large volumes of fluid must be taken on long journeys
- Endurance athletes must be meticulous in their preparation for fluid intake in competition. They should know what fluid to use, where it will be, and must practise drinking in racing situations

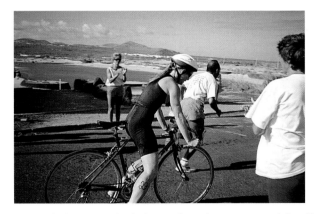

Figure 7.3   Athletes competing in heat and sun face many potential problems

Exposure to the sun can also be harmful both in the short term (sunburn can severely handicap an athlete) and the long term (premature skin ageing, abnormal pigmentation, and skin cancers). The incidence

141

of malignant melanomas in the UK is increasing; athletes may be at a greater risk because of their prolonged exposure. Sudden exposure with burning causes more damage than gradual exposure without burning. Exposure should be gradual, with the use of high Sun Protection Factor suncreams (SPF>15–20). Athletes should use shade when possible. Athletes in outdoor watersports must use waterproof sun creams and reapply them frequently – the effect of even the best creams will be reduced after 1–2 hours.

Heat illnesses

A variety of problems are caused by exercise in the heat. The concept of these as a continuum, or progression of a single disorder is no longer

---

Prevention and management of heat illnesses

- Appropriate preparation and fitness level reduces the risk. Acclimatisation should begin prior to travel to hot environs with the use of extra clothing, a hot room or a heat chamber
- Acclimatisation (up to 10–14 days) will increase the athlete's ability to cope in heat with the training load, increasing by 10% per day during this period
- Adequate hydration is essential throughout exposure to hot climates. Use of electrolyte balanced sports drinks should be encouraged
- Appropriate clothing and protection from the heat and sunshine should be used when possible
- Trained personnel should be available to diagnose and treat immediately any hyperthermic athlete
- If in doubt an intravenous infusion should be set up

---

thought to be valid. Prevention of heat illnesses requires a good fluid intake – small amounts (120–150 ml) are taken frequently (every 15–20 minutes) of a fluid which contains no more than 5% carbohydrate. The presence of a small amount of electrolytes in the fluid may help absorption. Salt tablets are unnecessary if salt is taken with a normal diet. Clothing should be white to reflect more radiant heat and loose enough to allow air to circulate. In some sports the wearing of protective clothing (e.g. American football or cricket) may make this difficult. Attempts should be made to increase heat loss whenever possible by loosening clothing and seeking shade.

Heat cramps

Short-lived episodes of painful cramps after prolonged exercise may be associated with electrolyte imbalance around an area of injured muscle. Treat by adequate fluid and electrolyte intake and a reduced intensity of training.

Heat syncope

Fainting after exercise is a result of venous pooling from sudden loss of the calf and foot muscle pump. It is commonly seen at the end of a race. Treat by walking or elevation of the legs and oral rehydration.

Heat exhaustion

This term is used for an excessive rise in body core temperature exacerbated by dehydration leading to weakness, reduced blood pressure but high heart rate with clammy skin. The effect is worse in highly motivated individuals in intense competition over relatively short distances. Treat by cooling and rehydration.

Heat stroke

This is an idiosyncratic reaction to exercise in the heat. Signs include dizziness, headache, nausea, tachycardia, and lack of coordination, fitting,

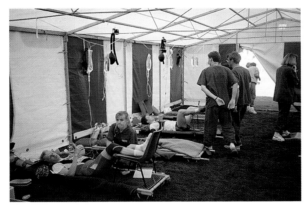

Figure 7.4   There should be no delay in treating athletes at on-site facilities

and loss of consciousness. The skin is pale and dry. The risk is of progression to multi-organ failure and death.

143

Treatment of heat stroke involves rehydration and cooling. Cooling may be rapid. Loss of heat by causing vasoconstriction of the skin does not seem to be a problem. Immersion in a cold bath is effective, but requires suitable facilities. Early transfer to hospital may be life-saving.

There should be no delay in treating heat illnesses and procedures should be carried out on site by trained personnel. A system of luke-warm water spray and fanned air increasing heat loss by evaporation is an effective way of lowering body temperature. If the symptoms are at all serious an intravenous infusion should be used. Core temperature, urine output, weight, cardiovascular status, and conscious level are closely monitored. Rectal temperature and not oral temperature must be measured in any case of heat illness. Access to resuscitation equipment is required as there is a risk of ventricular fibrillation.

Cold environments

In the UK we are accustomed to cold, wet weather, but prolonged exposure can lead to hypothermia. Hypothermia can strike in many sports, and rugby players may show early signs at the end of a rugby game in cold, wet conditions with extra time played. During the last few miles of a marathon, runners are at risk. Symptoms and signs include confusion, slowness of thought, weakness, and disorientation. Assessment must include core temperature measurement. Athletes showing signs of imminent hypothermia should be removed from the field of play. The patient must be rewarmed as quickly as possible, although it is during this phase that there is the greatest risk of ventricular fibrillation. Warming can be achieved by transferring the patient to a warm site, giving warm fluids, and reducing heat loss by insulation. Drying can be important in cold, wet conditions where the water will add to the heat loss by evaporation.

Diet and fluids during travel

Although this subject has been dealt with earlier under various headings, there are some problems specific to team travel that require emphasis. It is not always easy when at home and in control for athletes to arrange their diet so as to satisfy the recommendations of 60% carbohydrate which apply. It is very much harder in a hotel abroad or in the athletes' village, where a lot of the food on offer will be different from that available at home. Education before departure can help to identify those foods high in carbohydrate and those that are high in fat for example. Some parts of the world supply food that does not contain the correct proportions (e.g. a high fat diet in parts of the USA) and it is helpful to get sample menus from hotels in advance to ensure there is enough carbohydrate, for example.

Fluid replacement has also been dealt with elsewhere in the chapter, but it must be remembered that the need for extra fluids starts on the plane, where a dry environment can lead to dehydration, and that thirst is a poor guide to the state of hydration. Dark urine indicates the need for more fluid, and if competition starts soon after arrival it is important to arrive hydrated. If it is possible it is useful to check fluid balance during training, for example by weighing before and after exercise, to identify those that sweat more and will therefore need more fluid more frequently.

Sometimes a special policy is needed to maintain fluid intake during certain sports where replacement during the game is difficult. Alcohol is not good, either as a fluid or as calories, since it acts as a diuretic, increasing fluid loss, and the calories are only available after metabolism by the liver and therefore are not useful during the exercise period.

Drugs and equipment

The drugs and equipment which need to be taken abroad with teams is dependent on the team and the medical problems of the team members, the sport and its particular risks, and most importantly the destination and the problems likely to be encountered there. Enquiry from the embassy of the destination country can give some information but risks are likely to be played down and information from the Travel Clinic at The Hospital for Tropical Diseases in London can be invaluable. There is also a computer program available from Pro-Choice called "Traveller" that lists the diseases (from a list of 13) that are prevalent in each of 200 countries, but the information is rather bland and not tailored to the particular needs of a team.

A simple test when preparing to go abroad is to list all the possible medical problems that could arise and check that treatment from your kit will be available for all of them. To check on any medical ailments that members of your party may suffer from, it is advisable to get all members to fill in a confidential medical questionnaire before departure. It is important to know in planning if you are likely to have asthmatics, diabetics, epileptics etc. in the party. In countries where access to drugs is limited a more comprehensive drug list will be needed.

Importation of drugs into some countries such as Japan is difficult and clearance with the country's customs, usually through the organising

Headings for the medical kit list

- Diagnostic tools (stethoscope, otoscope etc.)
- Resuscitation tools (airways, disposable mask etc.)
- Surgical tools (suture kit, scissors etc.)
- Records (notebook, pen etc.)
- Drugs: tablets
- Injections (including infusion set)
- Inhalers
- Topical drugs
- Suitable waterproof container and suitable clothing

Drugs list guidelines – headings used to plan drugs taken

- Gastrointestinal
- Antacids, antidiarrhoeals, anti-emetics, ?H₂-blockers
- Laxatives, haemorrhoid treatment
- Analgesics
- Minor: paracetamol and aspirin
- Intermediate
- Strong, ?injectable
- Anti-inflammatories, migraine
- Antibiotics: wide range of activity spectra including any specific to destination
- Topical, antiviral, antifungal
- Anti-allergy etc: antihistamines, steroids, ENT sprays
- Asthma treatments
- ENT and eye: antibiotics, anti-inflammatories, throat treatments
- Gynaecological: progesterone, oral contraceptive (including post-coital), anti-monilial
- Topical: anti-inflammatory, antipruritic
- Hypnotics and sedatives

committee of the games or competition, or the embassy, before departure is advised. A list of the drugs being carried and their purpose, on official headed notepaper, is essential to reduce delays at the customs.

The equipment taken will depend on the destination and the local availability of full medical back-up. Obviously stethoscope, otoscope, sphygmomanometer, and thermometer are essential, but it may be useful to take disposable vaginal speculae and other more specialised equipment. It is always useful to take suture kits, and it is also sometimes worth taking intravenous infusion sets in some circumstances (e.g. on trips to India).

Vaccinations are, of course, essential for many destinations and forward planning to ensure maximum safety cover is advisable. Up-to-date information can be obtained from the Department of Health and is regularly distributed to General Practices in the UK.

Malarial prophylaxis may involve a daily dose (e.g. of Paludrine) and it is possible to get the drugs packaged together in strips for daily use by the team, which aids compliance.

Travel to countries where traveller's diarrhoea is common clearly carries risks, and there is debate as to whether the prophylactic use of antibiotics is of value. Current advice from the Travel Clinic of the Hospital for Tropical Diseases suggests that a daily dose of ciprofloxacin (250 mg) will reduce the risk. Cheaper alternatives are Septrin (co-trimoxazole) (trimethoprim is less effective alone because of the high incidence of resistance) or doxycycline, but both carry risks of side effects. A study of treatment with a single dose of 500 mg of ciprofloxacin immediately after the first loose stool suggested this can cut the episode short from an average of 50 hours to just 20. This avoids the expense and risk of non-compliance with regular prophylaxis.

Commonsense in the choice of food and its source is the most important element of prevention of diarrhoea, and prophylaxis makes this no less important. Athletes should be worried if there are risks from the water supply; bottled water is usually available and should be used for drinking as well as toothbrushing etc. Salads will be washed in the tap water and so should be avoided unless additional preparation is adequate. Seafood is especially prone to infection, as is reheated food, and eating "off the beaten track" should be discouraged. If prophylaxis is not used, then appropriate treatment for the likely pathogens is important, such as metronidazole for Giardia in parts of Russia and India, and ciprofloxacin for enteropathic *Escherichia coli*, as well as non-specific antidiarrhoeals.

As most of the drugs and equipment will not be available during the travelling period, it is useful to carry a small travel kit containing a few basic drugs including an analgesic, an anti-emetic and an antidiarrhoeal, an antihistamine, possibly an antacid and a hypnotic for long flights, and a few plasters and dressings.

A sewing kit is another helpful piece of equipment, to mend kit etc., as well as a good pair of scissors.

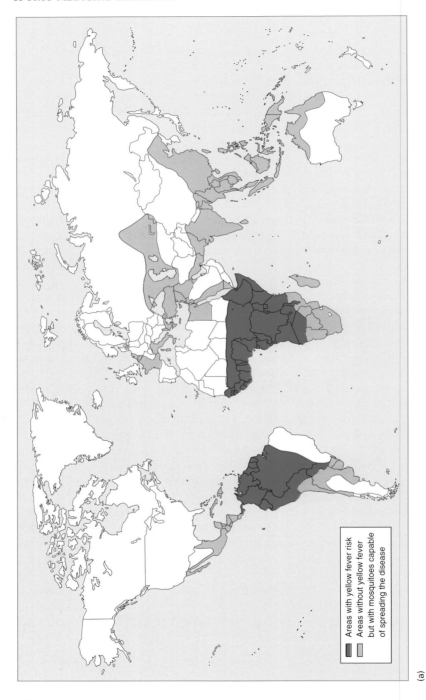

Figure 7.5

Areas with yellow fever risk
Areas without yellow fever but with mosquitoes capable of spreading the disease

(a)

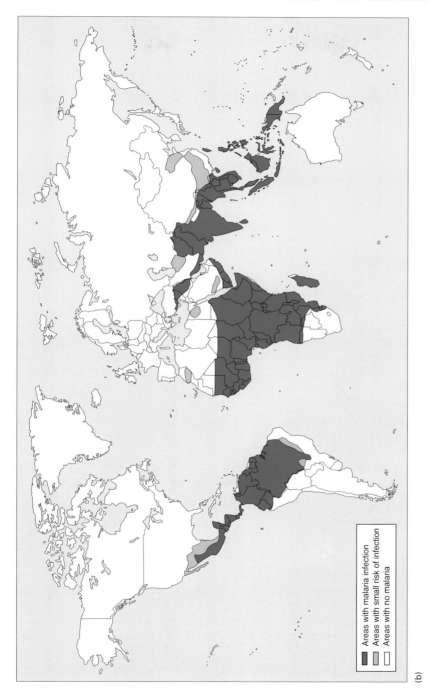

Figure 7.5   Forward planning is essential for travel to areas requiring vaccination (adapted from International travel and health: Vaccination requirements and health advice 1966, *Geneva: WHO)*

Areas with malaria infection
Areas with small risk of infection
Areas with no malaria

(b)

149

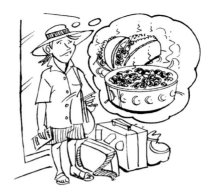

Figure 7.6   Competitors abroad should make sensible food choices

Doping

The team doctor has certain responsibilities with regard to doping. Firstly, the doctor should educate the athlete as to what is banned and what is allowable in terms of medication. Problems can arise from areas such as cold remedies and certain herbal remedies that contain stimulants such as ephedrine. Some asthma treatments are only allowed in inhaler form, such as beclomethasone, while salbutamol now requires an annual certification. A few athletes may have to alter treatments slightly to avoid any risk of a positive drug test. It is obviously important also to teach the dangers of many of the banned drugs and strongly discourage athletes from using anything to gain short term benefits without consideration of the long term dangers.

Secondly, the team doctor should educate the athlete about the testing procedure, which may vary slightly from country to country, and from competition to competition. This will reduce the anxiety naturally associated with drug testing. There is nothing more frightening for an athlete who has never been through the procedure before to be met with a doping control officer brandishing a pot and asking for urine to be passed under direct vision. Worries can be reduced by clear explanations beforehand. The athlete is allowed to have a representative with them when being tested and we believe this person should be a member of the medical team if at all possible.

The doctor must be available for sympathetic advice on all aspects of doping control and therefore must be well informed. In some circumstances the doctor will be part of the process for informing an athlete of a positive dope test, and a policy for this situation must have been thought through with all the relevant officials beforehand.

150

Ethical considerations

The team doctor will sometimes be placed in a difficult situation when, for example, an athlete informs the doctor of a problem that affects the athlete's ability to compete. Communication and openness are important and this sort of information must not be passed on to the manager without the permission of the athlete. Yet responsibility to the team and management make it essential that it is not brushed under the carpet. Usually open discussion with all parties involved will resolve any conflicts.

A relationship must exist with the selectors such that if the doctor decides that a team member is unfit to compete, that member does not do so. That decision requires confidence between the doctor and the team management. If the situation is not so clear-cut, then discussion of the risks and advantages with the athlete and the selectors should be considered, but the doctor should have no involvement in the actual selection process. The physician will be interested in the long term interests of the athlete while the management may be more interested in the short term interests of the team, and occasionally these may conflict.

Clearly the doctor will do his or her best to ensure any athlete is fit to compete, but may occasionally be asked to mask an injury. This raises the question of when (if at all) it is justified to give local anaesthetic before competition. Risks may be minimal, if for example local injection is given to a local bruise to gain full function, but even here there is a risk of reducing the natural defences. Often anaesthetising a soft tissue injury will make it more likely that the injury is made worse by exercise. Informed consent – with the athlete knowing and understanding the risks and implications – must be gained first. For many competitions it is then necessary to inform the organisers of the administration of the drug, and for what reason. Careful monitoring of the situation is then essential. There will be many occasions when the risks are too high and you must resist pressures to "give it a go". Again, you are responsible for the continuing health of the athlete as well as the team's interests.

Clear records are essential, not just for medicolegal reasons but for later referral or further management, and analysis of data when preparing for the next trip. Keep one line records for most minor things, coded for easy analysis, and full page entries for major and continuing problems. Writing records beside a rain-drenched pitch is not possible, but at the soonest possible time a short note of what occurred and what treatment was given is required. For a lot of problems a note to the athlete's GP on return home will ensure good continuing care.

151

Forward planning

When planning to travel abroad, it is useful to make a few contacts with the local medical services as early as possible, even before departure if

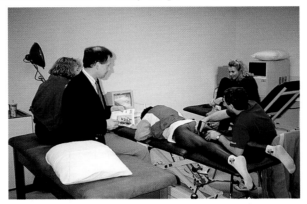

Figure 7.7   A major event clinic located beneath a stadium. Facilities of this standard may not always be available

appropriate. Find out what services will be provided on site – Will there be an ambulance present? Will there be local doctors and physiotherapists available at major games? It is useful to know in advance where the nearest hospital is in the event of a serious injury, and whether you will be able to order X-rays etc. and what specialist services are available. There is an ever-increasing number of doctors around the world who have undergone some sports medicine training in the UK and who will be keen to help and can give useful advice on using the local services.

You will need to know where to replenish supplies if you are away for long periods – can you buy drugs over the counter or will you need to get them through a hospital? How easy is it to get bottled water and sports drinks? These points considered before departure will make the trip run more smoothly.

Forward planning checklist

- Up-to-date vaccinations
- Identification of athletes with medical problems
- Education of athletes about destination
- Drugs approved by country of destination
- Knowledge of facilities available
- Travel kit arranged
- Kit list appropriate to destination and sport

Forward thinking and forward planning may result in you providing the best possible medical support for your team. The checklist (see Box opposite) may help.

Acknowledgements

Figure 7.1, 7.5, and 7.6 are reproduced with permission from Walker E *et al.*, *ABC of healthy travel*, 5th edn. London: BMJ Publishing Group, 1997.

Bibliography

Aschoff J, Fatranska M, Giedke H, Doerr P, Stamm D, Wisser H. Human circadian rhythms in continuous darkness: entrainment by social cues. *Science* 1971;**171**: 213–15.

Antal LC. The effects of the changes of circadian body rhythm on the sports shooter. *Br J Sport Med* 1975;**9**:9–12.

Czeisler CA, Kronauer RE, Allan JS. Bright light induction of strong resetting of the human pacemaker. *Science* 1989;**244**:1328–33.

Minors DS, Waterhouse JM. *Circadian rhythms and the human.* Bristol: John Wright, 1981.

Neilsen B. Thermoregulation during work in carbon monoxide poisoning. *Acta Phys Scand* 1971;**82**:98–106.

Reilly TJ. Circadian rhythms in muscular activity. In Marconnet P, Komi PV, Saltin B, Sejeested OM, eds. *Muscle fatigue mechanisms in exercise and training.* Basel, Karger, 1992, pp. 218–22.

Reilly TJ, Mellor S. Jet-lag in student rugby league players following a near maximal time zone shift. In Reilly TJ, Lees A, Davids K, eds. *Science and Football.* London: E & FN Spon, 1988, pp. 249–56.

Salam I, Katelaris P, Leigh-Smith S, Farthing M. Randomised trial of single dose ciprofloxacin for travellers' diarrhoea. *Lancet* 1994;**334**(8936):1537–9.

Sutton JR. Physiological and clinical consequences of exercise in heat and humidity. In: *Oxford textbook of sports medicine*, 2nd edn. Oxford: Oxford University Press, 1998.

Walker E, Williams G, Raeside F, Calvert L. *ABC of healthy travel*, 5th edn. London: BMJ Publishing Group, 1997.

Wever RA. *The circadian rhythms of man.* New York: Springer-Verlag.

8 Management of acute injuries

DONALD AD MACLEOD AND W STEWART HILLIS

Introduction

The management of acute injuries and illness in a sporting context invariably challenges the attending medical team to demonstrate innovative approaches, often in a difficult environment, to deal with a wide range of clinical problems. Individual activities such as hill walking can be associated with varied and potentially lethal environmental conditions where the doctor is facing a very different agenda from a colleague looking after an indoor athletics match or watching a junior football match when a player or spectator collapses.

The care of acute injuries and illness occurring during sport and exercise is an expanding field of clinical practice which is often directly in the public eye. Public expectations, frequently expressed by the media, are rising.

Preparation

The Taylor Report gives firm recommendations regarding medical facilities required at licensed sports stadia, but it mainly applies to football. Any doctor can be called on to provide "Good Samaritan" care, but a doctor agreeing to provide medical cover at a sporting event, for a team or an individual, must be prepared to deal with a wide range of predictable problems – each sport has a pattern of identifiable injuries – as well as the unexpected. The doctor can also play a significant role in injury prevention by ensuring all participants are appropriately prepared for an event.

154

● Know the activity	Research the patterns of injury and illness as well as the regulations controlling the activity
● Know the participant(s)	Prior knowledge of the injury or medical problems of participants aids planning
● Know your support	Clarify what first aid, paramedics, and rescue services are available
● Know the environment	What medical facilities are available? Is the venue safe? Will the weather affect the event? Is there an appropriately equipped First Aid room?
● Know the responsibilities	Are you responsible for officials, VIPs? Are you acting as "crowd doctor"? If involved in doping control, is there an adequate facility?
● Know your chain of command	The patient/doctor relationship is an absolute priority, but it is important to clarify relationships with the coach, officials, and management

First aid/resuscitation

The vast majority of injuries in sport and exercise are minor, but serious injuries, collapse, and illness can occur, when first aid and resuscitation may be life-saving.

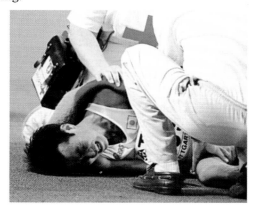

Figure 8.1 Fist aid and resuscitation can sometimes be life-saving

Collapse during sport or while exercising may be due to the activity or coincidental medical problems. Both situations will inevitably result in secondary complications, such as a hill walker who is injured as the result

155

of a fall but who will also inevitably be exposed to a windy, wet, and cold environment.

The first aid and resuscitative equipment that an experienced doctor will ensure is available will vary with the venue, the activity, perceived risks, and the support services available. The sophistication of equipment present at, for example, motor racing will vary with the competence of the medical staff, but should include cardiac monitors, defibrillator, chest drains, suction apparatus, intubation equipment, intravenous fluids, appropriate drugs, and a range of splints.

Doctors involved in sport must be capable of carrying out effective cardiopulmonary resuscitation (CPR) and maintaining an adequate airway. Management of the airway, breathing, and circulation with cervical and thoracolumbar spinal control (A,B,C with spinal control) must be given absolute priority. Assessing conscious levels and potential spinal injuries are key skills expected of a doctor in sport (see Table 8.1).

Table 8.1 Planning equipment: major injury and collapse

1st priority		
A trained doctor with appropriate support		
Airway	Cervical collar	Environmental protection
Suction	Spinal board	Communication
2nd priority		
Oxygen	Sandbags	Documentation
Analgesics	Splints	Diagnostic aids
		torch
		thermometer
		sphygmomanometer
		BM stix
3rd priority		
Supplementary drugs	IV access	Transport

Cardiopulmonary resuscitation

Collapse without the possibility of an associated injury is best managed according to standard resuscitative procedures. These procedures must be modified if injury such as a blow to the head may have caused the collapse, to ensure constant support and stabilisation of the spine while trying to achieve an effective circulation of oxygen and blood to the brain. This may require the use of the spinal recovery position (upper limb flexed under the head and neck, see Figure 8.3) or an appropriate rigid cervical collar and spinal board, stabilisation of fractures, especially of the pelvis, ribs, and lower limbs, in conjunction with elevation of the lower limbs if appropriate or feasible. External haemorrhage should be controlled by direct pressure, wherever possible.

On-field assessment

The great majority of acute injuries in sport and exercise affect the soft tissues and joints:

- Skin, skin appendages, and bleeding
- Muscle and the musculotendinous junction
- Tendons, their attachments and sheaths
- Ligaments and their attachments
- Joints, especially ankle, knee, shoulder, and digits.

The doctor must also be able to diagnose and initiate treatment for less common injuries such as concussion, eye, nose, and mouth injuries, fractures, and subluxations or dislocations.

On-field assessment of an injured player, especially in team games or a public venue, requires a calm structured approach. The mad dash to the injured player's side followed by immediate treatment indicates that a thorough assessment has not taken place. The time needed for an assessment will vary with different injuries, for example a cut compared with possible concussion. It should be established with the referee or officials controlling an event that an adequate assessment can take place prior to removing the player from the field of play.

- Observe – self and others
- History – injured player and other participants
- Demonstration – function and coordination
- Examination – local, regional, and general
- Working diagnosis
- Decision re. management

The doctor may have observed the mechanism of the injury but the doctor's assessment should be supplemented by asking the injured player or other observers what happened. On-the-spot examination should assess function and coordination on the basis of what the player can demonstrate before a "hands on" assessment takes place. Examination requires adequate exposure of the injured part prior to inspection, palpation of the damaged structures, and assessment of resisted movements. Stability and coordination should be included in all assessments. The doctor should wear sterile, talc-free gloves when assessing wounds or injuries to the eyes, nose, and mouth.

With all injuries, occasions will arise when a specific anatomical diagnosis cannot be reached on the field. The player should not be allowed to continue in the event (training or competition) in these circumstances, and a more detailed assessment should be carried out off the field.

157

Head injury

On-field assessment of a player who has clearly been or is unconscious, even if only for a few seconds, is straightforward. The player cannot continue to participate in exercise or sport and requires careful ongoing medical care.

An unconscious player who only responds to pain, or has a Glasgow Coma Scale score of 10 or less, has a serious head injury requiring rapid evacuation to hospital. The unconscious player's airway is always the number one priority.

Assessment of conscious levels

Immediate
Alert
Voice – responds to voice
Pain – responds to pain
Unresponsive

(Modified Advanced Trauma Life Support)

Planned

Function	Response
Eye opening	4. Spontaneous
	3. To voice
	2. To pain
	1. Unresponsive
Best verbal response	5. Appropriate
	4. Confused
	3. Inappropriate words
	2. Incomprehensible sounds
	1. Silent
Best motor response	6. Obeys commands
	5. Localises pain
	4. Withdraws from pain
	3. Flexion reflex
	2. Extension reflex
	1. None

(Glasgow Coma Scale)

Assessment of concussion is much more difficult because the player will make light of "seeing stars" or "being dazed". A careful history with structured questioning may identify a transient loss of consciousness,

Assessment of concussion

Physical
  Eyes
  Speech
  Coordination/balance

Intellectual
  Orientation
  Memory
  Calculation

amnesia, disorientation, or a recent similar injury. Examination should be directed to assessing powers of concentration, reaction time, and coordination. The doctor's responsibilities for a concussed player include ensuring that the player receives continuing supervision.

The management of acute spinal injury

Sport and leisure activities are responsible for a significant proportion of serious spinal injuries – fractures, subluxations and dislocations, or acute disc prolapse, all of which can occur with or without cord or nerve root injury. Symptoms may vary from a transient burning pain radiating to a limb, to spinal pain, with impaired neurological function – quadriplegia, paraplegia, cauda-equina lesion or damage to a nerve root.

Spinal pain, paraesthesia or impaired motor function must be managed as a potential disaster. Most patients with serious spinal injury sustained during sport or leisure activities are conscious and will give an appropriate history. All patients unconscious as a result of injury must be assumed to have an associated spinal injury and managed as such. This includes near-drowning. Diving into shallow water is the most common cause of quadriplegia in sport and leisure activities in the UK.

An injury to the spine, spinal cord, or nerve roots must not be aggravated by inappropriate immediate assessment and handling. Airway, breathing, and circulation must always take priority with the unconscious subject but spinal control must be maintained while carrying out A, B, C.

The patient should, ideally, be managed supine irrespective of the level or nature of the injury, with a rigid cervical collar or spinal board. The patient should be stabilised with sandbags and strapped to a suitable spinal stretcher. This may require "log-rolling" a patient, a procedure which should only be carried out by sufficiently experienced personnel. The only

159

exception to these recommendations is the patient who may vomit, who should be maintained in the spinal recovery position, which can be used with or without a collar or board (Figure 8.2).

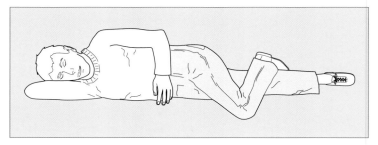

Figure 8.2 The spinal recovery position

Extreme care must be taken to ensure that a patient with a suspected spinal or neurological injury is not left lying for any length of time on an uneven surface because pressure sores develop very rapidly in anaesthetic skin. This includes smoothing folds in clothing, removing keys from pockets etc.

Oxygen and a non-steroidal anti-inflammatory drug should be given to try and minimise oedema formation, which may aggravate the initial damage to nerve tissue.

The on-field medical bag

No one medical bag can give comprehensive support for all injured or ill participants in sport or exercise. The equipment required on the field or at the touchline will vary with the experience of the doctor, the activity, the venue, and the availability of trained support. The doctor, and anyone helping at the touchline, must be able to lay their hands on any piece of equipment without delay. The doctor should liaise with the physiotherapists or trainer to ensure that between them they have a full supply of all equipment required, including dressings, eye drops, an oral airway etc.

The priority for any medical equipment in the on-field bag relates to A, B, C with spinal control. The minimal acceptable equipment is a range of oropharyngeal airways. A rigid cervical collar may not be practical in the on-field bag, but the doctor can stabilise the spine while an appropriate collar is provided.

Two separate water containers are among the most useful items of equipment in the on-field bag. One contains iced water for cleaning intact skin or applying to minor contusions sprains and strains. The other is for

---

The on-field medical bag

A,B,C with spinal control:	oropharyngeal airways: stiff collar
Water dispensers:	drinking
	cleaning
	cold application
Bleeding control:	sterile, talc-free gloves
	sterile dressing
	topical adrenaline
	haemostatic gauze
	sterile saline
	topical antiseptic
Pain relief:	crushed ice
Eye care:	sterile saline
	torch
	mirror
Medications:	personal requirements, e.g. inhalers for asthma
Equipment:	scissors
	tongue depressors
	sterile container
	tapes – stretch, non-stretch
	bandages – compression
Refuelling:	carbohydrate and electrolyte drinks (isotonic)
Other:	personal choice
	spare equipment

---

drinking water or an isotonic sports drink. This container should be designed to ensure hygienic use of the dispenser. Fluid replacement can help prevent injury and illness.

Minor concussion is a risk in many sporting activities. The on-field medical bag does not require any specific equipment for managing a player with possible concussion. "Smelling salts" to revive the player with a potential head injury are inappropriate.

All sport recognises the risks of external bleeding. The on-field medical bag must facilitate hygienic, if not fully sterile, assessment and control of bleeding from abrasions and wounds with sterile saline, dressings, and talc-free gloves for the doctor. This may not prove possible, for example with a bleeding nose, intraoral wounds, and a proportion of lacerations, when the player will require further treatment in an appropriate facility with good lighting and sterile equipment.

The management of wounds on and off the field should follow standard clinical practice:

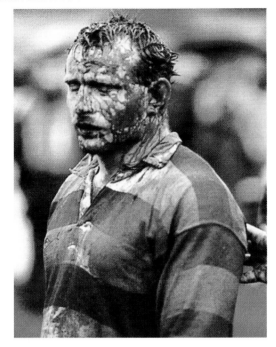

Figure 8.3 All external bleeding must be controlled, either on or off the field (Reproduced from McLatchie G, Harries M, Williams C, King JB. ABC of sports medicine. London, BMJ Publishing Group: London, p. 32.)

- Assessment and control of bleeding by direct pressure.
- Thorough irrigation and cleaning with placement of a secure sterile dressing.
- Minimal wound excision, if applicable, with removal of all dead or devitalised tissue and foreign bodies.
- Wound closure with sutures or staples.
- Occasionally, antibiotics may be required.

Bleeding players are no less liable to wound infection or tetanus than the general public. Tetanus prophylaxis must be checked and updated where necessary.

The majority of minor contusions, sprains, and strains, after careful assessment, will respond to time and topical ice, cold water, or cold spray. A sprained ligament, strained muscle or tendon that requires the application of support taping or compression bandaging is significant enough to merit assessment off the field before an accurate working diagnosis can be made.

Eye injuries are common in sport and can be difficult to assess. The on-field medical bag should, with the help of a torch, mirror, and sterile saline, allow the doctor to deal with a foreign body or displaced contact lens. A

162

direct blow or graze affecting the eye resulting in visual disturbance must be assessed in an appropriately equipped, clean, and well lit facility.

A broken or avulsed tooth must be handled very gently, cleaned, and kept moist in saliva (under the player's tongue), sterile saline, or milk, and dental care is required straight away. Similarly, a displaced tooth requires immediate dental help.

The on-field bag will carry personal requirements for individual players such as approved asthma inhalers, or spare contact lenses. The bag should also contain energy or electrolyte supplements for use during endurance events. In addition, most doctors will carry their own favourite or most useful items of equipment.

Provision of care off the field

The equipment for A,B,C with spinal support, splints for fractures, and stretchers to ensure safe evacuation from the event to a sheltered environment should be readily available, with sufficient trained personnel to offer assistance. In certain circumstances, full resuscitative support will be advisable with suction, oxygen etc.

Touchline support should include the provision of a clean, warm, well lit and properly equipped facility for detailed assessment of patients and appropriate treatment to be started. Hot and cold running water is necessary. This facility should be restricted for medical use and should have good communications.

Review of an injured player will allow a working diagnosis to be defined more accurately and appropriate management initiated. This may involve immediate referral to hospital of an unconscious player or players with a suspected spinal injury, haemarthrosis, or eye injury.

The initial management of most sprains and strains should be within the competence of sports doctors with adequate touchline facilities. Supplies of crushed ice, stretch and non-stretch tapes, self-adherent compression bandages, shaped elastic tubular bandages and compression garments, chiropody felt, compression pumps, and facilities for elevation will cope with most musculotendinous and ligamentous injuries.

Care of wounds and abrasions requires separate clean facilities, sterile stitching/stapling equipment and dressings, including non-adherent gauze, swabs, and permeable membrane dressings. A range of antiseptics will be necessary, as well as copious sterile saline for wound cleansing. Doctors should not treat wounds in facilities which would not be acceptable at a health centre or in an accident department.

Assessment of corneal abrasions will require topical staining (fluorescein) facilities, antibiotic drops, and eye pads. Imbedded foreign bodies or suspected orbital margin and eye injury requires specialised care.

The range of drugs necessary will vary from resuscitative drugs to mild analgesics, depending on the doctor and what injuries or illnesses will be treated at the event. Secure storage facilities and appropriate stock control are essential for all drugs.

Drugs, food supplements, herbal remedies, inhalations, and topical applications prescribed by the doctor must meet the requirements of International Olympic Committee regulations on doping control, plus any additional requirements laid down by the relevant governing body in sport. Clear guidelines should be given regarding the potential presence of banned substances contained in proprietary medicines which sportspeople may obtain as supplementary therapy.

The range of medicine required by sportspeople during training or competition can be subdivided into categories:

- Pain relief – acute, recurrent, or overuse injury, headache.
- Gastrointestinal – heartburn, dyspepsia, diarrhoea.
- Skin conditions – fungal infections, cold sores, abrasions.
- Disturbed sleep – hypnotics.

Pain relief for significant injuries on the field or in the medical room must be a priority. Splinting fractures and reducing or adequately supporting subluxations, dislocations, or traumatic haemarthrosis will require an appropriate range of equipment. Adequate analgesia thereafter will vary with circumstances. Rapid, effective pain relief can be achieved by the sublingual route using non-steroidal anti-inflammatory drugs. Oral and intramuscular treatments are second best but may be sufficient for most minor injuries. Inhalation of nitrous oxide and titrated small doses of intravenous opiates are rapidly effective for serious injuries, but may be contraindicated if a head injury is present.

Non-steroidal anti-inflammatory drugs (NSAIDs) are widely used by sports participants and exercisers. They are most rapidly effective if given sublingually and this is the initial route of choice for acute soft tissue injuries. NSAIDs have analgesic, antipyretic and anti-inflammatory properties which are present in variable proportions. The anti-inflammatory properties reduce tissue oedema by blocking release of vasodilating and permeable prostaglandins (PG) E_2 and I_2, without reducing the accumulation of inflammatory cells needed to initiate healing. The short term use of NSAIDs can be justified in acute injuries to reduce oedema, but their continued or long term use as an analgesic for sports injuries is questionable because of the side effects of these drugs on the gastrointestinal tract, aggravation of asthma, renal damage, or blood dyscrasias.

The value of ice compresses as an analgesic is frequently underestimated. Appropriate application of ice compresses for 20 minutes every 2–3 hours

164

will have a potent analgesic effect, as well as minimising bleeding and oedema.

The role of local anaesthetic injection in acute injuries is variable – appropriate for suturing wounds; inappropriate for soft tissue strains, sprains and minor joint injuries or fractures if intended to allow the athlete to return to, or participate in, a subsequent event before healing has occurred.

The management of muscle strains

The assessment and immediate management of an acute muscle injury highlights many aspects of soft tissue injury.

Muscle is disrupted by a direct blow or during eccentric and concentric contraction when muscle fibres tear. The disruption results in a gap between torn muscle fibres which fills with blood, oedema and adjacent muscle goes into spasm. The disruption may be minor, i.e. a few fibres, or complete. The amount of bleeding will relate to the portion of fibres torn and the dynamic blood supply of exercising muscle. The blood can extravasate with early bruising if the muscle sheath is disrupted, or be confined within the muscle.

Muscles most commonly tear at their musculotendinous junction, but direct blows and a proportion of indirect injuries affect the muscle belly.

On-field assessment and establishing a working diagnosis of players with a muscle injury is based on the doctor observing the mechanism of injury, for example a direct blow, which is confirmed on history, demonstration of impaired function, and palpation. The player should **rest** the injured muscle to minimise tissue disruption by bleeding and oedema as this will facilitate recovery.

The muscle should also be treated locally for 36–48 hours by continued **rest**, the application of **ice packs** for 20–30 minutes every 2 or 3 hours during daylight hours, **compression** using appropriate bandaging (with the sulcus around bone prominences filled with shaped compressed wool chiropody felt) or the intermittent air compression pump, and **elevation** where practical, such as elevating the foot of the bed. In addition, the player should be given a short course of NSAIDs starting within 2 hours of injury.

During the first 1–3 days it is important to undertake repeated examination to gauge the degree of muscle disruption and localisation of the haematoma. Any suggestion of a total disruption requires urgent hospital assessment and a large loculated or intramuscular haematoma may also benefit from aspiration or evacuation.

165

Summary

Participants in sport and exercisers will inevitably face risks. The management of acute injuries or illness at an event, either "on the field" or "at the touchline" is not a casual responsibility that can be accepted without careful planning on the basis of appropriate clinical experience, knowledge of the activity, and constant alert observation of what is happening.

Rapid but thorough assessment of injuries, steps to minimise tissue damage, prevention of a second injury, achieving an accurate diagnosis,

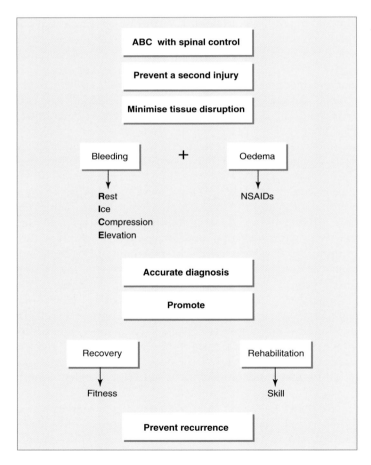

Figure 8.4   Management of sports injury: a summary

initiating treatment, and careful documentation with good communication are the key activities undertaken by a doctor providing sports medicine cover at any form of sporting or leisure activity (see Figure 8.4).

9   Lower leg injuries: calf, ankle, and foot

ROGER G HACKNEY AND
GRAHAM MN HOLLOWAY

Introduction

The foot and ankle are wonderful weight-bearing structures which have been rather neglected in comparison with more "glamorous" joints such as the knee and shoulder. This is despite the fact that ankle sprains are the most common injury in sport and the general population. Structures of the foot are largely subcutaneous, and hence a knowledge of anatomy

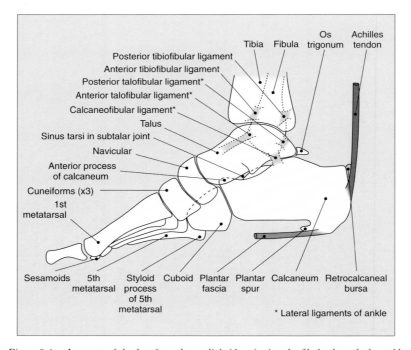

Figure 9.1   Anatomy of the foot from the medial side, viewing the fibula through the ankle

is vital if sites of injury are to be identified and appropriate management instigated.

Footwear

Sports shoes have advanced considerably over the past 20 years, running shoes in particular. Some of the advances have been beneficial, some contribute to injury. The following general advice can be offered on choosing new footwear:

1. Select a pair of shoes from a reputable retailer which offers expertise in your sport.
2. You should be permitted to try running in the shoes on an appropriate surface.
3. Unless you know you have an abnormality of gait which requires correction, avoid elaborate (often expensive) shoes.
4. Avoid shoes which have spent a long time on the shelf.

Training shoes: assessing used footwear

Running shoes become "broken in" to adapt to the runner's gait. This frequently exaggerates any gait abnormality. Look at the shoes on a flat

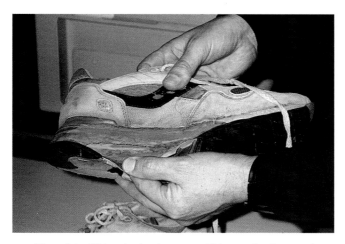

Figure 9.2   This pair of trainers was still in use after five years!

surface to gauge the change in shape of the shoes. Look at the athlete wearing used shoes and if possible running in them. In particular, assess the degree of pronation and the rapidity with which the motion takes place.

169

The wear of the sole of the shoe gives an indication of the type of gait of the runner. Most heel strike and toe off from the hallux.

The following further advice can be offered regarding used shoes:

1. Running shoes lose, on average, 50% of their shock absorbency in 500 miles. Do not continue to use shoes for running on hard surfaces after this distance.
2. Have at least two or three different pairs of running shoes available, and switch between them on a regular basis.
3. Run on appropriate surfaces for the soles.
4. Throw the shoes away when the heel becomes worn.
5. Throw the shoes away if the support on the medial side becomes beaten down.
6. Do not use shoes over a year old.
7. Do not walk about in old running shoes. Shoes with an altered shape should be discarded.
8. Over-tightening of laces can lead to pain on the top of the foot.
9. Trim heel tabs if they impinge upon the achilles tendon with the foot plantarflexed.

Gait analysis

Gait analysis is an increasingly popular way of looking at running injuries. The result is frequently prescription of a pair of orthoses. Although the effect of appropriate alteration of gait can be dramatic in reduction of pain, orthoses tend to be overprescribed and their value can be questionable. Overpronation can be speedily assessed by asking the athlete to stand and then bend the knees to 90 degrees with the heels on the ground. Observe for flattening of the medial longitudinal arch. Look at the patient from the front and behind, then ask the patient to stand on tip toes. Examine the mobility of the midfoot and the height of the arch. With the athlete lying prone, legs over the end of the couch, hold the heel in neutral. Light pressure under the lateral border of the foot will give an indication of the degree of forefoot varus/valgus.

Instead of resorting immediately to sports orthotics, sticky-backed "surgical felt" can be placed on the undersurface of the insole from the training shoes to provide a temporary, custom-made orthotic. The felt can be trimmed and contoured for comfort. When the forefoot fails to correct to neutral, the orthotic support needs to be extended along the medial border of the foot.

Injuries

Shin splints

This is a general term used to cover all the causes of shin pain, more particularly anteriorly. There are several possible aetiologies.

Medial tibial stress syndrome; medial tibial periostitis

This is thought to be caused by excess stress of the origin of one or more muscles of the calf, i.e. soleus, tibialis posterior, or flexor digitorum longus. The periosteum or lining of the lower and middle thirds of the bone is inflamed (periostitis).

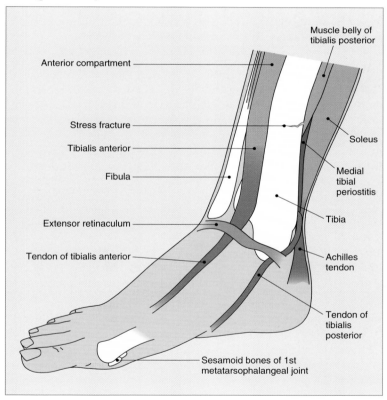

Figure 9.3 Differential diagnosis of shin pain

History Sufferers include athletes from any sport involving running. The pain is felt along the medial (inside) border of the tibia and comes on with

171

activity, but eases with rest. The pain can be sore enough to prevent running and produce a limp. Medial tibial periostitis is associated with altered training, increased mileage, hard surfaces, poor training shoes, and poor running technique, especially with fatigue. Sufferers are almost always overpronators, although the syndrome is also found in those with a pes cavus.

Examination   The sore area is palpated around the junction of the upper two thirds and lower one third of the medial border of the tibia. The most tender area is just on or adjacent to the medial border of the tibia. On standing, look for pronation and pes cavus. Always ask to see the training shoes.

Investigation   X-rays show little; the cortex may be thickened. Bone scan shows a *diffuse* uptake along the medial border of the tibia.

Treatment   Treatment is by control of pain with relative rest, local massage, and analgesics. New training shoes are nearly always recommended. Training errors – usually excessive mileage, too much too soon – must be corrected. Biomechanics can be improved using insoles, usually a medial heel raise for correction of overpronation.

Return to running should be gradual, on soft ground, over short distances, with new training shoes, and with a stretching programme for the lower limb.

Surgery may help if conservative measures fail. Muscle origins are released from the periosteal attachment.

Stress fractures

There is a constant turnover of normal bone as a reaction to the various stresses placed upon it. When repeated microtrauma overcomes the healing mechanism, a fatigue fracture develops. Fatigue fractures of metal are a similar process of repeated minor stresses leading to total failure. Stress fractures may complete across the bone if ignored; they are then very difficult to heal. Bone abnormalities may be responsible. The female triad of amenorrhoea, poor nutrition, and osteoporosis may be implicated.

History   Pain is of gradual onset, which may follow or occur in endurance events. The pain becomes severe, causing a limp, with pain at night and rest as well as on exercise. There is usually a history of a sudden change in training.

Examination   One place in particular is more sore than the rest. Tapping the bone reproduces the soreness, usually at the junction of the mid and lower third in adults. The site is usually higher in children.

Investigation   As for periostitis. Plain X-ray will not show a stress fracture for *at least* 3 weeks. Bone scan shows an intense hot spot. MRI scan shows oedema.

Treatment   With care! RICER (Rest, Ice, Compression, Elevation, Rehabilitation). Correct abnormal biomechanics, training errors, and poor footwear. Pain is an indication to stop the activity.

Compartment syndrome

The calf muscles are enclosed within tight fascial compartments. Exercising muscle demands an increase in blood supply, which occupies space. If the compartments do not stretch sufficiently, then tissue pressure within the compartment rises to above the normal levels. This affects transfer of nutrients and waste across the capillaries, causing local pain and fatigue. Increased pressure also cuts venous outflow, further increasing intra-compartment pressure, leading to a vicious circle. Pain is from ischaemia (lack of tissue oxygenation), waste build-up, and stretching of the compartment.

Chronic compartment syndrome is not usually severe enough to affect nerves and major blood vessels within a compartment. This is in contrast to an acute compartment syndrome with the swelling and bleeding from trauma, i.e. a fracture of the tibia. In the latter situation, there is intense

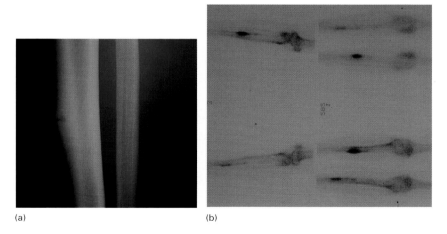

(a)   (b)

Figure 9.4   (a) Stress fracture of the distal tibia; (b) bone scan of distal tibial fracture

173

pain on moving the toes into dorsiflexion or plantar flexion. This demands immediate surgery or the muscle will die and lead to a contracture (Volkman's). This can occur in sports injuries as an acute event from trauma and from highly motivated individuals trying to "run through" their pain.

All four compartments of the calf can be affected by chronic compartment syndrome. By far the most common is the anterior compartment, then deep posterior, lateral, and superficial posterior compartments.

History   The pain develops after 15 minutes running and worsens unless rested. With rest, the pain subsides to leave a residual ache. There is no pain at rest. The site of pain is usually fairly well localised over the appropriate compartment. A dull, poorly localised ache in the calf may be all that is felt in deep posterior compartment syndrome.

Examination   The individual may have bulky muscle groups. The anterior compartment is tense after exercise, while the deep posterior compartment has deep pain but little to palpate. Small muscle hernias are often seen as bulges in the anterior compartment on tensing the muscles. These should be regarded as attempts at auto-decompression and must not be repaired.

Investigation   Investigation is based on clinical competence from the history and examination. Pressure studies are diagnostic, but not widely available.

Treatment   Chronic compartment syndrome is worth a trial of rest and a gradual return to activity if a provoking episode such as hill running can be avoided. Cross training with a bicycle is effective in maintaining cardiovascular fitness. Surgery works well. The problem with deep posterior compartment syndrome is making the diagnosis. Do not repair muscle hernias.

Other causes of chronic calf pain

- **Chronic calf sprain:** Muscle pulls in the calf which have been mismanaged by attempting a too early return to sport and repeating the injury.
- **Nerve entrapment:** Superficial peroneal nerve, into lower calf and dorsum of foot. This nerve may be damaged by incorrect surgery.
- **Popliteal artery entrapment:** Rare. The artery is trapped by the medial head of gastrocnemius, and gives symptoms of intermittent claudication, very similar to chronic deep compartment syndrome. Foot pulses are

reduced on exercise and dorsiflexing the foot. Requires specialist surgical treatment.

- **Effort thrombosis:** Very rare. Continuous pain and swelling in the calf.
- **Muscle exertional pain:** Follows unaccustomed, usually eccentric, exercise. May last two weeks.
- **Fibula stress fracture.**

Heel pain

The differential diagnosis of heel pain is surprisingly varied, and includes achilles tendon pain, achilles "tendonitis", insertional pain, Haglund's syndrome, retrocalcaneal bursitis, plantar fasciitis, stress fracture, nerve entrapment both local and proximal, and posterior impingement

The achilles tendon (tendo achillis, TA)

The achilles tendon is a common source of pain in sportsmen and women. Pain in and around the tendon away from the insertion may be due to inflammation of the paratenon, or internal degeneration of the tendon itself.

Paratendinitis   The condition presents as an acute episode following excess exercise, with severe pain and swelling around a length of the tendon. Crepitus, a crackling sensation in the tissues, is present on movement.

Tendinitis   This is a misnomer, as the suffix "itis" means inflammation, and the condition is rather one of degeneration. Tendinosis is more accurate. The TA becomes thickened and painful. The inside of the tendon becomes degenerate and forms scar tissue.

Bursitis   A bursa is a sac of fluid over a bony prominence whose function is to allow a tendon or skin to glide smoothly. They have the potential to become inflamed and painful. There are two bursae associated with the TA. The retrocalcaneal bursa lies between the TA and the calcaneum, and is an important cause of heel pain. The other bursa is associated with the pump bump, and lies under the skin.

Sever's disease   The growth plate at the back of the calcaneum can be affected by chronic traction from the TA in active children. Damage can occur, but this usually settles with rest from the aggravating activity and a graded return to sport.

175

Achilles tendinitis/paratendinitis

History As above. The pain is usually of a gradual onset associated with a new pair of shoes or errors of training. Pain occurs with exercise and leaves a residual aching and stiffness. Morning stiffness and pain on allowing the foot to hang dependent are characteristic.

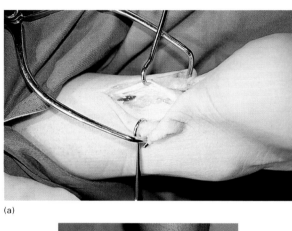

(a)

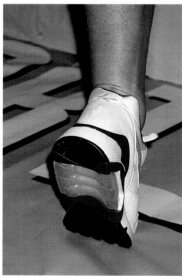

(b)

Figure 9.5 Achilles tendinitis: (a) mucoid degeneration in the tendon; (b) heel tabs are often responsible for this problem

176

Examination There is a painful nodule 2 inches above the insertion and swelling. The site of pain is important. Pain at the insertion suggests retrocalcaneal bursitis. Pain medially suggests excess pronation. Pain may be relieved partly by tightening the tendon. Assess calf and hamstring stretching. Assess the stretch with the knee straight and bent. Examine the shoes. Crepitus is prominent with paratendinitis.

Investigation Intratendinous damage is seen well on ultrasound and MRI scan. X-ray the heel for retrocalcaneal bursitis to look for a posterior bony prominence.

Treatment There are a large number of conservative treatments that can be applied to injuries of the achilles tendon. My own (RGH) experience with maintaining an international running career in the presence of a tendon with central degeneration bears witness. Treatment includes:

- Pain control with ice, ice cube massage of the nodule, calf massage and stretching, and NSAID gel.
- It is important to maintain fitness, but relative rest can include cycling and swimming.
- Use a heel raise in the shoe.
- Calf stretching with knee straight and bent. Hamstring stretches.
- Assess for overpronation, poor shoes, training errors (e.g. excess or sudden use of a synthetic track in spring).
- Electrotherapy may be useful for acute paratendinitis, e.g. ultrasound, laser.
- Cut down the heel tabs on the back of the shoes.
- Rehabilitation with control of foot motion, new shoes, progress from walking pain-free to skipping, running short distances on soft ground.
- Steroid injection. (I [RGH] am against the use of steroid around the TA, with the possible exception of retrocalcaneal pain. The risk of rupture of the tendon increases and leakage of steroid under the skin causes atrophy.)

Surgery has much to offer for TA pain after at least a 3–6 months trial of conservative treatment. Too many authors in the literature do not use a sufficient period of conservative treatment. Tissue handling should be extremely sensitive as poor wound healing is a major complication. The scar tissue is excised and the tight paratenon removed. Removing bone from around the insertion may be necessary. The threshold for surgery is less for retrocalcaneal pain, where a significant amount of bone is removed with scar tissue.

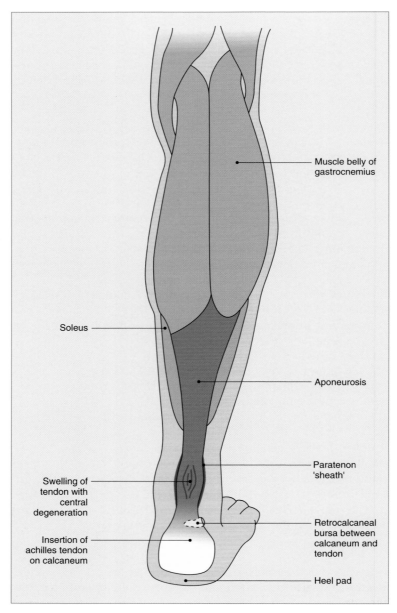

Muscle belly of
gastrocnemius

Soleus

Aponeurosis

Paratenon
'sheath'

Swelling of
tendon with
central
degeneration

Retrocalcaneal
bursa between
calcaneum and
tendon

Insertion of
achilles tendon
on calcaneum

Heel pad

Figure 9.6   Anatomy and pathology of achilles tendon

Achilles tendon rupture

This is a serious injury still missed in up to 25% of cases.

History A middle aged subject, typically a squash player, feels and hears a crack as his or her tendon snaps, and is then unable to walk properly.

Examination The athlete can plantarflex the foot using other muscles whose tendons wind round the malleoli. There is often not very much swelling or bruising. The gait can be surprisingly normal after a few days. A gap in the tendon may be palpated.

The diagnosis of a delayed rupture will also be picked up using the following tests:

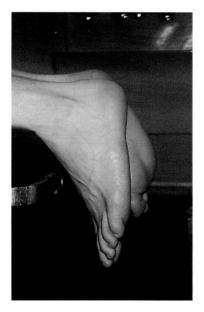

Figure 9.7 Right achilles tendon rupture: the Angle of Dangle. Note that the contour of the achilles tendon on the left (ruptured) looks normal

The Angle of Dangle (Figure 9.7): Lie the patient prone with feet hanging over the edge of a couch. The injured foot will hang vertically down, the normal foot will point out from the table slightly due to the muscle tension in the intact calf.

Calf squeeze test: Gently squeezing the bulk of the calf muscle in a normal limb will cause the foot to plantarflex. This does not occur with a TA rupture.

179

Investigation   Partial ruptures can occur, though they are less common and a specialist diagnosis. Ultrasound and MRI scan will confirm the diagnosis of a rupture, but the diagnosis should be made clinically. If in doubt, refer.

Treatment   The best results for an acute rupture of a TA in a sportsperson are obtained by surgical repair followed by early mobilisation. Care needs to be taken with handling soft tissues as poor wound healing can be a problem. Mobilisation in a proprietary walking boot with a 20 degree block to extension gives a very rapid return to sport with a low incidence of recurrence of rupture.

Delayed diagnosis needs careful assessment. The tendon heals long or with a gap. In that case surgery can borrow from tissue elsewhere to plug the gap and give a sound repair. A partial rupture may need surgery to remove poorly functional scar tissue and strengthen the remaining tendon.

The tendon which heals long defunctions the calf. Early experience with surgical shortening [RGH] indicates return to function is possible.

Tendinitis around the ankle

Flexor hallucis longus

The long flexor of the great toe is often inflamed in dancers. It is injured as it passes in a tunnel behind the posterior talus. Injury causes inflammation, swelling, and nodule formation which leads to binding and even triggering. Irritation may be caused by an enlarged os trigonum. Treat with rest, NSAIDs, and physiotherapy. Correction of dance technique and footwear causing excessive use of hallux is very important. If treated early, surgery is not required. Steroid should be avoided. Surgical release is frequently curative if the condition has become chronic.

Tibialis anterior, peroneal tendons, tibialis posterior

All these tendons can become inflamed as they pass across the ankle. The diagnosis is made by palpation of the sore tendon and reproduction of pain on stressing. There may be crepitus. A search should be made for the cause, a training error or something as simple as overtight shoe laces. Tibialis anterior may be injured in hill running, the peronei by an ankle sprain and tibialis posterior in overpronation.

Plantar fasciitis

The plantar fascia is a dense sheet of tissue which derives from the time in evolution when the TA extended to the toes. Its function is to provide support for the arch and in the special fat within the sole that provides shock absorbency.

History Plantar fasciitis occurs when the fascia is stretched. It usually occurs at the attachment to the medial tubercle. The pain spreads into the foot and into the TA. The heel is painful to walk on and may be sore at night and in the morning. The onset may be gradual, or start with a sudden tearing sensation in the arch of the foot. The condition tends to last a long time.

Examination Tenderness is rather diffuse, but firm palpation on the anterior part of the medial tubercle of the calcaneum is most sore. Observe for overpronation or pes cavus. The calf stretch is often poor.

Investigation The diagnosis is clinical, but X-ray may show a plantar spur. This is a bony projection out from the base of the calcaneum. The plantar fascia does not attach to the spur, and it is something of a red herring.

Treatment Pain control is by avoiding footwear which aggravates the symptoms, or partial weight-bearing with crutches for severe cases. Apply ice and NSAID gel. Training shoes will need replacing. Alter training patterns, avoiding excess hard ground and insufficient cushioning in the footwear. Correct overpronation and provide an arch support. Strapping the arch can provide excellent relief of pain (see Chapter 21). A night splint to keep this foot at neutral dorsiflexion prevents the early morning stiffness of plantar fasciitis. Stretch the calf muscles, use local massage and stretching of the foot muscles/ligaments. Shock absorbing heel pads can be helpful. Do not expect a rapid response, several weeks may be needed.

Injection of local anaesthetic and steroid should be directed from the lateral side and not straight through the heel. This is because the steroid causes atrophy of the septae of the heel, dramatically reducing the shock absorbency and leading to heel pain. The needle should be advanced over an area whilst the steroid is being injected, needling the sore part.

Surgery removes the degenerative tissue around the plantar fascia, and releasing the fascia which then heals long. The bony heel spur lies deep to the fascia, which is released to gain access to the spur. The spur itself can fracture, but is only rarely the cause of heel pain. The spur is generally removed at operation, although more for the benefit of showing the patient the change on X-ray.

Stress fracture of the calcaneum

Stress fracture of the calcaneum is uncommon. It presents as gradual onset of deep heel pain, worse on weight-bearing, partly relieved by rest with the

181

foot elevated. Squeezing the heel between the hands of the examiner is a useful diagnostic tip. The diagnosis may be confirmed by plain X-ray, the fracture will show as a hot spot on bone scan, but can be defined on MRI.

The plantar spur can stress fracture in rare instances, this shows on a bone scan.

Nerve entrapment in heel pain

Both the medial calcaneal branches of the posterior tibial nerve, and the first branch of the lateral plantar nerve can become trapped giving rise to heel pain. The diagnosis is suspected by recognising that the heel pain is more diffuse and associated with some alteration in sensation of the skin of the heel. The pain spreads into the medial side of the ankle and along the foot, and laterally for the lateral plantar nerve. Tapping along the path of the nerve may reproduce the patient's heel pain with a pins and needles type quality.

Tarsal tunnel syndrome occurs more proximally where the posterior tibial nerve is trapped around the medial malleolus. The athlete complains of a burning sensation in the sole of the foot associated with walking or running.

Correction of overpronation may give some relief.

If symptoms justify, then surgical release gives relief. The medial calcaneal nerve is trapped under the aponeurosis of abductor hallucis, the plantar nerve deep under the plantar fascia.

Ankle ligaments

The ankle is the most commonly injured joint in sport. Injuries of the ligaments around the ankle (see Figure 9.1) account for the majority of these, in particular the lateral ligaments. There are numerous other ligaments around the ankle which can be injured

Acute ankle sprains: lateral ligaments, inferior tibiofibular syndesmosis

Three lateral ligaments, thickenings of the joint capsule, are described. The anterior talofibular ligament (ATFL) runs from the anterior part of the lateral malleolus forwards to insert upon the talus. The middle ligament, the calcaneofibular (CFL), passes inferiorly and *posteriorly*, crossing the subtalar joint to insert on the calcaneum. The posterior talofibular ligament (PTFL) runs back from the fibula.

Lateral ligament sprains

There are three degrees of injury with increasing severity. The excess inversion injures the ATFL first, the tearing extending posteriorly from there.

- **Grade 1:** A stretching of the ATFL with no disruption of the ligament. Presents with mild bruising and tenderness and little difficulty weight-bearing.
- **Grade 2:** A moderate injury with a complete tear of the ATFL and some damage to the CFL. Range of motion is restricted with significant pain and swelling. The ankle may be unstable and will not permit normal weight-bearing or going onto tip toe.
- **Grade 3:** Complete tearing of both the ATFL and CFL. If the tear extends to involve the PTFL, the injury may be caused by dislocation. There is pain, swelling, and an inability to weight bear.

Injuries to the ligaments of the inferior tibiofibular syndesmosis frequently occur in association with lateral ligament injuries. The tear may run proximally into the interosseous ligament. These must not be missed.

History The athlete feels the ankle give way and rotate suddenly, associated with a painful popping or tearing sensation around the lateral malleolus.

Examination Look at the site of the swelling. Careful palpation will confirm the diagnosis. Severe bone pain indicates the need for an X-ray. The inferior tibiofibular joint, 5th metatarsal, and peroneal tendons must be examined.

Anterior draw sign: The anterior draw sign (Figure 9.8a) is performed with the lower limb supported over the edge of the couch, the foot in slight plantarflexion, the heel cupped in the examiner's palm. The heel is then pushed up towards the toes, and the degree of movement compared with the normal side. A positive test indicates rupture of the ATFL, as this is the only part of the ligament passing anteriorly.

Talar tilt: The talar tilt test (Figure 9.8b) attempts to tilt the talus out of the ankle joint. The foot is moved carefully into inversion, the examiner's opposite hand feeling the movement of the talus as it emerges from under the lateral malleolus.

The anterior draw sign will be positive in grade 2 and 3. If the ligament is torn, then this test will not be painful; the patient must be reassured of this! The talar tilt will be painful, but may not be sore in grade 3, even in the acute situation.

Injuries of the inferior tibiofibular ligament can be detected by the external rotation test, where the foot is externally rotated, stressing the ligaments, causing pain.

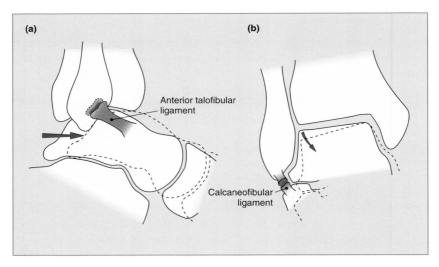

Figure 9.8   (a) Anterior draw sign: rupture of anterior talofibular ligament; (b) talar tilt sign: rupture of calcaneofibular ligament

Investigation   Plain X-ray must exclude bony injury of the fibula and 5th metatarsal. The width of the inferior tibiofibular joint should be noted. Stress films and arthrography are unreliable and are not necessary in the acute situation. Damage to the dome of the talus can be seen on MRI scan.

Treatment   Grade 1 and 2 injuries are treated with early protected weight-bearing in a brace followed by functional rehabilitation. The rehabilitation aims to restore proprioception and the strength and speed of reaction of muscles stabilising the joint. Return to sport can be achieved within 2 weeks, possibly with the assistance of protective strapping or bracing to improve proprioception. Avulsion of bony flakes should be managed as ligament injuries.

The management of grade 3 injuries has fluctuated between functional rehabilitation, incarcerating in plaster, and surgical repair of the ligament.

A plaster cast will cause random healing of the ligament with scar tissue and muscle wasting, and it aggravates the loss of proprioception which then requires longer to regain. Surgery has not been shown to convey any advantages in the acute situation; the athlete has all the risks of surgery and no benefit.

The recommended treatment is functional rehabilitation; the authors prefer using the Aircast brace which allows plantarflexion and dorsiflexion, but prevents inversion and eversion.

Inferior tibiofibular ligaments

Injuries of the inferior tibiofibular ligaments require care in their management. The presence of swelling anterolaterally over the inferior tibiofibular joint indicates an injury. External rotation of the foot stresses the ligament and causes discomfort. Mild injuries may be treated by cast bracing; more severe injuries do require immobilisation in a plaster cast for 6 weeks or more, depending on the severity of the injury. Significant widening of the inferior tibiofibular joint seen on X-ray requires surgical fixation. Palpate the proximal fibula to avoid missing the Maisonneuve fracture which indicates a diastasis (separation) of the ankle mortice.

Fracture of the base of the 5th metatarsal

This can be missed if there is insufficient care in examination. Symptoms eventually focus onto the avulsion injury of the insertion of peroneus brevis. These usually heal with a period in plaster for comfort. A fracture of the proximal part of the shaft is often called a Jones fracture. The fracture is on the tension side of the bone which means that the fracture often fails to heal. The quickest way to ensure healing is immediate surgical fixation, particularly in athletes.

Medial ligament sprains

Isolated injuries are rare. Assess for a syndesmotic injury or fibular fracture. The medial ligament injury is treated by cast bracing. The Maisonneuve fracture of the proximal fibula requires exclusion as this represents a very serious injury when associated with a medial ligament tear.

Fractures of the ankle

Bony tenderness indicates the need for an X-ray. If a fracture is seen, then specialist referral is necessary. Many fractures require operative fixation to reduce bony displacement. The rationale behind this is that the talus has only to move 1 mm on X-ray to reduce the "fit" of the joint by 49%. Accurate reduction gives the best chance for optimal healing and avoidance of osteoarthritis.

Chronic lateral ligament instability

Sadly, treatment for acute ankle injuries is neglected for many sportsmen and women, who are dismissed with a length of tubigrip. Continued early attempts to return to activity lead to further episodes of injury and a chronically unstable ankle.

185

History   The athlete reports the ankle giving way when walking on uneven ground, twisting or stepping off a kerb. The ankle swells with each episode and becomes chronically sore.

Examination   The anterior draw and talar tilt signs are positive. If either is negative, then a search through the differential diagnosis should be made. Standing on one leg with eyes open, then closed, reveals the proprioceptive loss as the athlete staggers on the affected side (Romberg's test).

Investigation   Stress views are usually positive, though not required, as with practice the draw signs are diagnostic. A plain X-ray may reveal damage to the talus.

Treatment   A programme of rehabilitation with a physiotherapist is the best means of treatment. Proprioception is regained with exercises to strengthen the calf muscles and retrain control of balance. The traditional wobble board is effective; a lump of foam can be used. The ankle will require extra help from a brace or taping to begin with. Rehabilitation should include a staged return to competitive sport.

Surgery is effective for those who fail a conservative programme. A variety of operations have been described, mostly with good results. The current vogue is for the Brostrum procedure, which is a reefing of the attenuated ligaments, with the Gould modification where the extensor retinaculum is included in the repair. A further period of rehabilitation is necessary following surgery.

Differential diagnosis

Peroneal subluxation   A history of a snapping sensation associated with the ankle giving way may be caused by the peroneal tendons snapping out over the lateral malleolus. The patient may not be at all aware of this subluxation. On examination, there is generally some swelling around the sheath of the peronei. When the patient attempts to resist forced inversion, the tendons can be seen to move out over the malleolus, reproducing the patient's symptoms. Treatment is surgical reconstruction of the retinaculum holding the tendons in place.

Osteochondral fractures of the dome of the talus (Figure 9.9)   When the ankle suffers an inversion injury, the talus impacts upon the lower end of the tibia. Lateral injuries are caused by inversion and dorsiflexion; medial injuries by inversion, lateral, and plantarflexion. These injuries frequently do not show on initial plain X-rays. Instead, they present over a year following the injury with continuing pain, swelling, and instability which

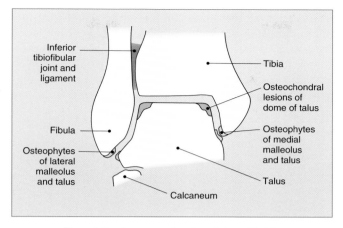

Figure 9.9   Anteroposterior view of the ankle joint

fails to respond to the usual measures for treating a chronically unstable ankle. Other symptoms include clicking crepitus and even true locking (from a loose body).

Investigation A radiolucency may be seen at the anterolateral or posteromedial dome of the talus. A CT or MRI scan will define the lesion better. The lesions can be visualised at arthroscopy. Four stages were described by Bernt and Harty:

1. Small area of compression.
2. Partly detached osteochondral fragment.
3. Completely separated fragment but still in place.
4. Detached, displaced fragment.

Treatment   Early and grade 1 lesions are treated by reducing weight-bearing either in a brace or plaster cast, and NSAIDs for 6–8 weeks.

Grade 2 lesions can be treated as above or by drilling through the fragment to encourage re-vascularisation and healing.

Grade 3 lesions are less likely to settle with non-operative treatment and may need pinning and grafting.

Grade 4 lesions should have removal of the loose body and debridement of the surface remaining. This can be achieved arthroscopically.

The technique of mosaicplasty, the grafting of bone and overlying articular cartilage from the knee, has something to offer treatment of Stages 3 and 4 which otherwise have a poor prognosis.

Other conditions Other conditions in the differential diagnosis include **sinus tarsi syndrome**, a strange condition causing pain in the sinus tarsi, between the talus and calcaneum following an ankle sprain, which can be treated by steroid injection into the canal or surgical exploration and debridement; and **missed fractures**, such as the anterior process of the calcaneum (see Figure 9.10).

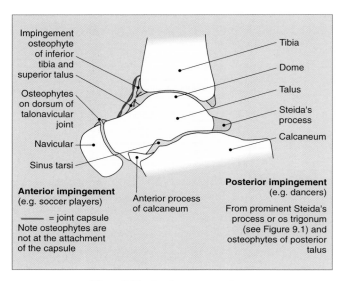

Figure 9.10   Impingement syndromes

Ankle impingements (Figure 9.10)

Repeated trauma to the ankle produces a synovitis and bony projections from the anterior tibia. Soccer players and dancers are the most frequent sufferers, hence "footballer's ankle". Repeated trauma to the anterior joint stimulates bony projections, exostoses, which further restrict movement. Anterior impingement may be associated with joint narrowing and osteophytes on the medial, lateral, and posterior joint, evidence of a degenerative disorder.

Anterior impingement

History The athlete complains of a restriction of dorsiflexion, together with an aching over the anterior joint line, usually lateral. There may be a history of an unstable ankle. Dancers frequently complain of a tight achilles tendon, but this is not the cause of the lack of dorsiflexion.

188

Examination   There is a restriction of dorsiflexion which becomes obvious on weight-bearing with the heel on the ground. There is anterior tenderness and an effusion, best seen at the back of the ankle, either side of the achilles tendon. There is thickening of the synovium and palpable osteophytes. Pain is reproduced by forced dorsiflexion.

Investigation   On plain lateral X-ray, a weight-bearing view in dorsiflexion demonstrates the impingement.

Treatment   Avoid irritating the joint by ceasing the activity which reproduces pain. A heel raise may allow some settling of the discomfort.

Ankle arthroscopy can be used to remove the irritated synovium, loose bodies, and osteophytes on the lower lip of the tibia. Experience is required to assess accurately how much bone has been removed arthroscopically, and whether full dorsiflexion has been regained. Postoperatively, it takes 3 months to regain full function. In the author's experience, the condition is frequently associated with ankle laxity or instability. The aetiology of the osteophytes may be due to anterior subluxation mimicking the anterior draw sign causing impingement osteophytes from repeated trauma. It is possible to stabilise the ankle and perform debridement at the same surgical sitting.

Other conditions

Bassett's ligament is an extra insertion of the anterior talofibular ligament which can cause irritation laterally. **Meniscoid lesions** are described as an entrapment of the synovium, which becomes swollen and catches between the fibula and talus. Both are arthroscopic diagnoses and treatment is shaving of the ligament/lesion.

Posterior impingement

A combination of soft and bony entrapment may occur, especially in dancers going *en-pointe*. It presents as posterolateral pain in full plantarflexion. Tenderness is felt behind the peroneal tendon and pain is reproduced by forced plantarflexion. X-rays in this position show bony impingement. It may occur with an accessory bone, the os trigonum, or a long posterior prominence, of the talus and is associated with tendinitis of flexor hallucis longus.

Treat by modification of activity, which may allow the pain to subside. Injection of local anaesthetic and steroid can give relief. Surgical clearance is a last resort.

Stress fractures of the foot

Stress fractures were first described in 1883 in Prussian soldiers, and termed "march fractures". Still the most common stress fracture, the metatarsal stress fracture is often found in athletes. As already described, these are fatigue fractures caused by overuse.

Metatarsal stress fractures

These injuries are more common in overweight athletes with biomechanical and gait abnormalities.

History There is insidious onset of foot pain which increases as training continues. Pain is worst on impact and eventually enforces rest. A snapping or clicking may indicate a completion of the fracture.

Examination Local bony tenderness is associated with swelling.

Investigation Plain X-rays may show a fracture, or callus after 3 weeks, but may require longer than this. Bone and MRI scan show positive within a day or two.

Treatment Rest from the aggravating activity is the only way of ensuring healing. Women may show a higher incidence, with the possibility of osteoporosis secondary to amenorrhoea.

Two particular metatarsal stress fractures deserve special mention. The base of the second metatarsal is held firmly in Lisfranc's joint and is a source of pain in dancers. The lesion is difficult to see on X-ray and requires a bone scan. The Jones fracture of the proximal shaft of the 5th metatarsal fails to heal. Delayed and non-unions are common, even when treated with a non-weight-bearing cast. Early fixation is recommended, possibly with bone grafting.

Stress fractures of the navicular and other tarsal bones

Tarsal stress fractures are more common than previously thought. They are often missed for months and are responsible for prolonged periods off training and competition. The navicular stress fracture is the most common.

History There is gradual onset of severe but diffuse aching in the mid-foot, worst on impact, becoming sufficiently painful to enforce inactivity.

Examination   Careful palpation of the navicular shows this to be the source of pain and swelling. A knowledge of surface anatomy is essential to identify the bone palpated. Observe for overpronation.

Investigation   Standard AP views may show the fracture line, but need a careful search and an index of suspicion. Special views can be requested. Bone scan is positive. CT scans show the fracture very well and aid management decision-making.

Treatment   Incomplete fractures seen early can be expected to heal with several weeks' rest, in plaster cast if necessary. Completed fractures, or those with sclerotic edges will not heal without open reduction, fixation, and bone grafting.

Conditions of the forefoot and toes in athletes

Conditions that may be encountered in the forefoot and toes of an athlete include the following:

- **Metatarsalgia** (pain of the metatarsal bones): Treat with a metatarsal pad behind the weight-bearing area.

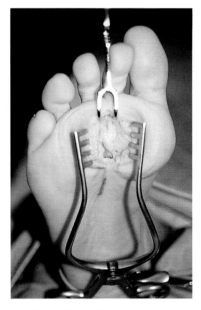

Figure 9.11   Morton's neuroma

191

- **Callosities:** A prominent metatarsal head bears an increase in the weight-bearing load. This leads to a callus and tenderness of the underlying bony prominence. Treat by a load-sharing pad behind the affected area. Surgery can be helpful, but may simply shift the load to another bone, with recurrence there.
- **Freiberg's infarction:** An avascular necrosis (loss of blood supply and bone death) of the metatarsal head which may be painful before any changes show on X-ray. Treat with a metatarsal pad to avoid load-bearing.
- **Morton's neuroma** (Figure 9.11): The digital nerve passes between adjacent metatarsal heads, and may become entrapped. This injures the nerve, which swells and forms a painful neuroma. Pain and electric shock sensations are felt along the sides of adjacent toes. In atypical cases the athlete may simply complain of a diffuse dull ache between the toes. In early cases, wearing looser footwear may settle the problem, otherwise surgical excision is needed.

Sesamoiditis

The sesamoid bones lie within the split tendon of flexor hallucis brevis. They are weight-bearing structures which can be palpated at the proximal half of the callus under the first toe. They are injured by impact, commonly in jumpers or runners. The bones may undergo fracture, stress fracture avascular necrosis or osteoarthritis against the overlying metatarsal. They are commonly bipartite. Bone scan will be positive with a true injury. Treatment is by avoiding weight-bearing, and a metatarsal pad. Steroid injection can be used but is painful. Surgical excision or shaving of the inferior surface of an arthritic sesamoid can be beneficial, but both sesamoids should not be excised.

Hallux rigidus

This is a disabling arthritis of the first metatarsal joint. It presents with a swollen joint, most painful on dorsiflexion, which is limited. Any running or jumping activity is affected. The athlete may be unaware of the limitation of movement, and comparison with the asymptomatic side must be made. Bony osteophytes are visible and palpable on the top of the joint.

X-ray shows a narrowing of the joint space, sclerosis, and osteophytes. Treatment is by rest and NSAIDs. If pain does not settle, then intra-articular injection of steroid can bring temporary relief but may accelerate the degenerative changes. Surgery to remove the bony osteophytes and inflamed synovium gives partial relief. A dorsal wedge osteotomy of the proximal phalanx increases the functional range of movement, and may be a better option for the athlete. Fusion relieves pain but is career ending.

Occasionally hallux rigidus may present via a secondary injury. The athlete may learn to externally rotate the foot to avoid dorsiflexion at push off, aggravating any functional pronation.

Turf toe

This is an American term which describes trauma to the first metatarso-phalangeal joint, usually occurring on artificial turf. The toe hyperextends with additional valgus or varus stress with some axial loading. There is a gradation of injuries from grade 1 to 3:

1. is a capsular sprain;
2. is a tear of the capsule and ligaments with pain on weight-bearing;
3. is a larger tear with possibly a fracture.

Dislocations or fractures may injure the volar plate.

Treatment is with pain relief followed by rest to allow the joint to recover. Improving footwear to reduce the flexibility in the forefoot is essential for prevention.

Marked displacement of the sesamoid bones identified on a weight-bearing X-ray should be referred to an orthopaedic specialist for surgical repair.

Hallux valgus, bunions, and bunionettes

These are bony prominences, commonly seen on the big and little toes. Poor fitting footwear may aggravate symptoms in an athlete.

Skin and nails

A black nail is caused by blood under the nail. Before the blood clots, it can be released by burning a small hole with a safety pin heated by a flame. Release of the fluid gives dramatic pain relief. The athlete should then examine footwear, which is too short.

Tumours

Tumours occur in sportspeople as well as in the rest of the population, and swellings must be taken seriously.

The Lisfranc joint

The Lisfranc joint lies between the tarsal and metatarsal bones. The joint is named after a surgeon in the Napoleonic army who described a fracture dislocation caused by the foot being caught in the stirrup as the rider fell from his horse. Injuries occur via direct or indirect force. The mechanism in sport is usually a fall onto a plantarflexed foot with the toes extended. Other mechanisms include a misstep or a blow to the heel with the weight-bearing foot in a plantarflexed position.

There are several grades of injury, from the frank fracture dislocation to the subtle ligamentous injuries. Recognition of the injury is important as they are often missed and are frequently the cause of prolonged discomfort. Clinically the patient complains of an inability to walk on tip toe with mid-foot pain and pain on passive abduction of the tarsometatarsal joint. Palpation will be tender.

Weight-bearing X-rays are essential. Very subtle malalignments of the base of the metatarsal bones are seen. Fleck fractures of the 2nd metatarsal, compression fractures of the navicular, and avulsion fractures should all alert to the possibility of a Lisfranc injury.

Treatment should not be delayed, and requires surgical reduction of displaced segments, or chronic pain is very likely.

10 Acute injuries of the thigh and knee

STEVE BOLLEN

Injuries to the thigh and knee include a range of problems from minor hamstring tears and contused thighs to career-ending and limb-threatening knee dislocations. To prevent long term disability and return sportsmen and women to the field as quickly as possible, it is important to be able to identify potentially serious problems and make sure they are referred early to an appropriate specialist.

The thigh

The musculature of the thigh is a common site of injury, either from a direct blow causing a muscle haematoma or myositis ossificans, or from excessive demand for power, causing tearing of a muscle.

Hamstring injuries

"Once a hamstring always a hamstring" is an old coaching saying, and hamstring injuries do have an annoying habit of becoming chronic. It is far better to aim for prevention rather than belated treatment, and the cornerstone of management is *appropriate* flexibility and strength for the activity involved, and a proper warm-up before competing or training.[1]

Assessing hamstring flexibility is essential in most sports that involve sprinting or kicking. Traditional sit and reach testing (Figure 10.1) is a poor assessment of hamstring tightness and improvements tend to occur in trunk flexibility rather than in muscle loosening. Straight leg raising is a useful test, but only for one specific area of the hamstring muscle tendon unit.[2] "90/90" testing, where hip and knee are held at 90 degrees before extending the leg, is an additional test and produces a tightness in a different part of the muscles. This can be done with the foot in internal or external rotation to isolate biceps femoris or the medial hamstrings.

195

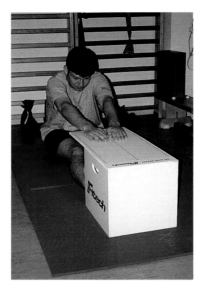

Figure 10.1   The sit and reach test is a commonly used measure of flexibility. Improvements in this measurement usually reflect increased trunk flexibility rather than improvements in the hamstrings

It is important to analyse which phase of activity and which part of the hamstrings are most at risk and then tailor stretching and strengthening programmes to a particular individual's demands. Quadriceps–hamstring imbalance is known to predispose to injury and is common in athletes who concentrate on quadriceps work to the exclusion of hamstring strength.[3]

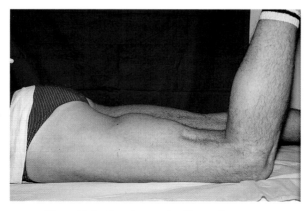

Figure 10.2   Complete proximal hamstring rupture

It is possible to completely rupture the muscle belly of a hamstring (Figure 10.2) and any dramatic failure during a sprinting event, associated with severe pain and a palpable gap in the muscle, should have an urgent ultrasound examination to confirm the diagnosis and then undergo surgical repair.

The far more common minor tearing produces localised pain and limitation of motion. Subsequent to this, muscle wasting occurs. This is not nearly so obvious as in the quadriceps and, unlike quadriceps weakness, does not lead to functional problems in day-to-day life. After the standard first aid measures have settled the immediate symptoms, the main feature noticeable to a sportsperson is the limitation of motion, and so it is not surprising that this is the area of rehabilitation that is usually concentrated on. It is, however, common to see "rehabilitated" sportspeople who have a profound hamstring weakness, and this will inevitably lead to further injury. This is one area where isokinetic testing, using machines such as the Cybex and Kincon, is invaluable as it can document hamstring weakness and hamstring–quadriceps imbalance and allow monitoring of retraining, particularly eccentric strengthening.

Differential diagnosis

Low back pain is frequently referred to the hamstring and buttock area. Mild low back pain may produce a lordosis with hamstring "tightness" or spasm as the major presenting symptom. The "slump" test is used to detect an element of nerve root involvement. The patient sits over the edge of a couch in a slumped position with a reverse lordosis. The affected leg is extended to the point of discomfort. Reproduction or exacerbation of the patient's pain by flexing the neck or dorsiflexing the foot indicates irritation of a nerve root. Investigations may show a variety of pathologies from pars defects to tears of the annulus of the intervertebral disc. The nerve irritation is treated conservatively by stretching and spinal mobilisations, and other lesions treated as appropriate.

Hamstring injuries

- Prevention is better than cure
- Stretching and strengthening should be tailored to individual needs
- Do not forget eccentric strengthening as well as regaining range of motion after injury

---

Rectus femoris tears

This relatively common injury often remains undiagnosed until the patient notices a "lump" appearing in the front of the thigh when tensing the

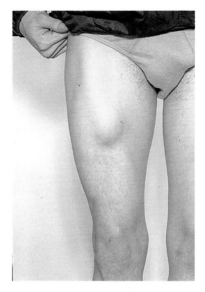

Figure 10.3   The typical appearance of a rupture of rectus femoris when tensing the thigh sometimes referred for an urgent opinion as a "tumour"

quadriceps (Figure 10.3). The injury occurs with a violent quadriceps contraction or when a kick is suddenly blocked by the ground or an opponent. Improper stretching techniques may be implicated (see Chapter 2).

The muscle is usually torn at the distal musculotendinous junction above the quadriceps tendon and presents with pain and swelling above the patella. Straight leg raising is preserved and so the injury is often missed in its early stages. Fortunately, long term disability is rare and the loss of power from this muscle is readily compensated for by the other, and more powerful, quadriceps muscles.

Thigh contusions: "corked thigh"

A direct blow to the thigh is a common event in many contact sports and may produce two types of muscular haematoma – intermuscular and intramuscular. It is important to differentiate these, as management is very different and inappropriate treatment may cause complications.

An intermuscular haematoma occurs in the area between individual muscles. It usually presents with poorly localised, painful swelling, which may move distally under the influence of gravity. Response to standard soft tissue injury treatment is swift and an athlete often returns to jogging after 3–4 days and may resume training once a full range of pain-free movement has been achieved.

An intramuscular haematoma occurs within a muscle belly. This produces pain and spasm, limited to the affected muscle. The haematoma can often be palpated as a tender, indurated swelling. Early mobilisation, heat treatment, and massage may cause rebleeding, which can occur for up to about 10 days post injury.

Treatment should be in three phases.[4] Phase 1 is to limit haemorrhage by rest. This is achieved by immobilisation in the maximum amount of flexion that is comfortable, ice, and elevation and is carried out over the first 24–48 hours.

In phase 2, passive, and gentle active, flexion–extension exercises are initiated. Progressive weight-bearing is started and when there is no pain or limp and 90 degrees of flexion is achieved, full weight-bearing is allowed. Once 120 degrees of pain-free flexion has been gained, phase 3, a return to participation in non-contact sports is begun. When full power, endurance, and motion have returned, the patient is allowed to return to contact sports.

It is possible for a thigh contusion to produce a compartment syndrome within one of the fascial compartments. Swelling, severe pain that fails to improve quickly with conventional treatment, and a tense compartment are indications for compartment pressure measuring. There is no disturbance of sensation as the nerves of the leg are extra-compartmental. If pressures are excessively raised when compared with the opposite side, a fasciotomy should be performed.[5]

Thigh contusions

- Important to differentiate inter from intramuscular haematoma
- Initially rest, ice, and immobilisation in flexion
- Steady build-up of activity depending on range of movement and symptoms
- Beware compartment syndromes

Myositis ossificans

As a complication of a thigh contusion, heterotopic bone formation may occur. Initially there will be localised pain, tenderness, swelling, and loss

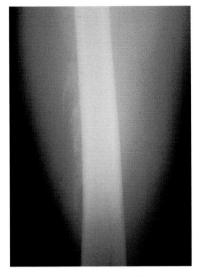

Figure 10.4   This fairly extensive area of heterotopic ossification in the thigh of a 12-year-old boy completely resolved over a period of 8 weeks

of knee flexion that fails to settle with conventional treatment. By 3–4 weeks post injury, a firm mass may be felt in the thigh and X-rays will show new bone formation adjacent to the femur.

Where this condition is suspected treatment should follow standard lines for soft tissue injury but with *avoidance of stretching*. Weight-bearing and mobility should be within the limits of pain. By 3–6 months post injury the bone mass will stabilise or even decrease in size. In the young, complete resorption may occur over a couple of months (Figure 10.4).

Occasionally the bony mass persists and may be painful and cause limitation of function. If conservative treatment fails, surgical excision may be indicated, but not until at least 6 months post injury when the bony mass should have finished maturing. A bone scan may be helpful in deciding whether the lesion is quiescent.

The knee

The knee is the most commonly injured joint in sporting activity.[6] This is perhaps not surprising when one considers its complexity and vulnerable position. In a study of a large series of knee injuries in the USA by

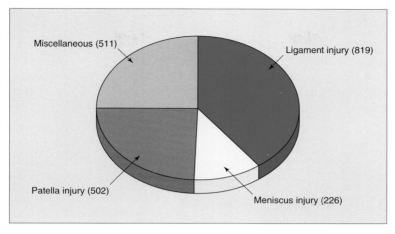

Figure 10.5   Distribution of diagnoses in a series of 1833 knee injuries (Myasaka et al, 1991[7])

Myasaka,[7] the distribution of diagnoses was as seen in Figure 10.5. It is interesting to note that ligament injuries were found to be more common than meniscal injuries. An acute knee injury is always worrying to a sportsperson and requires a prompt diagnosis and appropriate management to avoid prolonged morbidity and a possible permanent place on the sideline.

It is no longer acceptable to apply a diagnosis of "internal derangement of the knee" (IDK or "I don't know"), or a "knee sprain" to an injured joint and every effort should be made to make a proper diagnosis and therefore an appropriately formulated treatment plan.

There is no substitute for a careful history and examination. The mechanism of injury, the speed of swelling, *exact* location of pain, limitation of movement, or feeling of instability will usually indicate the diagnosis and examination will confirm it. Conventional radiographs are useful to identify osteochondral and avulsion fractures and it must be remembered that "small flakes often indicate big injury".

Diagnosis of knee injury has been helped by the advent of magnetic resonance imaging (MRI) which gives excellent images of the soft tissue structures of the knee. MRI is not infallible, however, and to a certain extent is radiologist-dependent for its interpretation. It certainly does not replace clinical acumen and has been shown to be less accurate than an experienced clinical examiner in diagnosing injuries such as anterior cruciate ligament rupture,[8] and often does not alter clinical decisions about treatment.[9]

201

First aid measures are the same as for any other soft tissue injury but I would recommend the addition of an adjustable, long leg, off-the-shelf brace with hinges that can either be locked at any angle or a limited range of movement allowed. One of these should be part of the first aid kit of anyone providing medical (or physiotherapy) cover for any sporting event where knee injuries may occur. They provide comfort for the patient and can minimise further trauma before definitive treatment can be carried out.

Acute knee injuries

- Apply conventional first aid
- If necessary, immobilise in a brace
- Take a careful history to establish likely diagnosis
- X-ray to exclude osteochondral or avulsion fracture
- Refer urgently to a knee specialist

Causes of haemarthrosis in acute knee injury include:

- Meniscal tear
- Cruciate ligament tear
- Patella dislocation
- Osteochondral fracture (large fragment may be replaced surgically to restore articular surface).

Extensor mechanism failure

This term covers patella tendon avulsion, patella fracture, and quadriceps tendon rupture. They are grouped together as they have a common mechanism of injury of a violent quadriceps contraction or sudden blocking of a kick, similar to that of a rectus femoris injury.

In adolescence it tends to affect the patella tendon, in middle years the patella fractures, and in late middle age the quadriceps tendon ruptures. Examination will reveal tenderness, swelling, and a palpable gap at the appropriate site. The patient will be unable to perform a straight leg raise – a simple test, often not performed and responsible for the soft tissue types of this injury sometimes being missed. X-ray will show a high patella when the patella tendon is torn or an obvious fracture of the patella. X-ray will be normal with a quadriceps tendon rupture.

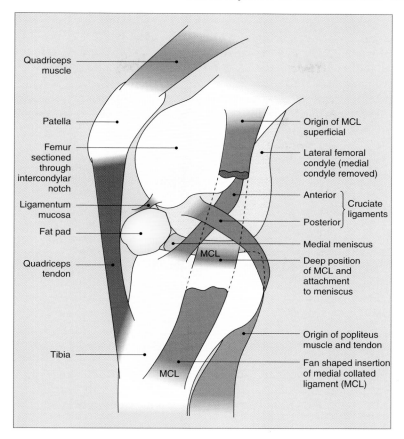

Figure 10.6 Lateral view of the knee

A complete rupture of any component of the extensor mechanism will require urgent surgical intervention to repair the torn tendon and medial and lateral retinaculae. Soft tissue disruptions require postoperative immobilisation in a plaster cylinder for 4 weeks, but a patella fracture openly reduced and fixed with tension band wiring may be mobilised early.

Patella dislocation

Acute patella dislocation sometimes presents a diagnostic problem as it often relocates spontaneously and patients present with a haemarthrosis and medial pain.

203

If a careful history is taken, however, the patient has usually felt the "knee cap" move out of place at the same time as the leg gives way. A careful examination will reveal medial *retinacular* tenderness rather than medial joint line or medial epicondyle tenderness, and there will be a positive apprehension sign.

The joint should be aseptically aspirated and a skyline and intercondylar X-ray obtained to exclude an osteochondral fracture which may be in the lateral gutter or intercondylar notch. Occasionally, the unwary may mistake a loose marginal fracture of the patella that has dropped down into the intercondylar notch, for an anterior cruciate ligament (ACL) avulsion.

If there is a loose osteochondral fragment it should be removed arthroscopically. The standard treatment then consists of a 4 week period of immobilisation in a plaster cylinder, followed by physiotherapy.

If the alignment of the non-injured limb is of the patella alta, genu valgum, genu recurvatum type, the likelihood of recurrent dislocation is in the order of 50% and a good argument for surgical repair of the medial retinacula ligament can be made.[10] If the alignment of the non-injured leg is normal, recurrent dislocation is about 20%.

Meniscal injuries

The menisci of the knee are cleverly designed structures to share the load-bearing through the joint surfaces. The menisci take 50% of the weight passing through the knee. Their location and function puts them at risk in

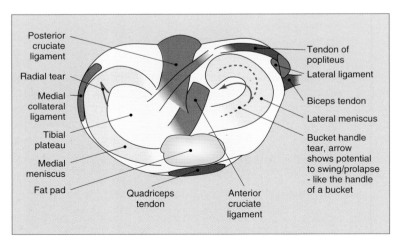

Figure 10.7   View of superior surface of the tibia

any activity involving weight-bearing and twisting, particularly if this is performed with the knee flexed.

There is usually a history of a weight-bearing/twisting injury. If a bucket handle tear is produced and flips into the centre of the joint there is immediate pain and an inability to straighten the knee. Undisplaced or stable peripheral tears, flap tears and horizontal cleavage tears have pain and swelling which occurs slowly and is often not noticed until the following day. Examination will reveal the presence of joint line tenderness on the affected side of the knee and an effusion if seen after about 12 hours post injury. McMurray's testing may produce a painful clunk from the joint line.

If the knee is locked, management should be by immobilising the knee in a brace, in the position of most comfort. With all tears, weight-bearing should be aided by crutches. Urgent referral to a specialist in arthroscopic surgery of the knee should be made.

Simple arthroscopic excision results in rapid recovery and can allow a return to playing within 3–4 weeks, although 6–8 weeks is more usual. The rate of rehabilitation depends on joint pain and swelling. Initially swelling should be controlled with standard techniques and range of motion and static exercises started. The patient then progresses through aqua-jogging, static cycling, and step machine before returning to running on soft surfaces and a progressive sport-specific programme.

Meniscal injuries

- History of weight-bearing/twisting injury
- Usually slow swelling over 24 hours
- Pain localised to joint line
- Joint extension may be blocked
- Refer early to knee specialist with arthroscopic skills

Many peripheral meniscal tears may be suitable for arthroscopic repair rather than excision, although the rehabilitation is much longer and healing rates in isolated tears are only in the order of 70%.[11,12] If a professional footballer has a cup final in the offing, it may be difficult to persuade him that the potential advantages of repair, in terms of delaying the onset of arthrosis in the dim and distant future, outweigh the immediate potential gains of excision and a more rapid return to playing.

205

Popliteus tendon avulsion

Popliteus tendon avulsion is a rare cause of acute lateral knee pain associated with a haemarthrosis.[13] The history is usually of an external rotation injury on a partially flexed knee followed by acute lateral pain and rapid swelling. Examination will reveal a large effusion, tenderness over the lateral epicondyle (above the joint line), restricted range of movement, and a stable knee. Plain X-ray may show a small flake avulsion fracture from the lateral condyle on the AP view.

Management requires arthroscopy to visualise the lateral gutter and then the anatomical replacement and fixation of the fragment, in order to prevent long term posterolateral laxity. If this is performed early, the long term prognosis is excellent.

Anterior cruciate ligament injuries

Rupture of the anterior cruciate ligament (ACL) is the commonest ligament injury in any sport that involves turning or changing direction of a weight-bearing leg (Figure 10.9). External rotation of femur on tibia produces the injury. The ACL is also vulnerable in jumping sports such as netball, when landing and turning. Acute valgus strains in contact sports or valgus/external rotation strains such as occur in skiing when bindings fail to release, can both cause ligament failure.

The common history is of a non-contact twisting injury, hearing or feeling a "pop" or snap (or feeling "something go"), and swelling that usually occurs very quickly, certainly within 4 hours. Players usually go off the field but sometimes try to rejoin the match only to have the leg collapse under them again.

If seen acutely, it is worth aspirating the haemarthrosis under aseptic conditions as this makes the patient more comfortable and examination easier. There is often a block to the last few degrees of extension, best appreciated by picking both legs off the examination couch by the big toes. Any larger block to extension, particularly if associated with joint line tenderness, should alert the examiner to the possibility of an associated meniscal tear.

A standard anterior draw test is largely useless in the acute situation and the two key parts of the examination are the Lachman and pivot shift tests.

The Lachman test is an anterior draw test performed at 20 degrees of knee flexion and, certainly in big legs, is easier to perform by draping the injured leg over the examiner's knee (Figure 10.10). One is feeling for the sudden stop of anterior translation that occurs in a knee with an intact ACL. The absence of a "hard end stop" is characteristic of ACL insufficiency.

206

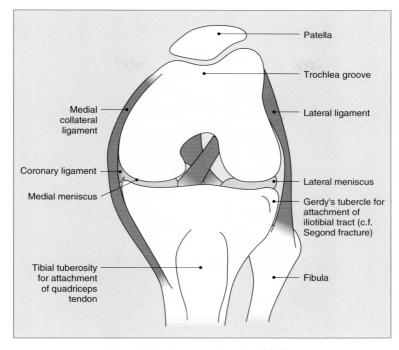

Figure 10.8   Anteroposterior view of the knee

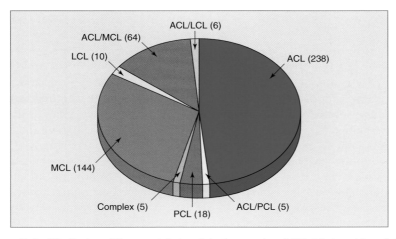

Figure 10.9   Distribution of ligament injuries of the knee: series of 500 injuries with pathologic motion (Myasaka et al, 1991[7])

ACL = anterior cruciate ligament; PCL = posterior cruciate ligament; MCL = medial collateral ligament; LCL = lateral collateral ligament

207

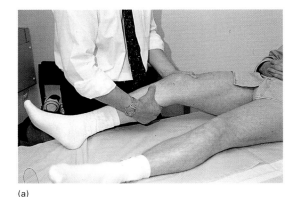

(a)

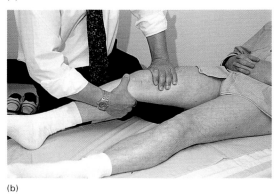

(b)

Figure 10.10   The standard Lachman test is easy to do in patients with thin legs but in the average rugby player it is much better to drape the patient's leg over yours, relaxing their muscles and allowing a much better appreciation of abnormal anterior laxity

A positive pivot shift test (Figure 10.11) present in the injured but not in the non-injured leg, is pathognomonic for a non-functioning ACL.[14] It requires a lot of practice to perform well, but the feeling of the joint subluxing out in extension and snapping back as the joint is moved into flexion (while applying internal rotation and a valgus load), is instantly recognisable to examiner and patient alike. Although sometimes uncomfortable for the patient, with an experienced examiner it does not require the giving of a general anaesthetic, a view that some orthopaedic surgeons still hold! In experienced hands, the diagnosis of ACL rupture has been reported to be 100% specific and 100% sensitive – better than MRI.[8]

An X-ray should be taken to exclude osteochondral fracture and to identify cases of ACL avulsion. It may show a small flake off the anterolateral

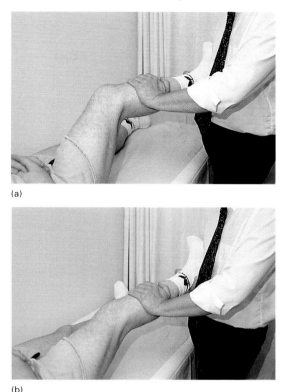

(a)

(b)

Figure 10.11   The pivot shift test requires a lot of practice to do well. In extension and applying a valgus load the tibia subluxes forward. As the knee is flexed, the iliotibial band passes behind the axis of rotation of the knee and suddenly becomes a flexor, reducing the tibia with a sudden jerk

tibia – the "Segond fracture" (Figure 10.12), commonly associated with ACL injury.

If the tibial spine is avulsed (Figure 10.13) the prognosis is good, as the energy of the injury is dissipated through the fracture and the ligament itself is frequently not attenuated. Under anaesthetic, a lateral X-ray in full extension should be taken. If the fragment reduces, a plaster cylinder is applied and maintained for 4 weeks. If the fragment is not reduced in extension, an open, or arthroscopic, reduction and fixation is performed.

In the absence of a tibial spine avulsion, treatment of "isolated" ACL injuries remains controversial. There is no doubt that some ACL-deficient knees become functionally unstable and with recurrent giving way episodes, further joint damage occurs and leads to accelerated

209

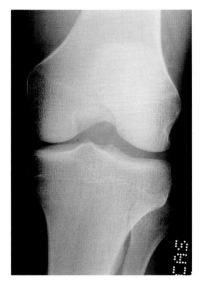

Figure 10.12 The small flake of bone off the lateral aspect of the tibia, or "Segond fracture" has a high association with a rupture of the anterior cruciate ligament

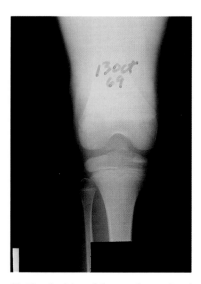

Figure 10.13 Avulsion of the anterior cruciate insertion

degenerative change.[15–17] Current evidence is weak that ACL reconstruction will prevent degenerative change occurring.[18] Also, there is undoubtedly a group (10–20%) of patients who can play high level sport without an anterior cruciate, although the knee does tend to decompensate with time.

Whatever the arguments about surgery, patients need early control of swelling and physiotherapy supervised rehabilitation with muscle and proprioceptive retraining. Counselling is important as patients need to appreciate they do not have, and never will have, a normal knee whatever surgical procedure may be performed.

Advances in ACL reconstruction (which can now be done arthroscopically) however, coupled with rapid rehabilitation utilising co-contractions, *closed* kinetic chain exercises (such as half squats, static cycling with a high seat, and step machine), and early full range of movement,[19] can reliably stabilise a functionally unstable knee with minimum operative morbidity.

Professional sportsmen warrant early reconstruction (not before 3–4 weeks post injury to reduce the complication of arthrofibrosis[20,21]), to minimise time away from earning their living, but it will take about 6 months from surgery utilising an autogenous graft, before returning to competitive sport. Other patients have to decide if instability is bad enough to undergo surgery.

In a large review of ACL reconstruction failures, 60% were due to "surgical error" – there is little margin of error in these procedures and they should only be carried out by surgeons who perform this type of surgery on a frequent and regular basis and have full and experienced rehabilitation back-up.

Anterior cruciate injuries

- Commonly non-contact, twisting injury
- Often hear or feel a "pop" or "snap"
- Swelling immediate or within 4 hours
- High incidence of instability in sports requiring sudden change of direction
- Surgery now more reliable and with less perioperative morbidity

---

Posterior cruciate ligament injuries

Posterior cruciate ligament (PCL) injuries usually occur with a blow to the front of the tibia or a fall on a flexed knee. They are often thought of as minor injuries and it can be possible to play on for a short while before

211

swelling occurs. There is often pain felt in the popliteal fossa made worse by knee flexion.

Clinical examination in acute cases will reveal a haemarthrosis and often tenderness in the popliteal fossa. With the knee at 90 degrees there will be a characteristic posterior sag. This may not be great and a careful comparison with the normal leg should always be made, with the knee in this position. A common mistake is to miss this and then interpret the increase in anterior draw, caused by the knee starting from a more posterior position (Figure 10.14) as a sign of anterior cruciate injury. There will be a soft end point

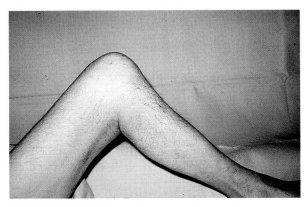

Figure 10.14   Rupture of the posterior cruciate ligament (Sag sign)

to the posterior draw. An X-ray should be taken to exclude an avulsion fracture.

If there is an avulsion fracture displaced by more than 2 mm, it should be surgically fixed back in place. Otherwise, the PCL rarely ruptures completely but attenuates within its substance, so conservative treatment allows the residual ligament to scar and tighten up. If seen acutely, the knee should be treated in a plaster cylinder or brace in extension for 4 weeks. Regaining flexion after this can be slow, but this method of treatment results in less residual posterior sag.

Posterior cruciate ligament injuries

- Commonly, a blow to the front of the upper tibia or fall on a flexed knee
- Often thought of as minor injury by the patient
- Exclude displaced avulsion fracture with X-ray
- With proper rehabilitation, "isolated" injuries rarely cause problems in the short term
- Reserve surgery for combined injuries and displaced avulsion fractures

---

Chronic, isolated PCL injuries rarely cause functional problems in the short term, providing adequate quadriceps strength is maintained.[22,23] In the longer term, patellofemoral osteoarthrosis will supervene, but so far reconstruction has not been shown to prevent this.

A combination of a PCL and posterolateral corner injury is a lot more serious and usually leads to functional instability. It is therefore important to pick out this subgroup and consider early surgery, depending on the patient's demands and expectations.

Medial ligament injuries

Medial ligament injuries occur with a sudden valgus stress to the knee and are common in contact sports. There is usually medial pain, knee swelling, and a reluctance to straighten the knee.

On examination there will be tenderness, which can be pinpointed most commonly above the joint line on the medial epicondyle and sometimes at the distal insertion of the MCL on the tibia. The knee can usually be gently persuaded into full extension, but this will increase pain.

Valgus stress should be applied both in extension and in slight flexion. Trying to apply a valgus load in flexion often causes rotation of the leg and this is frequently interpreted as joint opening by the inexperienced. This problem can be overcome by sitting the patient and applying the load across the ball of the foot in line with the femur – Bollen's test (Figure 10.15).[24]

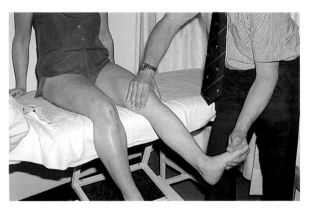

Figure 10.15 Applying a varus or valgus load by grasping the foot across the metatarsal heads and aligning these with the shaft of the femur, eliminates the tendency for the femur to rotate. The knee is fixed on the edge of the couch with the finger and thumb on the joint line, allowing an accurate assessment of joint opening

Opening of the joint in full extension indicates injury to the posterior oblique ligament with an associated injury of the ACL. If opening in flexion occurs, it may come up against a firm stop, indicating a grade 2 tear, or there may be no stop, a grade 3.

It is paradoxical that with the most severe, grade 3, tears there may be little pain and no effusion, due to complete tearing of the capsule destroying nerve endings and letting the haemarthrosis leak out of the knee and into the soft tissues of the leg. The initial severity may therefore be overlooked and only when extensive bruising appears in the calf a few days later is it appreciated that something serious is amiss.

Treatment of grade 1 tears is functional as there is no instability of the joint. Local physiotherapy and progressive retraining within the limits of discomfort may allow return to sport within 6 weeks.

Grade 2 tears should be treated with bracing to protect the medial complex from valgus stress while it is healing. Off the shelf, long leg braces are useful but in my experience many players will remove them as they begin to feel better, or when they want a bath etc. Cast bracing has the advantage of not being removable except by saw and this is usually immediately noticeable to the treating surgeon! The ligament tear usually firms up over a 4–6 week period.

Bracing does not mean the patient has to stop all activity, and indeed joint motion is beneficial for increasing the strength of the healed ligament. Providing the cast brace is applied to allow sufficient knee flexion, activities such as cycling, step-ups, step machine, and weight training are all possible and should be encouraged.

Grade 3 tears can be treated along similar lines as above but the brace is locked at 20 degrees for the first 2–3 weeks, to allow the ligament to "stick down", before commencing active rehabilitation. This is especially important when the posterior oblique ligament has also been torn.

In isolated MCL tears there is no evidence that surgical intervention produces better functional results. Indeed it has been shown to delay recovery and provide a weaker strength repair.[25-27]

There is a variation of MCL injury which can occasionally lead to a diagnostic dilemma. With a combination of a twist and valgus strain the deep part of the medial ligament (between the medial meniscus and tibia) can be injured.[28] This produces joint line pain, an effusion, and pain on twisting and turning, i.e. almost identical symptoms to a medial meniscal tear. The slight increase in medial laxity (in the order of 3–4 mm) is difficult to detect clinically and the principal physical signs are of joint line tenderness and pain on McMurray's testing. Arthroscopy reveals lifting off of the medial meniscus from the tibial plateau when a valgus stress is applied and often granulation tissue can be seen beneath the posteromedial aspect of the meniscus (Figure 10.16). Pain on sporting activity may persist for several months, but the prognosis for recovery is always good.

Combined injuries of the ACL + MCL are serious and produce terrible results if not treated adequately. There is some experimental evidence that

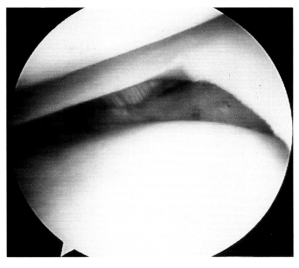

Figure 10.16   Granulation tissue beneath post-medial aspect of meniscus

the MCL does not heal well in the presence of instability produced by ACL insufficiency. In practical terms, however, if the knee is properly protected from repeated giving way and excessive anterior draw in a cast brace, the MCL appears to heal adequately. Young, active, and high risk groups warrant delayed reconstruction of the ACL after bracing the MCL for 4–8 weeks post injury, to allow swelling to settle and regain full range of motion.[29]

Occasionally, pain at the proximal origin of the MCL becomes prolonged and unresponsive to standard treatments. This usually heralds the development of a Pellegrini–Stieda lesion, seen on X-ray as calcification

Medial ligament injuries

- History of a valgus strain
- Pain and tenderness, usually on the medial epicondyle
- The most severe injuries may have least pain and no swelling
- Bruising with local swelling. The bruising may track down to the calf
- Conservative treatment results in faster and stronger healing

on the medial femoral condyle (Figure 10.17). A cortisone injection into the painful spot may help but symptoms often persist for months.

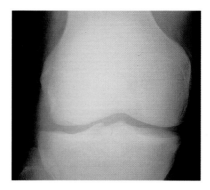

Figure 10.17   Calcification at the attachment of the proximal MCL indicates the development of a Pellegrini–Stieda lesion

Complex ligament injuries

Complex ligament injuries are invariably the result of high violence occurring in contact sports. They usually occur in collisions or when an opponent or team mate falls across the knee of an outstretched leg.

The player is usually aware that something serious has happened and that the knee has "come apart" with the sensation of structures within the knee tearing or snapping. As with severe MCL injuries, pain may be slight after immediate symptoms have settled.

If the knee has dislocated and not spontaneously reduced, it is a surgical emergency and requires prompt reduction under general anaesthetic, followed by an on-table arteriogram to exclude associated popliteal artery injury. If the vascular status is satisfactory immediate reconstruction of all injured structures, followed by a period of postoperative continuous passive motion, can produce good results (Figure 10.18).

Other serious injuries should be immobilised and referred early to an appropriate knee specialist. If the lateral structures have been injured it is essential to check the function of the lateral popliteal nerve prior to surgery. Loss of function has a poor prognosis as it is usually due to a stretching of the nerve producing an axonotmesis.

Reconstruction of complex ligament injuries is highly demanding, technical surgery and thus not for the occasional ligament reconstruction surgeon. After reduction and immobilisation patients should be immediately referred to a local centre of expertise.

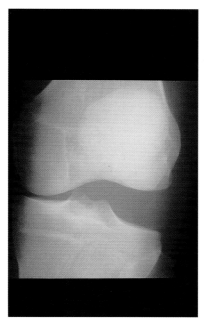

Figure 10.18   Complex ligament injuries can produce dramatic knee instability. It was probably not necessary for the orthopaedic registrar to take this X-ray to confirm lateral laxity! At operation, this patient had ruptured the iliotibial band, the lateral ligament, the popliteus tendon, the whole lateral capsule, biceps femoris, and the anterior cruciate ligament. Six months after reconstructive surgery of the lateral complex and ACL, he has a virtual full range of motion and a stable knee and is talking about returning to playing football

References

1 Agre JC. Hamstring injuries. *Sports Med* 1985;**2**:21–33.
2 Gajdosik RL, Rieck MA, Sullivan DK, Wightman SE. Comparison of four clinical tests for assessing hamstring muscle length. *J Sports Physiother* 1993; **18**:614–19.
3 Knapik JJ, Beauman CL, Jones BH, Harris JM, Vaughan L. Preseason strength and flexibility imbalances associated with athletic injuries in femal collegiate athletes. *Am J Sports Med* 1991;**19**:76–81.
4 Ryan JB, Wheeler JH, Hopkinson WJ, Arciero RA, Kolakowski KR. Quadriceps contusions – West Point update. *Am J Sports Med* 1991;**19**:299–304.
5 Rooser B, Bengtson S, Hagglund G. Acute compartment syndrome from anterior thigh muscle contusion: a report of eight cases. *J Orthop Trauma* 1991; **5**:57–9.
6 Nicholl JP, Coleman P, Williams BT. *Injuries in sport and exercise.* London, Sports Council, 1991.
7 Myasaka KC, Daniel DM, Shore ML, Hirshman P. The incidence of knee ligament injuries in the general population. *Am J Knee Surg* 1991;**4**:3–4.
8 Gelb HJ, Glasgow SG, Sapega AA, Reilly PJ, Sokolow PP, Torg JS. Clinical value and cost effectiveness of MRI in the management of knee injuries in sports medicine practice. *Proceedings AAOS* 1994, p. 117.

9 Wertheim SB, Gillespie S, Klaus RM, Frederick RW. The role of MRI in the treatment of knee injuries. *Proceedings AAOS* 1994, p. 118.

10 Cash JD, Hughston JC. Treatment of acute patella dislocation. *Am J Sports Med* 1988;**16**:244–9.

11 Tenuta JJ, Arciero RA. Arthroscopic evaluation of meniscal repairs – factors that affect healing. *Am J Sports Med* 1994;**22**:797–802.

12 Horibe S, Shino K, Nakate K, Maeda A, Nakamura N, Matsumoto N. Second look arthroscopy after meniscal repair. *J Bone Joint Surg* 1995;**77B**:245–9.

13 Nakhostine M, Perko M, Cross M. Isolated avulsion of the popliteus tendon. *J Bone Joint Surg* 1995;**77B**:242–4.

14 Lucie RS, Wiedel JD, Messner DG. The acute pivot shift: clinical correlation. *Am J Sports Med* 1984;**12**:189–91.

15 Fetto JF, Marshall JL. The natural history and diagnosis of ACL insufficiency. *Clin Orthop* 1980;**147**:29–38.

16 Satku K, Kumar VP, Ngoi SS. ACL injuries – to counsel or operate?. *J Bone Joint Surg* 1986;**68B**:458–461.

17 Kannus P, Jarvinen M. Conservatively treated tears of the ACL. *J Bone Joint Surg* 1987;**69A**:1007–12.

18 Daniel DM, Stone ML, Dobson BE, Fithian DC, Rossman DJ, Kaufman KR. Fate of the ACL-injured patient. *Am J Sports Med* 1994;**22**:632–44.

19 Paessler HH, Shelbourne KD. Biological, biomechanical and clinical approaches to the follow up treatment of ligament surgery of the knee. *Sports Exerc Injury* 1995;**1**:83–95.

20 Shelbourne KD, Wilckens JH, Mollabashy A, Decarlo M. Arthrofibrosis in acute ACL reconstruction. The effect of timing on reconstruction and rehabilitation. *Am J Sports Med* 1991;**19**:139–47.

21 Waselewski SA, Covall DJ, Cohen S. Effect of surgical timing on recovery and associated injuries after anterior cruciate ligament reconstruction. *Am J Sports Med* 1993;**21**:338–47.

22 Parolie JM, Bergfield JA. Long term results of non-operative treatment of isolated posterior cruciate ligament injuries in the athlete. *Am J Sports Med* 1986;**14**:35–8.

23 Torg JS, Barton TM, Pavlov H, Stine R. Natural history of the posterior cruciate deficient knee. *Clin Orthop* 1989;**156**:208–16.

24 Bryant JD, Bollen SR. Elimination of femoral rotation in clinical testing for varus/valgus laxity of the knee. *Clin Biomech* 1993;**8**:329–31.

25 Woo SL-Y, Inoue M, McGurk-Burleson E. Treatment of the medial collateral injury 2. Structure and function of canine knees in response to differing treatment regimes. *Am J Sports Med* 1987;**15**:22–9.

26 Indelicato PA. Non-operative treatment of complete tears of the medial collateral ligament of the knee. *J Bone Joint Surg* 1983;**65A**:323–9.

27 Reider B, Sathy MR, Talkington J, Blyznak N, Kollias S. Treatment of isolated medial collateral injuries in athletes with early functional rehabilitation. *Am J Sports Med* 1994;**22**:470–7.

28 Bollen SR. The sportsman's coronary – injury to the deep part of the medial collateral ligament. *J Bone Joint Surg* (in press).

29 Shelbourne KD, Patel DV. Management of combined injuries of the anterior cruciate and medial collateral ligaments. *J Bone Joint Surg* 1995;**77A**:800–6.

11   Chronic knee pain

GRAHAM MN HOLLOWAY AND
ROGER G HACKNEY

The knee is the largest joint in the body, is superficial and vulnerable to injury. The stability of any joint depends on the bony contours of the articular surfaces, its supporting ligaments, and the strength of the controlling muscles. The knee is not simply a hinge joint but has a certain amount of rotation. The articular surfaces impart little stability; the ligaments are vital, but so too are the controlling muscles which must maintain congruity of the patella throughout the range of flexion and extension with varying degrees of tibial rotation. Any disturbance of the normal patellofemoral tracking commonly causes pain at the front of the knee or patellofemoral pain. This is a common problem, causing chronic restriction of function and is frequently very difficult to treat. It is not adequate to make a diagnosis of anterior knee pain but to try to determine the underlying problem as several distinct causes have been identified.

Diagnosis

Effective treatment depends on accurate diagnosis. Diagnosis relies on the history, clinical examination, and further investigations. Clinical signs in chronic knee pain are few and often subtle; great importance therefore is laid on the history.

There follows a suggested approach to the problem, and this clinical history can be expanded as necessary depending on the patient's response.

1 Is there a history of injury? Cruciate injuries and minor meniscal tears are often missed at initial examination after the injury. They may present some time later with pain or instability. Anterior knee pain may follow a direct blow to the patella.

2 Is it referred pain? Is there a history of hip pain or stiffness or low back disorder? Establish early the possibility of the pain being referred from elsewhere; do not leave it as an afterthought. Referred pain from the hip

219

is common – consider Perthes disease, slipped upper femoral epiphysis and early osteoarthritis.

3 Any other joints affected? Sportspeople are not immune to generalised arthropathies. A history of bilateral anterior knee pain is unlikely to be traumatic and much more likely to be due to overuse or an underlying biomechanical problem.

4 Any swelling? Localised soft tissue swelling suggests bursitis, or a Baker's cyst, or a ganglion. Generalised swelling suggests an effusion which is likely to indicate an intra-articular problem. Local bony swelling can be an osteochondroma or Osgood–Schlatter's disease.

5 Any locking (a block to full extension)? Locking may be true – when associated with a definite unlocking episode – or 'spurious', which unlocks gradually and is often associated with chondromalacia. True locking may be due to an old meniscal tear, or a loose body from osteochondritis dissecans, or a shearing injury of the articular surface. Pain and restriction of flexion is often associated with degeneration of the posterior horn of the meniscus.

A generalised reduction in movement may indicate early osteoarthritis.

6 Any giving way? Instability or a loss of confidence in the joint may be due to:

- Mechanical damage, i.e. collateral or cruciate injury or meniscal tear.
- Muscle weakness or imbalance
- Reflex inhibition of quadriceps muscles by pain often seen in patellofemoral dysfunction
- Loss of proprioception – usually associated with ligament damage.

7 Where is the pain? Ask the patient to point to the area of maximum pain. This may be specific, i.e. joint line (meniscal tear, osteophyte), above the lateral joint line (iliotibial band friction syndrome), below the medial joint line (stress fracture, pes anserine bursitis), tibial tuberosity (Osgood–Schlatter's), or patella tendon.

Pain is more diffuse and generalised around the patella in most patellofemoral problems. Pain may occur in the popliteal fossa as well. Posterior knee pain is common and non-specific – may be meniscal, bursa, tendon, joint capsule etc.

Differential diagnosis of knee pain

Medial knee pain

- Chronic medial collateral ligament spasm
- Medial collateral ligament bursitis
- Pes anserine bursitis
- Stress fracture medial tibial condyle
- Plica syndrome
- Pellegrini–Stieda syndrome (chronic tear femoral attachment of medial collateral ligament)
- Medial meniscus degeneration
- Osteochondritis dissecans
- Osteoarthritis

Lateral knee pain

- Iliotibial band friction syndrome
- Popliteus tendinitis
- Cystic lateral meniscus
- Tear lateral meniscus
- Chondromalacia lateral tibial plateau
- Osteoarthritis

Anterior knee pain

- Osgood–Schlatter's disease (traction apophysitis of tibial tuberosity)
- Sinding–Larsen–Johansson disease (traction apophysitis of lower pole of patella)
- Patella tendinitis
- Infrapatella bursitis
- Suprapatella bursitis
- Plica syndrome
- Patellofemoral subluxation
- Excess lateral pressure syndrome
- Patella malalignment
- Hoffa's syndrome (fat pad entrapment)
- Osteochondritis dissecans
- Osteoarthritis

8 *When does pain occur?* Is it just associated with activity? Is there pain at rest? Meniscal degeneration pain is often worse at night when the weight of the bedclothes can add to the discomfort. Rest may include prolonged sitting, e.g. driving, sitting in the cinema – as with patellofemoral pain.

221

Does it occur with every step (i.e. iliotibial band friction syndrome, joint degeneration or articular damage)?

Pain going up and down stairs or rising from a sitting position: suggests Hoffman's syndrome.

Pain on twisting and turning: meniscal damage, chronic ligament deficiency, articular cartilage degeneration. Constant unrelenting pain may be due to reflex sympathetic dystrophy, chronic osteomyelitis or osteosarcoma.

9 Aggravating factors? Patellofemoral pain and extensor mechanism problems are worse descending stairs, when the quadriceps are working eccentrically.

Squatting is painful with meniscal degeneration and patellofemoral problems. Kneeling is painful in many conditions and running aggravates knee pain in most conditions and is non-specific.

10 Is it only present during one sport (i.e. "breaststroker's knee", a chronic spasm of the medial collateral ligament)?

11 Relieving factors? If rest does not improve the symptoms you must exclude a non-sporting cause, i.e. tumour, infection, rheumatological disorder etc.

12 Is the pain the same in different sports shoes or in bare feet?

Sporting history

Always take a full sporting history. Understand the repetitive movements that the sport requires as this may give an indication as to the source of the problem. Because 70% of chronic overuse injuries are due to errors in training, correction of technique may be the only treatment necessary. Ascertain whether there has been any unaccustomed exercise or sudden alteration of training.

Note the time spent training, the equipment used, and the environment and surface. Note the type and age of footwear and whether it is appropriate for the sport.

Clinical examination

Time spent on taking a good history may save time on clinical examination and it will allow you to make a preliminary diagnosis which can be confirmed by more specific clinical tests and possibly further investigations. Routine clinical examination should be methodical and sequential: **look, move, feel**. It must include assessment of the range of movement, active, passive, and resisted. Observe whether there is muscle wasting – measure thigh circumference if necessary. Check for effusions and locate areas of tenderness before progressing to specific tests.

Common overuse injuries

Some of the more common conditions, and description of their diagnosis and treatment, follow.

Iliotibial band friction syndrome (Figure 11.1)

This is a runner's knee problem due to repetitive friction between the iliotibial tract and lateral femoral epicondyle. It is most common in the

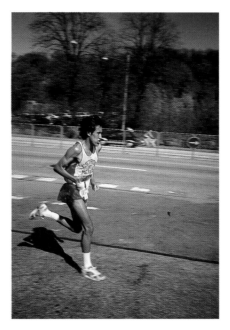

Figure 11.1   Iliotibial band in athlete

right knee in the UK because running facing the traffic the right leg is the "downhill" leg on cambered roads. Also common in cycling and following hill training.

223

1. Pain develops during a run.
2. Pain is present when bending the knee and worsens with increased distance and time. It cannot be run through. The athlete can walk stiff-legged.
3. Predisposing factors:
   - Tight iliotibial tract
   - Genu varum
   - Hyperpronation
   - Lateral pelvic thrust when running
   - Excess running on cambered roads.
4. Clinical features:
   - Local tenderness over the lateral femoral epicondyle, above the joint line, possibly with crepitus on movements in the acute case
   - Tight iliotibial tract on Ober's test: with the patient lying on the unaffected side with the leg flexed at the hip, the affected leg should adduct to the couch
   - Rennes' test – pressure on lateral epicondyle causes pain whilst doing a weight-bearing squat at 45°.
5. Treatment:
   - Discontinue aggravating exercise. Rub ice on tender point
   - Only walk with a straight leg until pain-free
   - Non-steroidal anti-inflammatory drugs are helpful
   - Do specific stretching exercises for the iliotibial tract
   - Local ultrasound may relieve pain
   - In recurrent cases local hydrocortisone injection is useful
   - Very rarely, resistant cases require release of the posterior third of the iliotibial tract
   - Reintroduce running gradually, keeping off cambered roads, and avoid hill running.

Popliteus tendinitis

An uncommon condition, it occurs in runners due to excess hill running. Lateral pain particularly when descending hills. Tenderness is just in front of the lateral ligament and may spread along the joint line and posteriorly into the popliteal fossa. It can be differentiated from lateral meniscus tear because there is no history of trauma or effusions.

Advise the patient to reduce training with no hill running, but may continue to run in water with an aquavest, non-weight-bearing. May respond to non-steroidal anti-inflammatory drugs or local injection of steroid.

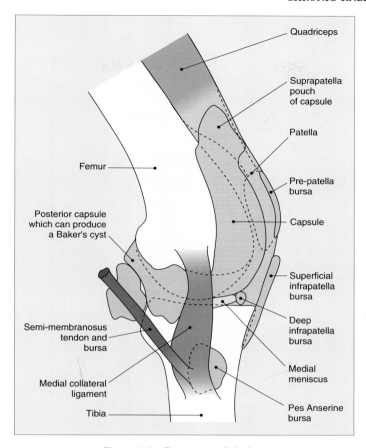

Figure 11.2   Bursae around the knee

Bursitis (Figure 11.2)

There are numerous bursae around the knee to allow free mobility of tendons and skin over bony prominences, ligaments, and other tendons. Excess friction can cause inflammation in any of these bursae.

The commonest sites of these problems are:

- Iliotibial band (see above).
- Prepatella bursa: usually following direct blow.
- Infrapatella bursa, superficial to patella tendon.
- Semimembranosus bursa, which lies between this tendon and the medial head of gastrocnemius: may be troublesome in rowers and runners.
- Pes anserine bursa between the medial hamstrings and the distal part of the medial collateral ligament: can be inflamed in long distance runners and swimmers.

225

- Deep infrapatella bursa between the distal patella tendon and tibia: may be a sequel to Osgood–Schlatter's disease due to altered biomechanics.

The principles of treatment for bursitis are first to reduce inflammation and secondly to prevent recurrence.

1. Rest, ice, non-steroidal anti-inflammatories.
2. Physiotherapeutic modalities, i.e. ultrasound, laser.
3. Commence stretching programme to relax all tight tendons etc.
4. Specific strengthening programme for muscles that need stretching.
5. Correct technique, modify training programme to reduce risk of recurrence.
6. Correct biomechanical abnormalities.
7. Injections of local steroid but beware:
    - *do not* inject into tendons or ligaments
    - prepatella bursa and infrapatella bursa is commonly infected – if there is any local induration or skin redness *do not* inject.

Pellegrini–Stieda syndrome (Figure 11.3)

Common in footballers and skiers following twisting injuries, it follows a valgus or external rotation injury of the knee which causes damage to the

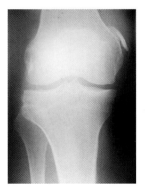

Figure 11.3   Pellegrini–Stieda syndrome

upper femoral attachment of the medial collateral ligament. Calcification or ossification may occur and be visible on X-ray. There may be a reduction in the range of movements. There is chronic pain over the medial femoral condyle and pain on kicking with the instep or on external rotation movements. The medial collateral ligament will be lax.

Treatment consists of:

1. Gentle stretching exercises and joint mobilising. No manipulation which would increase damage, causing more bleeding and scarring.

2. Local ultrasound.
3. Medial hamstring strengthening exercises to dynamically stabilise the medial joint line.
4. Proprioceptive exercises to improve joint position sense.
5. Return to sport when the joint is pain-free and functionally stable.

Patella tendinitis (jumper's knee)

The injury is commonly seen in sports involving high stress to the extensor mechanism of the knee especially when there are repetitive eccentric contractions of the quadriceps muscles. It is seen in jumping sports, basketball, and volleyball, but also in kicking sports and weight-lifting.

Pain is felt anteriorly and is insidious in onset. It starts as an aching after running or sport, and gradually worsens and becomes sore during sport. The pain is aggravated by climbing up or down stairs. The knee feels weak.

Tenderness is localised to the lower pole of the patella where the patella tendon is attached. There may be localised thickening. Resisted knee extension is painful.

The tendon becomes thickened and cystic degeneration may occur in the deep fibres of the tendon. In the acute situation there is oedema and some inflammation of the paratenon sheath, but as with achilles tendon, the chronic condition is one of degeneration rather than inflammation. In this condition the weak fibres may rupture and if untreated may progress to total tendon rupture. The diagnosis can be confirmed by ultrasound scan or MRI scan (Figure 11.4).

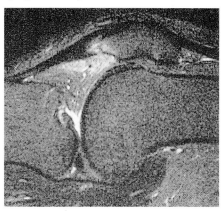

Figure 11.4   Patella tendinitis (MRI scan)

Treatment consists of:

1. Rest (which may need to be prolonged).
2. Ice for acute pain, heat is better when pain is more chronic.

227

3. Ultrasound.
4. Non-steroidal anti-inflammatories.
5. Stretching of hamstrings and quadriceps.
6. Correct patella malalignment with strapping or patella brace if necessary.
7. When pain-free, commence isometric strengthening.
8. Use of strap below patella around patella tendon – Chopart's strap.
9. Progress to concentric activity, i.e. cycling.
10. Increase weight-bearing activity gradually, avoiding jumping and sudden deceleration. Introduce eccentric training cautiously.
11. Chronic cases may respond to paratenon steroid injection but *not into tendon* (Figure 11.5).
12. If cystic degeneration becomes established, conservative treatment is unlikely to cure and surgical excision of all necrotic and diseased tendon is required.

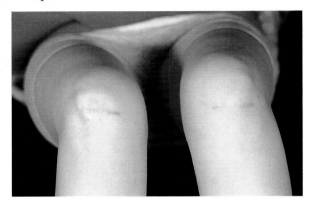

Figure 11.5   Steroid injury to patella tendon

Quadriceps tendinitis

The condition occurs in older age groups and is uncommon. There is a similar degenerative process to patella tendinitis, but affecting the quadriceps expansion above the patella. Treatment principles are the same as for patella tendinitis.

Osgood–Schlatter's disease (Figure 11.6)

This is a traction apophysitis of the tibial tuberosity due to overuse. It classically occurs in 13–16-year-olds and is more common in boys. Associated with repetitive high stresses in the extensor mechanism of the knee such as in kicking sports and mountain biking and in sudden

228

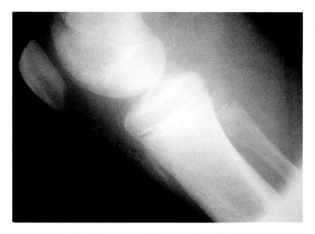

Figure 11.6   Osgood–Schlatter's disease

deceleration sports, i.e. squash. The excess stress on the patella tendon attachment to the tongue epiphysis of the tibia causes fragmentation with callus formation and gradual enlargement of the tibial tuberosity. There is pain at rest and during activity.

Clinical examination shows:

- Tender swollen tibial tuberosity, frequently bilateral
- Pain on resisted knee extension
- Tightness of quadriceps and hamstrings is common
- X-rays seldom necessary as the diagnosis is straightforward.

Treatment principles are:

1. Total rest is only necessary in the most severe cases.
2. A modification of sporting activity usually suffices, reducing frequency of sport and eliminating sports which are identified as provoking symptoms. Swimming and gentle cycling are usually permissible.
3. Institute a general flexibility programme concentrating on quadriceps and hamstring stretching. Do these gently to avoid producing pain.
4. Immobilisation should not be necessary.
5. *Do not inject.*
6. Persistent problems after skeletal maturation may benefit from excision of loose fragments of the tibial tuberosity.

Most cases occur in association with a growth spurt when bone is growing fast and muscles and tendons become tight. For prevention, during growth spurts a gentle stretching programme should be started and frequency of active sport reduced unless flexibility is maintained. Strengthening exercises should not be done if the musculotendinous units are tight.

229

Sinding–Larsen–Johansson disease

This is a traction apophysitis affecting the lower pole of the patella. It occurs in 11–13-year-olds. The causes, pathology, and treatment are the same as for Osgood–Schlatter's disease.

Plica syndrome

There are four named plicae in the knee which are normal vestigial remnants of embryonic membranes that divided the knee into separate cavities. They are present in 65% of normal people but occasionally can get trapped between patella and femur to cause pain. They can then become thickened and act like taut bands rubbing the medial femoral condyle joint surface. The commonest to cause symptoms is the medial plica, less commonly the suprapatellar plica.

The clinical picture includes:

- Pain in the front and medial side of knee, worse on activity.
- May be a painful arc from 15 to 40 degrees.
- Tenderness and sometimes a palpable band 1 cm medial to patella; tenderness spreads on to medial femoral condyle.
- May be visible on axial MRI scans

Treatment consists of:

1. Rest and avoidance of aggravating factors.
2. Non-steroidal anti-inflammatory drugs may help.
3. Specific stretching of patella retinaculum.
4. Correct patella tracking by strengthening vastus medialis. Avoid exercises through the painful arc.
5. If injection of a little local anaesthetic into the most tender area helps the pain it is worth injecting a little steroid.
6. Gradual return to sport.
7. Persistent problems require evaluation by MRI scan to exclude other intra-articular and extra-articular causes.
8. Arthroscopy will reveal the thickened plicae, which can be resected.

Patellofemoral joint disorders

The patellofemoral joint is subjected to enormous forces because of the long levers of the tibia and femur, and the retropatella surface is subject to forces equal to five times body weight when running. This is why the retropatellar articular cartilage is the thickest in the body. When the knee is straight the patella lies above the femoral articular surface. During flexion the patella has to get into the trochlear groove and then descends to end up adjacent to the intercondylar notch at full flexion. The area of weight-bearing on the patella changes during this movement. The movement requires fine control by the quadriceps musculature and if control is not good the patella does not track properly, causing areas of high and low pressure which can cause pain and further inhibit the muscles. The stability of the patella is therefore crucial.

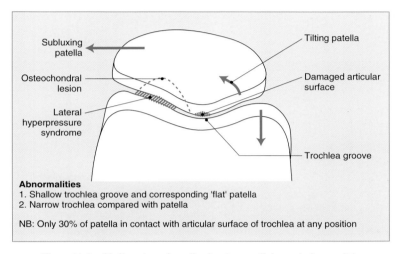

Figure 11.7   Skyline view of patella showing patellofemoral abnormalities

Patellofemoral joint stability depends on:

1. The bony contours, particularly the trochlear surface of the lateral femoral condyle which if underdeveloped will predispose to patella dislocation or subluxation.
2. Supporting ligaments, in this case the medial and lateral patella retinacula.
3. Muscular control by the quadriceps. Most of the quadriceps muscles insert via the quadriceps expansion into the superior pole of the patella. Because they arise from the femur their action is in line with the femur. The patella tendon, however, runs distally and laterally from the patella to the tibial tubercle, subtending an angle known as the Q angle. The vastus medialis obliquus inserts directly into the upper third of the medial border of the patella and controls the tracking of the patella by preventing it from being pulled laterally by the action of the rest of the quadriceps.

It is the key to understanding and managing patellofemoral pain (Figure 11.7).

231

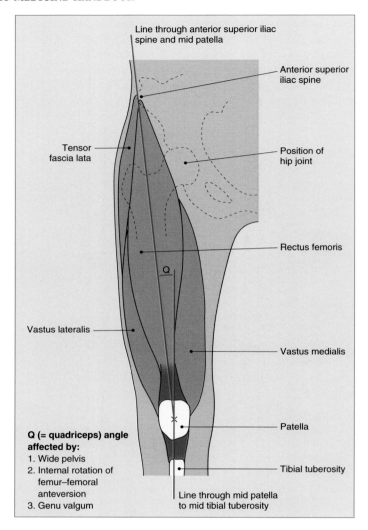

Line through anterior superior iliac spine and mid patella

Anterior superior iliac spine

Tensor fascia lata

Position of hip joint

Rectus femoris

Q

Vastus lateralis

Vastus medialis

Patella

Q (= quadriceps) angle affected by:
1. Wide pelvis
2. Internal rotation of femur–femoral anteversion
3. Genu valgum

Tibial tuberosity

Line through mid patella to mid tibial tuberosity

Figure 11.8   The Q angle

Patellofemoral joint tracking problems can be considered as due to:

1. Poor congruity or lax retinacula allowing patella subluxation or dislocation.
2. Tight lateral retinaculum causing maltracking and high lateral pressure syndrome.
3. Poor muscle control due to weak, uncoordinated quadriceps, especially vastus medialis obliquus, the lower, horizontal portion of vastus medialis.

232

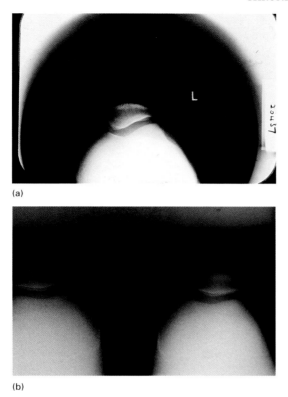

(a)

(b)

Figure 11.9   Patellae in groove

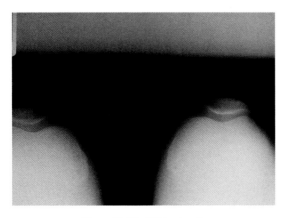

Figure 11.10   Tilting patella

233

4. Biomechanical problems such as persistent femoral anteversion leading to internal femoral rotation, compensatory external tibial torsion which causes an increase in the Q angle, and genu valgum. There may be external tibial torsion and hyperpronation – the so-called "miserable malalignment syndrome".

Clinical examination is based on *look, move, and feel*.
Look for:

- Quadriceps wasting, especially of the vastus medialis
- Patella tilting, rotation and subluxation
- Q angle at 20 degrees knee flexion: males less than 10 degrees, females less than 15 degrees (Figure 11.8)
- Squinting patellae due to internal rotation of femurs secondary to persistent femoral anteversion or weakness of hip external rotators
- External tibial torsion
- Examine feet for hyperpronation.

Move:

- Check range of hip movements, especially range of rotations with the hips extended. In persistent femoral anteversion there is excess internal rotation and limited external rotation
- Watch active knee movements for hitches in rhythm
- Test resisted movements for strength
- Test for generalised ligament laxity
- Check flexibility of quadriceps and hamstrings and iliotibial tract.

Feel:

- Shape, size, and position of patella
- Tenderness around patella and retropatellar surface
- Patellofemoral crepitus on movements
- Tightness of medial and lateral patella retinaculum
- Pushing patella laterally during flexion to look for apprehension in presence of subluxation
- Presence or absence of effusion.

Investigations comprise:

1. Plain X-rays, likely to be normal but exclude osteochondritis dissecans etc.
2. Skyline patella views show congruity of bony surfaces and patella tilt or subluxation (Figures 11.9, 11.10, 11.11).
3. Video gait analysis may reveal biomechanical abnormalities.
4. Isokinetic muscle testing may help prescriptive rehabilitation programme.

5. MRI scanning – axial views to show articular cartilage damage, intra-osseous oedema etc.

Treatment principles are:

1. Relieve pain.
2. Improve muscular control and coordination.
3. Correct patella maltracking.
4. Correct biomechanical errors.

General treatment of patellofemoral pain

1. Rest from sport, avoid kneeling, squatting, and stairs.
2. Non-steroidal anti-inflammatories.
3. Local heat.
4. Strengthen quadriceps with static straight leg raises.
5. Specific vastus medialis obliquus exercises.
6. Gentle introduction of dynamic quadriceps exercises, concentric before eccentric.
7. Correct maltracking with patellar stabilising brace or specific patella taping. Taping involves careful application of non-elastic tape around patella to control lateral glide, tilting, or rotation so that a half squat can be done without pain. The tape is left on during activities and changed when it loosens or symptoms return. It often makes the strengthening exercises more comfortable and easier.
8. Stretching programme for calves, hamstrings, quadriceps and hip muscles.
9. Correction of muscle imbalances around the hips.
10. Corrective orthoses if significant foot hyperpronation or supination.

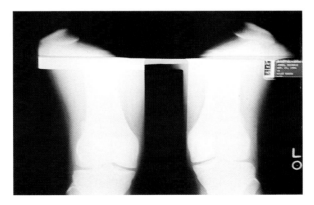

Figure 11.11   Bilateral patella subluxation.

Patella subluxation

This is most common in the presence of congenital joint laxity.

1. The patella is often small, very mobile, and sits high above the joint line – patella alta.
2. Subjectively the knee feels unstable and can often be dislocated at will.
3. Patella apprehension test is positive – pushing the patella laterally during knee flexion causes pain and apprehension.
4. Retropatellar surface may be tender.
5. If recent injury there may be tenderness over the stretched medial patella retinaculum.

High lateral pressure syndrome

Due to a tight lateral retinaculum, the patella is pulled laterally during flexion in spite of adequate vastus medialis obliquus (VMO). The patella subluxes and tilts over the lateral trochlear articular surface. There is high pressure on the articular surface which thins and patellofemoral osteoarthritis is the end result. Diagnosed by palpation of the patella which cannot be displaced medially due to the tight lateral retinaculum. The patella may be lower than normal – patella baja. There is retropatellar tenderness and frequently an effusion. Treatment in the early stages is by stretching of the lateral retinaculum, correction of patella tracking with tape. If symptoms persist, surgical lateral release will allow the patella to medialise.

Surgical treatment

1. Arthroscopic evaluation may show chondromalacia patella, a softening with fibrillation of the articular surfaces. This is often present in asymptomatic knees and seldom causes symptoms. Loose flaps of articular surface can be shaved.
2. A tight lateral retinaculum can be released.
3. Significantly thickened asymptomatic plicae can be excised.
4. In persistent patella subluxation or maltracking surgical realignment can be done. Medialisation of the patella tendon and reefing of the medial retinaculum will correct the Q angle. Proximal realignment of the patella is an alternative.
5. Macquet's osteotomy – lifting the anterior tibial cortex forwards advances the tibial tubercle so that the retropatellar pressures are reduced.
6. Patella resurfacing procedures using carbon fibre pads have had varied results.

The majority of patients with anterior knee pain or overuse problems can be adequately treated by correction of sporting techniques, modification of the training programmes, and simple conservative measures. It requires patience to recover from many of these injuries. Progression of exercises should be gradual and well controlled. Surgery should be the last option.

It is not sufficient just to treat the symptoms, but to identify the cause. Once you can eliminate the cause, the patient can return to their sport knowing that the risk of a recurrence has been substantially reduced.

Prevention is better than treatment.

12 Pelvic and groin pain

ROGER G HACKNEY

Introduction

The groin is an ill defined anatomical area lying between the abdomen and the thigh. Groin injuries are not especially common, accounting for roughly 5% of patients attending sports injury clinics. In the game of soccer, however, injury to this area is more common than this figure suggests. Groin injuries justify their reputation for being difficult to treat, and are responsible for a disproportionately large proportion of time lost from competition and training.

Chronic groin pain in sportspeople has a very large number of possible causes from the specialties of orthopaedics, urology, general surgery, and gynaecology. When considering an athlete with groin pain, it is important to remember to retain an open mind and not concentrate solely on sporting causes of groin pain (Table 12.1).

Table 12.1 Differential diagnosis of groin pain

Musculoskeletal causes
Adductor muscle sprain acute, chronic
Osteitis pubis
Hip joint; osteoarthritis, tears of the acetabular labrum, loose bodies
Psoas muscle and tendon pathology
Low back problems, spondylolysis, disc problems

Abdominal/genital causes
Sports hernia
Testicle inflammation, infection, tumour, benign or malignant
Prostate gland
Bowel problems, appendicitis, large bowel
Hernia

Gynaecological causes
Ovarian causes of pain
Vaginal prolapse

Adductor muscle sprain

The adductor group of muscles run from the pelvis into the femur. They bring the leg across towards the midline. The most common injury to the groin is a sprain of the adductor muscles. These occur when sudden abduction (away from the midline) stretch applied to the hip joint results in a sprain at the musculotendinous junction of the adductors. Common mechanisms are in a football tackle or sliding on a slippery surface. The pain and swelling can be easily located to the adductor muscles.

Examination There is adductor spasm, with localised tenderness and swelling at the site of injury.

Investigation MRI or ultrasound scans may show a haematoma in grade 2 or 3 sprains.

Treatment This is as for any muscle sprain, with the RICER principle (Rest, Ice, Compression, Elevation, Rehabilitation). Stretching is an important part of the rehabilitation, and a variety of stretches affecting different parts of the muscle should be used.

The problem may become chronic with repeated injury. Ultrasound scan may show changes in and around the tendon. A comprehensive rehabilitation programme should be used, but if after 2–3 months the injury has not settled, then division of the tendon with removal of scar tissue gives good relief.

Chronic pain in the adductor muscles is not only caused by recurrent sprains. If there is no history of repeated injury then the diagnosis must be questioned. The most likely cause of the pain is a sports hernia.

Other muscles around the pelvis

The rectus femoris, rectus abdominus, pectineus, and sartorius are all susceptible to injury. The diagnosis must be confirmed by careful examination and pain relief followed by rehabilitation as described in Chapter 22.

Sports hernia

The syndrome of a weakness of the posterior inguinal wall without a readily palpable hernia causing chronic groin pain is surprisingly common. The pain from this syndrome is diffuse and quite variable in distribution, but the diagnosis can be made from the history and examination. The condition does not respond well to conservative measures, including prolonged rest.

Despite a number of reports in the scientific literature, the syndrome only recently achieved widespread recognition. The syndrome of an early direct inguinal hernia in sportsmen can be treated with surgical repair to give excellent results. The average duration of symptoms to presentation in my patients averages 20 months with a range of 6 weeks to 5 years. Excellent results can be achieved with surgical repair, over 80% returning to competition and all patients reporting improvement.

A wide variety of sports have been associated with this injury. It is most common in soccer.

History The groin pain may be of gradual onset, or develop after a sudden tearing sensation. The initial pain is often not severe enough to prevent the player from completing his match or event, but becomes an unpleasant nagging ache during the next few hours. Soccer players frequently suffer adductor muscle pulls but notice that this pain is felt more strongly and deeper than the "groin strains" he has had in the past.

The player becomes unable to train between matches, and the groin pain comes on earlier in a game. The soccer player is substituted as the symptoms progress. The groin pain becomes progressively more severe to the stage where pain is felt at rest with a painful limp on walking.

The pain is diffuse and ill defined. Early symptoms include pain around the insertion of the adductors, midline, and the inguinal region. Pain usually centres upon the inguinal region but may spread laterally along the inguinal ligament, proximally into the rectus muscles, and even across to the opposite side and distally into the perineum.

A history of reproduction of pain on coughing or sneezing is very helpful in making the diagnosis. Testicular pain is a feature in about 30% of cases to the extent where this has led to investigation for testicular abnormality. Testicular pain may be due to irritation of nerves running through this area; certainly nerve entrapment in this region has been reported as a cause

---

Symptoms found in history of a sports hernia

- Deep aching groin pain after sport
- Pain on kicking, sprinting, or twisting and turning, and sit-ups
- Unable to train between matches
- Pain felt in the groin spreading to midline, between legs and out to the side
- Pain in the testicles and low back
- Coughing and sneezing reproduce pain
- Unable to lift both legs from the bed when lying flat

of chronic groin pain. Patients undergoing surgery to their testicles do not note any improvement nor does the enforced rest relieve symptoms. Surgery to the inguinal canal produces immediate testicular relief.

Examination Examination findings depend upon how much rest and treatment the sportsman has received. The pain disappears on prolonged reduction of athletic activity, only to recur with the same intensity on resuming training.

There is adductor spasm with tenderness around the belly and origin of the group. However, the tenderness is not the true site of the pain. The symphysis pubis and pubic tubercle of the affected side are tender to palpation. The inguinal rings and cough impulse must be assessed via the scrotum, as external examination usually fails to detect a hernia. In the UK the lack of an obvious hernia has frequently led to the denial of any pathology when sufferers have been referred to a general surgeon who has not come across this condition. The area around the enlarged external inguinal ring is tender. The most useful part of the examination is when the mid inguinal canal is palpated. The patient usually confirms that the pain is worst there and his pain is aggravated by coughing. In severe cases this is an extremely painful procedure. The cough impulse is felt over a wider area and is diffuse, more of a bulge than the normal side. The testes should be formally examined to exclude local pathology.

Findings on examination

- Adductor spasm with patient lying on his back, and feet together with hips and knees flexed. One leg will not lie down as far
- Local tenderness of adductor muscle and origin
- Pubic symphysis and tubercle tenderness
- Examination of the hernial orifices via scrotum, and assessment of cough impulse
- If the cough impulse is not significant then the patient should exercise until the pain recurs then repeat the examination

---

Investigation Plain X-rays may show osteitis pubis.

Herniography has been used to detect the sports hernia. It may be useful for deciding whether bilateral symptoms are due to bilateral hernias or spread of pain. Herniography shows a generalised distension of the anterior abdominal wall extending around to the perineum. Real time, dynamic ultrasound can detect hernias in skilled hands.

Treatment Patients report a long term failure of all conservative treatment. These included stretching and strengthening exercises from physiotherapists in addition to electrical modalities. Local anaesthetic and steroid injections provide no lasting relief, if at all. Rest settles the pain, but it returns rapidly on resuming sport. Surgery is very effective.

Operative findings   Operative findings are more pronounced the more longstanding the condition. There is a weakening and thinning of the fascia where the abdominal wall meets the inguinal ligament. The weakness can amount to a direct hernia. With a short duration of symptoms the defect seems to be more to the medial end of the inguinal canal. The repair tightens up the weaknesses, drawing down good tissue to strengthen the attenuated tissues.

Return to sport   Early return to sport may cause an increase in recurrence. Soccer players have been known to undergo multiple surgical procedures. I recommend that patients gradually return to activity with stretching and non-weight-bearing exercise such as swimming or cycling after 3–4 weeks. Running commences at 4–5 weeks, with daily training usually possible at 6 weeks. A number of sportsmen report pulling in the groin during this period, which gradually settles. I tell them to expect this, and attribute this to settling down of the repair. It is important that rehabilitation following surgery includes stretching and strengthening exercises of the muscles around the pelvis. Full sit-ups are banned for several months as this can lead to the return of symptoms.

Aetiology

Several theories of causation of the sports hernia have been described. A reduction in internal rotation of the hip joint produces a shearing force across the pubic symphysis from continued adductor pull. Shearing across the pubic symphysis leads to stress on the inguinal wall musculature. The anatomical defects in the wall, i.e. the inguinal rings, may account for the predominance of this condition in the male. The stretching of the conjoined tendon and transversalis with tearing of these structures from the inguinal ligament accounts for the pain. An alternative theory is that it is simply a chronic stretching of the posterior inguinal wall due to the excess demands of sport. Anatomical texts have described variability in the depths of fossae outlined in herniography. It may be the case that those who fall victim to this syndrome are predisposed by naturally deep fossae.

Osteitis pubis

The name osteitis pubis means inflammation of the pubic symphysis. This is despite the fact that inflammation is not a histological finding!

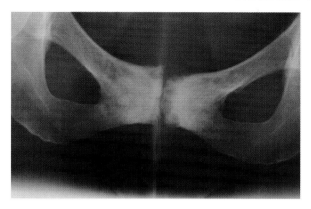

Figure 12.1 Osteitis pubis

The incidence of changes to the pubic symphysis on X-ray is higher in sportsmen, especially soccer players. Symptoms attributed to osteitis pubis are very similar to those produced by the sports hernia. X-ray changes lag behind the symptoms, although bone scans or MRI scans will show changes earlier. I do not consider that osteitis pubis is itself a common cause of groin pain; the pain tends to be more in the adductor region. Osteitis pubis is associated with the sports hernia. However, in rare cases it is possible for the changes to become so severe that instability between the pubic bones develops. An X-ray standing on one leg will show movement across the symphysis of greater than 4 mm. Surgical fusion of the joint may be curative.

Sacroiliac joint

This joint is the subject of much debate as to whether it is a source of pain in sportspeople. In my experience pain in the region of the sacroiliac joint may be associated with groin pain. Certainly bone scans have been hot in acute onset of symptoms, and the cause may be a stress fracture of the ridges of the joint surfaces. Changes in the sacroiliac joint have been described in soccer players with osteitis pubis, which may account for the associated low back pain. Manipulative therapists report reduction of groin pain on treating the sacroiliac joint. If the pubis symphysis does become unstable, even temporarily, in osteitis pubis, then there must be increased movement across the sacroiliac joint. I do not formally treat the sacroiliac joint in looking at groin pain, but use physiotherapy in the form of muscular control of the pelvis in the general management of pain in this region.

Psoas tendon

The psoas muscle is the largest in the body, running from the lumbar spine across the pelvis over the hip joint into the top of the shaft of the femur. It flexes the hip joint and rotates the leg internally when the hip is extended. When the hip is flexed, the psoas produces external rotation. The psoas tendon is a thick flat tendon as it crosses the hip joint, protected from rubbing by a fluid sac or bursa. The tendon can become tight across the hip.

History A clunk is felt deep in the groin when the leg is rotated and flexed, for example as the trail leg crosses a hurdle. The clunk or snap can give rise to a deep ache. Occasionally the bursa becomes inflamed, causing a psoas bursitis. Psoas tendinitis is particularly common in hurdlers and martial arts exponents but can be found in any sportsperson.

Diagnosis of psoas tendinitis
● History of clunk or click in groin associated with ache
● Clunk caused by sport aggravating the pain
● Pain and clunk reproduced by stretching the psoas tendon
● Pain aggravated by flexing the hip from a position of extension and external rotation.

Examination Stretching the psoas tendon can reproduce the pain felt by those suffering this injury, and is used as a diagnostic test. The patient lies supine with the pelvis overlying the edge of the couch. The unaffected leg is flexed, knees to chest. The injured leg is extended, the examiner pushing the leg into further extension. This will reproduce the pain. Asking the patient to flex his hip against resistance makes the pain worse. In severe cases of sports hernia, this stretch is also painful, but the patient does not recognise the pain produced as the pain which he suffers.

Treatment A programme of stretching has a very high success rate. Occasionally supervision by a physiotherapist is required. The commonest reason for failure of stretching is a poor technique, which when corrected gives the desired result. Surgery to divide the tendon when stretching fails is rarely indicated but very successful.

Differential diagnosis

Other causes of clicking or clunking around the hip are:

● Psoas tendinitis or bursitis
● Loose bodies within the hip joint

244

- Tear of the acetabular labrum
- Trochanteric bursitis.

Trochanteric bursitis

The tensor fascia lata is a muscle arising from the iliac crest which partly inserts into the deep fascia around the thigh, the fascia lata. There is a thickening behind the greater trochanter which can flick over that bony prominence irritating a protective bursa. The sensation is quite different from the deep clunk in the groin of the psoas. The diagnosis is made by reproducing the pain behind the greater trochanter by pressing as the hip is flexed.

Treatment Initial treatment is stretching of the muscle and tendon. Local massage with a non-steroidal anti-inflammatory gel will help pain relief. This generally gives good results, but local injection of corticosteroid is occasionally required. As a last resort, surgical release can be very effective.

Hip joint pathology

Hip joint pain

- General nagging ache in groin
- Aggravated by sport, running, or martial arts
- Associated with stiffness of hip joint
- Pain referred to anterior thigh and knee
- May be a history of hip problems as a child.

Osteoarthritis of the hip joint

Perhaps because this is predominantly a disease of the elderly, it is often missed as the cause of groin pain in sportspeople. A history of a general aching in the groin associated with stiffness and exacerbation of pain at the extremes of range of movement is typical.

The stiffness is usually worst in the morning. The pain is worst on exercise, with an aching afterwards.

Examination The arthritic hip has a reduced range of motion in all planes. The sportsperson has pain at the end of the range of external rotation and abduction in particular. There will be a diffuse tenderness deep in the groin. The athlete usually presents before an altered gait develops.

245

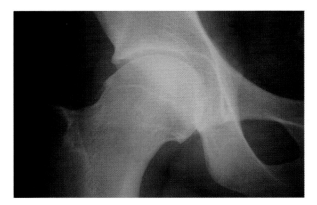

Figure 12.2   Early osteoarthritis of the hip joint

Investigation   A plain X-ray will show very early changes which include increased subchondral sclerosis, slight reduction in joint space, and curtain osteophytes around the femoral head. Subchondral cysts appear later. The findings may be quite subtle and need careful inspection. MRI scan may help confirm the diagnosis, although both MRI scan and bone scan are frequently normal or minimally changed. Arthroscopy of the hip may confirm the diagnosis.

Treatment   There is little that can be done to improve osteoarthritis at this stage. Moderation of activity is the key to management. Avoiding impact and contact sports and certain kicks in martial arts is essential. These patients require very careful counselling.

Acetabular labral tears

The acetabular labrum is a thick rim of dense fibrous tissue which provides extra stability. The labrum can tear, producing a flap which can interfere with the joint, giving a deep, painful clunk.

Arthroscopy of the hip is a well recognised technique which would confirm any changes of the articular surface in osteoarthritis. Loose bodies can be removed and any tears of the labrum can be trimmed arthroscopically.

Dislocation and subluxation of the hip joint

Dislocation generally requires a high degree of trauma, but subluxation has been described in adolescents with congenital hyperlaxity. Symptoms include a snapping or popping felt in the groin followed by aching. This is rare and requires a high index of suspicion.

246

Stress fractures of the pelvic bones

Stress fractures are a result of repetitive microtrauma which overcome local healing mechanisms. Pelvic stress fractures account for 1–2% of the total, but can be far more significant in terms of the harm they can cause. Fractures occur in the pubic rami or the proximal femur and, most seriously, the femoral neck.

The symptoms of a severe, deeply felt pain in the groin are of gradual onset. They follow an increase in training load or a long distance race. Weight-bearing is painful, and pain occurs at rest and at night. A sudden worsening may indicate a completion of the fracture. With this story athletes must be investigated urgently and *not* told to "run through" the pain.

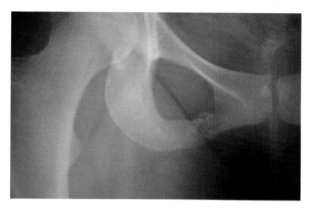

Figure 12.3   Pubic stress fracture

Investigation   The most common stress fracture of the pelvis involves the pubic rami. As with all stress fractures, the diagnosis can be made by plain X-ray after 3 weeks, but earlier on technetium bone scan or MRI scan.

Treatment   Stress fractures of the pubic rami can be treated with adequate rest in the expectation that they will heal without complication. The athlete can continue to exercise in non-weight-bearing sports when the stress fracture has settled sufficiently to allow walking. Stress fractures of the femoral neck are either seen on the superior or inferior surfaces of the femoral neck. The biomechanics of the femoral neck produce compression on the inferior aspect and tension on the superior surface. With rest, compression fractures can be expected to heal. Tension fractures, however, will complete across the femoral neck if the athlete continues to walk. This is an extremely serious situation as the fracture will not heal normally, and there is a risk that the femoral head will die. If the fracture is seen before completion then prophylactic fixation is necessary. If the fracture completes

247

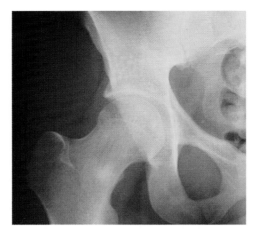

Figure 12.4   Stress fracture of the femoral head

then reduction and fixation must be performed. However, in published series no displaced fractures healed to produce a normal hip. In the worst case, the patient requires joint replacement.

Hip diseases of childhood: slipped upper femoral epiphysis and Perthes disease

In adolescents, groin pain may arise from disorders of the growing femoral head. They present with groin, thigh, and knee pain. The range of movement must be assessed and frog lateral X-rays taken. There is an interesting suggestion that the incidence of subclinical slipped upper femoral epiphysis may be increased with sporting activity.

Spondylolisthesis

Pain referred from the back may cause groin pain.

History   A diffuse pain which may or may not arise from the lumbar spine. Confusingly, there may be no back pain at all. The diagnosis is considered by excluding other causes of groin pain, and recognising that the pattern of pain does not fit any of those described in this chapter.

Examination   There is no local tenderness in the groin that can be palpated to reproduce the patient's pain. Back signs are very variable.

248

Investigations X-rays of the lumbar spine, particularly the oblique view, show the defect of the pars interarticularis. Bone scan or MRI will help determine whether the lesion is active. Trial injection of local anaesthetic and steroid under X-ray control will be diagnostic.

The spondylolisthesis is usually of L5.

Treatment Injection of local anaesthetic and steroid can also be therapeutic. Screw fixation of the spondylolisthesis will lead to abolition of groin pain.

Abdominal and pelvic organs

Appendicitis produces pain in the lower right abdomen. Acute onset of pain in this area with nausea, vomiting, and bad breath requires urgent medical consultation. The grumbling appendix may cause recurrent pain in the lower abdomen, but is felt above the groin region and very deep.

Prostate pain is generally felt deep in the perineum, and may be associated with pain on passing urine or blood in the sperm.

Urinary tract infections present with burning on passing urine. The discomfort associated with this may spread from the groin to the back.

Gynaecological causes of groin pain

A runner with a history of having two children reported a dragging sensation in the groin and between her legs which only occurred when she ran over 10 miles and was followed by an aching for some while afterwards. She was found to have a grade 1 prolapse. One gynaecologist refused to accept this as a cause of her symptoms, but she responded well to repair.

13 The lumbar and thoracic spine

MALCOLM TF READ AND ROGER G HACKNEY

Introduction

Spinal injuries account for up to 20% of sports injuries. Low back pain (LBP) is common in athletes and the general population. LBP is more common in high demand sports. Fortunately, the majority are self-limiting and settle within a few weeks. The significance of appropriate training of the musculature controlling the spine and correct posture is becoming more widely appreciated. Severe injuries causing damage to the spinal cord can have catastrophic results.

Injury prevention in sport

The doctor or physiotherapist who looks after the athlete has as much a responsibility for preventing injury as for treating the injuries that occur. Injury prevention depends on a knowledge of how injuries occur and what factors influence them. The incidence of spinal injury from contact sports has been reduced by altering the training methods and the rules of the game, and ensuring their enforcement.

Anatomy and biomechanics

The spine is made up of bones (the vertebrae) and soft tissues (ligaments and muscles).

The spine is comprised of 7 cervical, 12 thoracic, 5 lumbar and 5 (usually fused) sacral vertebrae. At the top, the cervical spine supports the head through the atlas (C1) while at the bottom the sacrum is anchored to the pelvis through stiff sacroiliac joints. A typical vertebra consists of a body, a ring, and three processes. The ring which surrounds the spinal cord is formed by the rear of the vertebral body, two pedicles with a transverse process to the side, a lamina either side at the back, and a central spinous process. In general the vertebral bodies increase in size from the top down. The anterior structures of the spine provide support for the trunk, the posterior structures function to protect neural structures and determine the direction of movement. The vertebrae articulate with one another via the intervertebral discs and the facet joints. The facet joints are about the size of the joint at the base of the thumb, and can be a significant source of pain.

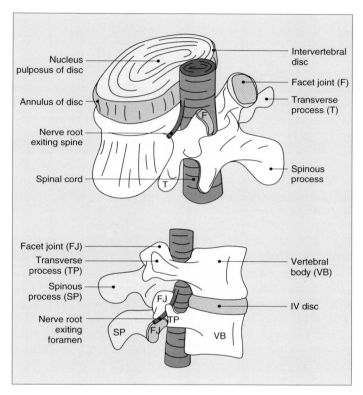

Figure 13.1   (top) Postero-oblique view of typical lumbar vertebra; (bottom) lateral view of adjacent vertebrae

Between each vertebra is an intervertebral disc which consists of an outer annulus which is predominantly collagen, and an inner nucleus pulposus. The central nucleus pulposus is composed of a matrix of protein, proteoglycans and water and acts as a very effective shock absorber – resisting compression and rotation, when constrained by the annulus fibrosus. In the lumbar spine the movements of flexion, extension and side flexion compress the disc on one edge and stretch the other. This movement pushes the nucleus pulposus towards the stretched surface; thus in flexion the nucleus pulposus will move posteriorly. As the annulus ages, the ability

251

to resist bulging is reduced and a tear of the annulus may result. *Intradiscal pressures are highest sitting and standing in a flexed position.*

The spinal ligaments and muscles act a little like guy ropes supporting a tent – and in doing so they help stabilise the spine. The spinal ligaments provide resistance to the extremes of range of motion and run the length of the spinal column, encasing the intervertebral discs. Their function is as a passive stabiliser of the spine whereas the spinal muscles act as both passive and dynamic stabilisers. The active anterior stabilisers of the spine are the psoas and the anterior abdominal muscles which are flexors and resist extension. The psoas works to flex the spine on fixed legs and will also extend the dorsal spine. The posterior paraspinal muscles are the active extensors of the spine. The curves of the shape of the spinal column are important in understanding the forces which might be applied to produce injury. The cervical spine is lordotic (concave when viewed from the side), the thoracic spine is kyphotic and the lumbar spine is again lordotic. The curves allow for a great deal of shock absorbency. The ideal posture places the head directly over the pelvis and feet, but having flexibility in the spine to move the centre of gravity of parts of the body and the whole body away from this position is essential for many sports. The anterior placement of the acetabulum to the spine allows for flexion at the hip, whilst maintaining spinal stability.

The reaction of bones and ligaments to an applied force is described as being anisotropic, which means that their mechanical properties are changed by the direction at which they are loaded. These tissues are also visco-elastic – if they are loaded slowly, they deform slowly; if they are loaded quickly, they are more resistant to deformity. A long bone such as the femur is excellent at resisting longitudinal compression forces applied rapidly, but poor at resisting rotational force. A vertebra is exceptionally strong in compression. For a given force, a rapid stretch applied to a ligament is less likely to cause failure than a slow stretch which goes beyond 4% of normal length.

Pain

Pain fibres are present in the annulus, ligaments, vertebral bodies, facet joint capsule, paraspinal muscles, neural tissues, and the sacroiliac joint. Pain in *any* of these structures can cause pain radiating from the lumbar spine into the sacroiliac buttock and the top of the hamstring. The precise determination of the source of pain is notoriously difficult. Compression of a nerve root gives pain in the distribution of that nerve, hence the term sciatica to describe nerve pain running the length of the back of the leg. This is a poor term which is widely misunderstood because pain from other sources radiating to the buttock and back of the thigh is often incorrectly called sciatica. Nerve root pain involving the 5th lumbar and 1st sacral roots affects the calf and sole of the foot respectively.

History

Back strains are produced by prolonged periods spent with the spine in a position of flexion. Excessive flexion forces may also lead to chronic low back pain. The pain may become continuous, but begins gradually and is characterised by periods of relief and exacerbation. The symptoms are mechanical, aggravated by exercise and relieved by rest, although morning stiffness is common.

Pain arising from an intervertebral disc – discogenic pain – is made worse by periods of prolonged sitting or standing. This corresponds with the measurably increased loads within the disc in these positions. Some patients will report a sudden severe incapacitating pain followed by leg pain after a seemingly minor twist. Any history of bladder incontinence, retention of urine, loss of control of the anal sphincter, or loss of erectile function in the presence of low back pain should prompt an urgent referral for a specialist surgical opinion.

Unremitting pain, worse at night, which wakes the patient, is suggestive of an infectious or neoplastic cause.

Activities involving extension and rotation of the spine may cause a spondylolysis, a stress fracture of the pars interarticularis. Pain aggravated by clinically stressing this movement is helpful in determining the diagnosis.

The spinal canal and/or nerve outlet foramen is narrower in some individuals than others. If this reduced space is restricted even more, by degeneration, disc prolapse, or other space occupying lesion, then the symptoms of spinal claudication may result. The typical story is of pain and paraesthesia in the lower legs brought on by walking or running, relieved by rest and forward flexion. Patients may be able to cycle without producing pain but not walk.

Examination of the spine

The examination begins by observing the patient walking into the treatment room and posture whilst standing and sitting. Watching the patient undressing can be very informative.

Standard examination follows the pattern **look**, **feel**, **move**, and **special tests**, beginning with the patient standing.

253

Posture

Look at the posture both standing and sitting. Good posture is highlighted by a gentle kyphotic curve in the thoracic region, and gentle lordotic curves in the cervical and lumbar spines. A patient with nerve root pain will stand with the affected leg flexed at the hip and knee with reduced weight-bearing on that side. Poor posture with slouching tends to result in the development of an increased thoracic kyphosis. A **scoliosis** is a lateral curvature to the left or right.

Scoliosis may be due to an abnormal spinal growth pattern, as a protection against pain, or can occur simply due to leg length discrepancy. It is relatively common in adolescence, with an incidence of 4% – girls more than boys – and it is typically painless.

The best test to demonstrate any rotational element of the curve is to ask the subject to bend forwards and place both hands together between the knees. A functional scoliosis will straighten. The chest wall may reveal asymmetry with a structural abnormality. An adolescent who appears to have a major scoliosis or where curvature is increasing should always be referred for a specialist opinion. An adolescent with a painful scoliosis may have a large disc protrusion or a more serious spinal disorder and should also be referred for an urgent specialist opinion.

Leg lengths

Leg lengths should be checked – both the true leg length anterior superior iliac spine (ASIS) to medial malleolus) and the apparent leg length (umbilicus to medial malleolus). Osteopaths are taught to call rotations of the ilium (anterior spine anterior, or posterior) as leg length discrepancies, so that often their description of a short leg does not reflect a true short leg but a possible functionally short leg. Only X-ray on a grid scale with pronation corrected is accurate for true leg length discrepancy.

Feel

In a patient with a **spondylolisthesis** there may be a palpable shelf in the lower lumbar spine where one spinous process (typically L5) sticks out backwards beyond the others (i.e. L4).

Spinal movements

The spine moves in forward flexion, rotation, extension, and lateral flexion (side to side bending). A simple method of quantifying the range of motion is to state the reach of finger tips in flexion and lateral flexion. There is normally a smooth rhythm of movement of the lumbar spine; patients with low back pain typically straighten the spine first, then as the last movement straighten the spine on the pelvis. A catch or sideways flick is an indication of mechanical disturbance.

The very stiff back may indicate ankylosing spondylitis (AS) or degenerative changes. It is common for AS patients to be unable to stand with their back against a wall and then to touch the wall with the back of their head – a useful screening test, as is an assessment of maximal chest expansion – suspect AS if chest expansion is less than 5 cm.

Extra spinal movement tests

There are two tests which provoke greater spinal extension than is normally tested and thus test for pain due to pathology in the facet joints or from pars interarticularis lesions. These are:

1. *The one-legged hyperextension test.* Stand on one leg, raise the contralateral knee towards the chest and lean back. Rotation adds greater strain.
2. Leaning backward, try to reach the opposite achilles tendon.

Hip movements

Pain from the hips may radiate to the buttock, groin, and knee; therefore all patients with spinal symptoms should be examined to exclude hip pathology. If hip pain is present it may be additional to the spinal problem but it warns the examiner that any manipulative manoeuvres which might be considered should not use the hip as a lever.

Dural stress tests

The straight leg raising (SLR) test is performed with the patient in a supine position, the examiner stabilising the pelvis with one hand and raising one leg by the heel with the knee straight with the other hand. The test is positive if it reproduces the patient's leg pain, particularly below the knee, or if it reproduces radicular symptoms such as tingling and pins and needles. If the test produces back pain only the test is considered negative for nerve root irritation. Pain produced at 70 degrees and beyond may be due to sciatic nerve deformation beyond the roots and may not be due to nerve root irritation but irritation outside the spinal column.

Two modifications can be added to the SLR test. When the extended leg is raised to a point just short of producing pain, dorsiflexion of the foot will reproduce the sciatic pain. In the second, the knee and hip are both flexed to 90 degrees and then the knee is slowly straightened. A positive test occurs if pain in the leg is produced.

The bowstring test was popularised by McNab. The straight leg is raised until pain is produced and then the knee is flexed slightly which reduces the symptoms. Finger pressure in then applied to the popliteal space over the popliteal nerve and causes painful radicular symptoms to reappear. Palpating the hamstring tendons is painless; protestation of pain provides information concerning the patient's reliability.

The Valsalva manoeuvre (exhaling against a closed glottis) also commonly produces lumbar pain with acute dural irritation.

The slump test involves examining the patient in the seated position with the knees hanging down and the patient slouched forwards (with an exaggerated kyphosis) with chin to chest. The knee is now extended while the hip remains flexed at 90 degrees. The patient may complain of leg pain or radicular symptoms and may try to extend the hip to reduce tension. Reduction of the pain by neck extension gives a positive result.

The well leg/cross leg raising test is carried out by elevating the extended unaffected leg. Reproduction of sciatic pain in the opposite (symptomatic) leg is strong presumptive evidence of a prolapsed intervertebral disc, particularly a large prolapse medial to the root.

The femoral nerve stretch test is performed with the patient in the prone position, by extending the hip with the knee flexed to 90 degrees. The well leg raising test can also be used with the femoral nerve stretch test.

The SLR and the slump test will usually be positive when there is a prolapsed intervertebral disc or adhesions of the nerve root or dura. SLR pain made worse with the SLR test but not with the slump test suggests peripheral nerve adhesions such as the so-called 'hamstring syndrome', where there is restriction of movement of the sciatic nerve either through the obturators or piriformis or a bowing of the nerve around the origin of the biceps femoris at the ischial tuberosity. The hamstring syndrome may be treated by nerve stretching techniques (adverse neural tension) or the resistant case by surgical release.

Nerve root irritation

It is important to look for signs of a nerve root irritation with reduced motor (myotome) power or altered dermatomal sensation during the examination. It is essential in all cases of back pain to examine for normal perineal sensation and normal sphincter contraction to ensure a serious spinal cord or cauda equina compression lesion is not missed.

Table 13.1 identifies the muscles and their nerve root innervation which should be checked during the examination.

Beware if more than two nerve roots appear to be involved. This is unusual with disc lesions, and other causes such as peripheral neuritis associated with diabetes or a neurological disorder, or a space occupying lesion in the spinal canal, should be considered.

Table 13.1 Muscle innervation

Muscle	Nerve root(s)
Psoas	L1/2
Quadriceps	L3/4
Tibialis anterior	L4
Extensor hallucis longus	L5
Extensor digitorum longus	L5/S 1
Extensor digitorum brevis	L5/S 1
Peronei	L4/5
Calf (tip toe)	S1
Hamstrings	(L5), S1/2
Glutei	S1/2
Anal sphincter[a]	S3/4

[a] Loss of control of urinary or anal sphincters or loss of perineal sensation (S3/4) requires **emergency surgery**.

Other mechanical derangements

Facet joint and sacroiliac joint

Clinically separating painful facet joints from sacroiliac joint dysfunction is very difficult and the following tests are not diagnostic but may be indicative. This is because all these tests stress both the facet joints and the SI joints at the same time.

Facet joint rocking   With the patient prone, the ilium is pulled posteriorly whilst the butt of the other hand holds down the transverse process of the L5 vertebra, thus allowing the facets of the sacrum to be impinged into the facets of the adjacent L5 vertebra. This is then repeated rocking L5 into L4 etc. The examiner tests each segment at a time and then assesses the other side.

Facet joint rolling   If there are no signs of dural tension then rolling the supine patient into a ball and taking both legs towards first one shoulder and then the other will gap the facet joints and if there is capsular irritation then this will produce pain.

Local palpation   The facet joints lie level with the gaps between the spinous processes, and local pressure about 2 cm from the midline may be tender. Rocking the spinous process only shows the dysfunctional level not the underlying cause.

The sacroiliac joint (SIJ)

The synovial SIJ has an auricular shape and although it does have a lining of articular cartilage it has an irregular surface and ligamentous attachments

within its joint. It moves in *rotational* plane by a few millimetres. The movement of the sacrum within the iliac wings is nutation, a nodding movement. The SIJ transmits impact loads up from the legs to the spine.
   The following tests may indicate SIJ dysfunction.

The Piedallu test   Place both thumbs on either side of one SIJ. Now ask the patient to raise the knee on the same side towards the chest. The posterior superior iliac crest should now rotate downwards in the normal way but may elevate or fix with SIJ dysfunction.

Pelvic spring   With the patient lying, distracting or compressing the anterior wing of the ilium will produce the opposite on the posterior structures. This is thought to be a test for the SIJ but quite obviously when one can reduce the pain from this test by supporting the L4/5 segments other structures must move. SIJ dysfunction is often seen in women both during pregnancy and around the time of the period, and it can often be reduced by sacral manipulative techniques and perhaps by sclerosant therapy.

Sacroiliac stress tests   With the patient supine the hip is flexed and a posterior compression and internal rotation force is applied. Pain over the SIJ is indicative. With the hip in full flexion and the force directed towards the opposite shoulder, the stress is thought to be sacrotuberous. In the mid-range, the stress is thought to be sacroiliac, and with the knee being in tension, towards the mid-opposite thigh, the stress is in the iliolumbar ligaments and is directed towards the SIJ.

Other tests

Abdominal palpation and auscultation   A history of pain brought on by walking and relieved by rest suggests claudication – either neurological or vascular. In the older person, especially with a history of vascular/cardiac problems, the abdomen should be checked for an abdominal aortic aneurysm.

Coccygeal palpation   A fall on the base of the spine may damage the sacrococcygeal ligaments. Sitting and full flexion are painful.

Rectal and vaginal examination   Intrapelvic lesions occur and any suggestion of intrapelvic or rectal causes should be accompanied by the relevant examination.

Investigations for low back pain

X-ray

Radiographs are the most common investigation performed. Plain antero-posterior X-rays may show bony abnormalities such as degenerative changes, spondylolisthesis (slippage of one bone against the next), Scheuerman's disease, traction spurs, fractures, and, of course, tumours. Reduced space between vertebrae is evidence of disc degeneration. Oblique X-rays show a spondylolysis and a spondylolisthesis. Any abnormality seen on an X-ray must be considered with *the whole clinical picture*. **They are rarely useful in the diagnosis of the cause of low back pain,** as normal, asymptomatic people have a similar degree of abnormal findings.

Bone scan

A bone scan involves injecting a radiolabelled substance, technetium 99, which is taken up by active bone into the blood. This is a non-specific test which demonstrates areas of increased bone turnover including abnormalities such as trauma, infection, inflammation, and tumour. An active spondylolysis may be picked up more accurately by a single photon emission computed tomography (SPECT) scan, a special form of bone scan.

Computerised axial tomography (CAT) scan

Useful in assessing fractures, tumours, and to a lesser extent the inter-vertebral disc. It will show a spondylolysis (especially if a reverse angle gantry is used).

Magnetic resonance imaging (MRI) scan

MRI scanning has become the gold standard investigation for many conditions throughout medicine. The commonly used scan gives a clear picture of the body as if a slice had been cut through it. MRI scanning detects varying amounts of water or fat in tissue, hence it will pick up oedema, excess tissue fluid produced by inflammation from any source, whether injury, infection, tumour etc. The scans still need to be interpreted in the light of the clinical picture. Otherwise normal, asymptomatic spines will show a range of abnormalities associated with pathological conditions. Gadolinium may be injected to differentiate between a disc prolapse and scar tissue.

259

Chronic disorders of the thoracic and lumbar spine

The common chronic disorders which are typically seen in sportspeople are summarised in Table 13.2.

Table 13.2   Disorders of the thoracic and lumbar spine commonly diagnosed in athletes

Typical age	Diagnosis	Associations
Child (up to 11)	Spondylolysis – a pars interarticularis fatigue fracture	Absent in newborn. Occurs in young gymnasts and ballet dancers, and possibly idiopathically
	Atlantoaxial instability	Down's syndrome
Adolescent (12–18)	Idiopathic adolescent scoliosis	Occurs in 5% of all children, commoner in girls, not painful and not related to injury. Should be referred for specialist orthopaedic opinion
	Scheuermann's disease	Growth disorder of the end plate of the vertebra; sometimes painful and may result in kyphosis
	Interspinous ligament compression syndrome	Occurs in gymnasts and acrobats with marked spinal hyperextension; gives perimenstrual backache
	Adolescent prolapsed IV disc	Painful scoliosis with restricted straight leg raise
	Spondylolysis (pars interarticularis fatigue fracture uni- or bilateral)	Occurs in young soccer players, gymnasts and butterfly swimmers, tennis players and cricketers
	Spondylolisthesis (forward slipping of one vertebra on another)	A small slip (grade I) may occur with a spondylolysis (above) and may result in a step in the spine on inspection and palpation
	Mechanical back pain	Causes include an annular disc tear, disc herniation, facet joint arthritis, tears of the posterior lumbar ligaments – the inter- and supraspinous ligaments, muscle injuries
	Spondylolysis pars interarticularis fatigue fracture	Cricket – fast bowling – and javelin throwing. Contact sports
		Possibly tennis serving
	Prolapsed IV disc	Flexion/rotational injury
	Ankylosing spondylitis	HLA B27 +ve in 40% of cases
	Sacroiliac joint sprain	Running, soccer, and sudden impact sports
Middle aged (40–54)	Prolapsed IV disc	Flexion/rotational injury
	Lumbar spondylosis	Degenerative changes in the facet joints and discs
Mature adult (55 +)	Spinal stenosis	Gives spinal claudication – leg weakness with pain on exercise
	Lateral canal stenosis	Gives sciatica aggravated by exercise and extension
	Degenerative spondylolisthesis	Forward slip of one vertebra on another with subluxation of the facet joints
	Paget's disease	Bone pain and spinal stenosis symptoms
	Metastatic deposits	Unremitting bone pain at rest and with activity

260

Spondylolysis and spondylolisthesis

These are common causes of low back pain in the athletic population. Never reported in the newborn, they seem to be a product of an upright posture. A spondylolysis is a defect of the pars interarticularis, classified by aetiology into:

1. Dysplastic.
2. Isthmic, subdivided into lytic, pars elongation, and acute fractures.
3. Degenerative.
4. Traumatic.
5. Pathologic.

A spondylolisthesis is a slippage of one vertebra against the next caused by a bilateral pars defect.

Physical activity is a major cause of isthmic spondylolysis. Gymnasts, fast bowlers in cricket, soccer players, and close family relatives of those afflicted all have a very much higher incidence compared with just 5% of the average population. The majority with spondylolysis and spondylolisthesis are asymptomatic, but the incidence of symptomatic lesions is higher in athletes. Symptoms include low back pain radiating to buttocks and hamstrings, and occasionally nerve root irritation leading to groin pain or more distal leg pain.

Initial investigation is by plain X-ray, the standard anteroposterior, lateral, and coned lateral are augmented by oblique views. Sclerosis, elongation, or a defect may be seen within the pars. Slippage may be unilateral, instability will be seen on flexion/extension views. Activity within the pars is confirmed by bone or SPECT scan. CAT or MRI scan provide only limited additional information. An injection of local anaesthetic under X-ray control may prove diagnostic if pain is abolished. Serial investigation may show a gradual elongation of the pars before a stress fracture develops. The classification depends upon the percentage slip of one vertebra against the next.

Treatment

Conservative The majority are asymptomatic. Young people frequently settle with appropriate rest from exercise together with back and abdominal strengthening exercises. Relief from hamstring pain is a good indication of resolution of symptoms or even healing of a spondylolysis. Symptoms may respond to local anaesthetic and steroid infiltration under X-ray control.

Surgical A symptomatic spondylolysis may require surgical fixation. Direct repair with internal fixation can be effective, although failure of bony union may result in recurrence of symptoms. Any degree of slippage is treated with

261

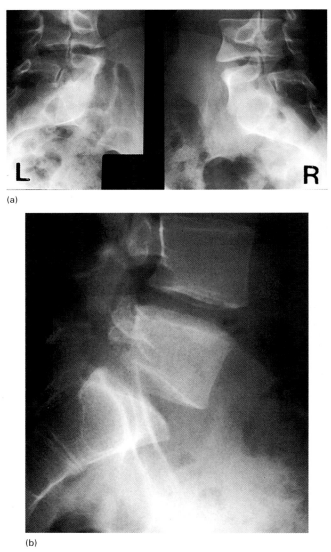

(a)

(b)

Figure 13.2   (a) Bilateral L4–5 and L5–S1 spondylolysis; (b) L45 spondylolisthesis – slippage of L4 on L5

fusion in situ. Spinal decompression may be required for any neurological symptoms.

Hamstring pain

Hamstring pain and spasm is frequently found in association with a spondylolisthesis. This is a product of a postural reflex to stabilise the

262

painful segment. The spasm is thought to be an attempt to readjust the body's centre of gravity which has slipped forwards. The pelvis is extended posteriorly.

Hamstring spasm frequently accompanies spinal pathology. The differentiation between local trauma in the muscle and a response to spinal pathology can be surprisingly difficult. A straight leg raise can give rise to pain from either source.

Causation of hamstring pain

- **Hamstring pathology**
  A history of a sudden onset of pain within the muscle associated with a specific movement
  Specific localised tenderness
  A history of bruising or swelling in the muscle
  Positive ultrasound or MRI scan
  Reproduction of pain with various hamstring stretches (see Chapter 2)
  Reproduction of pain with various hamstring isometric tests
- **Spinal pathology**
  History of altered sensation in the calf/lateral side of the foot
  Associated low back ache
  Spinal movements restricted
  Pain eased by spinal mobilisation/stretches
  Positive slump test. (Sit the patient erect on the edge of a couch with legs dependent. Extend the painful leg to the point of pain. Ask the patient to slouch (slump) with neck flexed, chin on chest. An increase in the pain with which the patient presents suggests a spinal cause of pain.)

Coccygeal pain

A ring cushion and occasionally posterior mobilisation of the coccyx may help as will steroid injections of the sacrococcygeal ligaments and, rarely, surgical excision.

Treatment of low back pain

Rest

As with any athlete, rest means relative rest, avoidance of aggravating activity. Analgesics, gradual mobilisation, and return to function via appropriate exercises will provide relief of symptoms within a few weeks for the vast majority of those with mechanical low back pain. Most backs

263

get better with conservative management and repeat scans show reduction in prolapsed discs over time.

Manipulation

There are various manipulative techniques – Cyriax, Maitland, Osteopathic, Chiropractic, Mulligans etc. – all of which may prove successful. It is probable that a disc lesion does not respond well to manipulation, whereas a facet joint or the facetal element of a disc problem will. SIJ manipulation can also be successful. There is discussion as to when mobilisation, which is a gentle rocking of a joint, finishes and manipulation which has an end point thrust begins. In practical terms this will inevitably depend on the patient, who will either be too sensitive to allow the joints to reach end point, and thus only permit mobilisation, or will relax enough to permit manipulation. However, one must be careful when assuming that we are absolutely symmetrical creatures, for too many manipulations to correct a non-painful, probably non-pathological asymmetry, can produce ligamentous laxity and further problems.

Traction

The idea is to pull the vertebrae apart so that a negative pressure effect is exerted on the disc, trying to reduce disc herniation. Traction can be given daily or every other day; the kilo-pull will be increased as required by the therapist. There may be short term relief, but little evidence of long term benefit.

Exercise treatment

Extension exercises (extension McKenzie) These may be carried out lying or standing, and either straight or with a side flexion. They should be used for patients aggravated by flexion movements. They should not be used for extension orientated problems. A trial of extension should be carried out to see if the pain peripheralises down the leg or develops in the leg during the trial.

Flexion exercises (flexion McKenzie) These are carried out by the patient pulling their knees to their chest and stretching the low back into flexion. This treatment is used to treat facet joint pain, and also for L5/S1 collar stud type disc prolapses. The addition of gapping rotations (rolling knees to one side or hanging one leg over the other) is thought to help painful facet joints, lateral canal stenosis, and SIJ pain. Care should be taken with flexion orientated problems.

264

Treatment based on adverse neural tension signs

These techniques have been popularised by physiotherapists who believe that a nerve trapped by a bony stenosis, adhesions, or scar tissue may be freed by gentle stretching techniques. These therapists are trained in eliciting the signs of adverse neural tension and the techniques for treating this condition.

Posture

Probably 80% of management of painful backs is the correct adjustment of posture for the individual, and correct posture may cure and prevent recurrences of many back conditions. Not every back responds to the same postural correction. Thus a flexion orientated problem will need extensions to improve and prevent disc creep. Facet joint pain and L5/S1 prolapsed intervertebral discs will require pelvic tilting to flatten the lordosis. However, the disc lesion may require pelvic tilt to start with, but as the disc regresses it will then require extension exercises. A thoracolumbar disc may have a compensatory low lumbar lordosis so that the adjustment of posture will be extension thoracolumbar, but pelvic tilt at the lumbosacral junction. Too much postural advice is given on general terms without taking into account the variations within and between backs. Some backs may have to be used in neutral, emphasising neither extension nor flexion.

Aids to posture

- **To increase extension**
  Sleep on hard mattress, floor, futon
  Kneel on chairs
  Low chair, high desk. Raise computer screen, sit with one knee drawn under chair
  "Wedge" cushion on chair. Cushion in small of back. Lumbar roll. Towel around waist at night
  Drive upright with bent arms
  Stand with weight towards balls of feet. Sit and stand tall. Slump in extension
  Stand with legs wide apart to lose height and lean pelvis into "washing sink", so forward lean is with extended spine
  Back in extension when bending or lifting

- **To decrease extension**
  Soft mattress
  Prop/sit on edge of table/bar stool. Use shooting stick
  Raise one foot 6–8 inches, i.e. foot rail in pub
  Stand with weight towards heels
  Back in neutral when bending or lifting

Lifting

Bending increases intra-abdominal pressure but, rather like a dam wall, the spine counteracts this by a convex surface (lordosis) so that a neutral to lordotic spine is required. Strong abdominal muscles will help to splint the spine in this position but too many types of abdominal exercises will harm the spine, i.e. straight leg raises force extension. Crunches force flexion and rotation. Too many diagrams show the spine during lifting being splinted and the knees and hips bent, but the buttocks tucked under the spine. Most people cannot lift from this position without flexing the spine. So the bent position must have an extended or neutral back but the buttocks should be pushed backwards, feet wide apart so that the forearms can be rested on the thighs. This is how weight-lifters lift, and how labourers in fields bend all day. This posture must be adopted for the slightest flexion load, even cleaning the teeth.

Training with weights

The back must be locked into neutral, preferably extension, even when sitting. The moment this position cannot be held, the exercise should stop. If the back is being thrown into the exercise then the muscles being trained have fatigued sufficiently for other muscles to be recruited and so the target muscles are no longer being trained. If extension cannot be held then the weight is too heavy or the person is in the wrong technical position for the exercise.

Leg length discrepancy

Most patients can adjust to 1–2 cm of shortening and do not require shoe raises or other treatment. However, bigger discrepancies have been associated with back symptoms long term and may benefit from specialist treatment.

Epidural injections

These injections appear to desensitise the nerve irritation over a few days rather than act as short term analgesics. An epidural will not reduce the mechanical prolapse, only inflammation or nerve sensitivity. The caudal epidural, popularised by Cyriax with 0.5% procaine, allows the patient to walk away and be treated as an outpatient. A stronger solution may be given for intense pain by providing some short term analgesia, but higher concentrations will result in some motor weakness. In the acute prolapsed disc there will be accompanying oedema which increases the pressure on the dura and nerve root, potentially increasing any damage and neuropraxia, so that the addition of a steroid to the solution should reduce the increased inflammation, pressure, and pain. It may also help to prevent long term adhesions. The epidural does not reduce a herniated disc, and it is important to continue to be alert for any neurological deterioration of the patient. Paravertebral blocks are used for lateral canal entrapment of the nerve root. An injection of hydrocortisone and local anaesthetic into the lateral canal may be achieved by a paravertebral approach.

Indications for epidural injections

- Night pain
- Acute, severe pain for short term relief
- Sciatica uncontrolled by other treatments except rest
- Chronic sciatica when the cause is root irritation
- For diagnosis when there is a suggestion of dural irritation

---

Local steroid injections

Perifacetal injections of corticosteroids often relieve the acute episode and may, when combined with local anaesthetic, allow earlier manipulation to be carried out. Osteoarthritis of the facet joints may improve, possibly by reducing capsular inflammation with a local anti-inflammatory agent. In these cases it is important to know that the facet joint has been injected and facetal injections should be done under X-ray control.

Sclerosant injections

These have been popularised by orthopaedic physicians, but without mainstream acceptance. A solution of dextrose sclerosant diluted 50/50 with anaesthetic may be injected into the posterior lumbar ligaments and SIJ. This is thought to be particularly useful for ligamentous pain such as the unstable pelvis, which has a positive pelvic spring test. It has also been used by some doctors to help stabilise a spondylolisthesis or an unstable vertebral segment.

Ligamentous pain is worse at rest, first thing in the morning, after sitting for a long time, and after standing for a long time. Clinical examination usually shows a full range of spinal movements but there may be aching at the end of the range. There are no accompanying signs of disc prolapse, facet pain or dural adhesions.

Indications for sclerosants Ligament laxity with a positive pelvic spring, SIJ symptoms, chronic facet joint pain.

267

Surgery

Localising the source of low back pain is notoriously difficult. Surgery for the spine must address the definitive problem. Indications include a prolapsed intervertebral disc, spondylolysis and spondylolisthesis, and a tight spine, termed stenosis. Spinal stenosis or lateral canal stenosis are treated by spinal decompression. Return to high level competitive sport is doubtful, as the spine may be rendered less stable without fixation.

The indications for treatment of a prolapsed intervertebral disc are:

1. Cauda equina syndrome: loss of bowel and bladder control or altered perineal sensation indicates compression of the sacral nerve roots and must be relieved surgically as an emergency.
2. Neurological deficit which fails to resolve: weakness of foot eversion or loss of power of dorsiflexion of the foot which fails to resolve with conservative treatment.
3. Intractable pain in the leg.

Back pain is not a good indication for discectomy. Modern techniques of microdiscectomy give rapid relief of symptoms with minimally invasive surgery. The technique is highly specialised and a spinal surgeon should be sought.

A fusion for spondylolysis and spondylolisthesis will usually resolve symptoms and allow a return to sport.

The concept of segmental spinal instability is gaining support. MRI scans are helpful in making the diagnosis. Spinal fusion may control symptoms; other forms of surgery to use artificial ligaments to regain stability are still under investigation and their use in athletes is experimental.

Sacroiliac joint (SIJ) pain

The concept of the SIJ causing chronic low back pain is not generally accepted amongst mainstream orthopaedic opinion. Referred pain from other structures is probably the commonest cause of pain over the sacroiliac joint, but problems undoubtedly occur in athletes. Symptoms may be acute or chronic. A bone scan may show increased activity which settles with time. The differential diagnosis includes the rheumatological condition of sacroiliitis with its various causes.

There is some evidence that a stress fracture within the joint may cause the pain in some athletes. Examination may reveal signs described earlier. Treatment includes manipulation and mobilisation, stretching and pelvis muscle strengthening exercises, and sclerosant, local anaesthetic, and steroid injections.

Injuries of the dorsal spine and chest wall

Acute injury to the paravertebral/scapular muscles causes local pain. Treatment is by conventional means with a period of rehabilitation to restore pain-free range of motion. These injuries may take 3–4 weeks to settle. Any pain persisting beyond this time should be reassessed.

The **differential diagnosis** of thoracic pain includes the following:

- Referred pain from the thoracic spine, intervertebral disc injury
- Costovertebral joint injury
- Referral pain from neck
- Intrathoracic causes such as myocardial pain, reflux oesophagitis, pleural injury
- Fracture of rib either primary from trauma or stress fracture, or secondary fracture
- Subscapular crepitus, the washerboard scapula
- Costosternal joint pain (Tietze's disease).

The thoracic spine is splinted by the ribs and hence has a restricted range of motion. Movement includes flexion both forwards laterally and rotation. Overload or trauma may cause dorsal spinal dysfunction. A common cause of problems are the facet joints and the costovertebral joints. It is unusual for a disc displacement to occur in the thoracic spine area. Many problems are postural in origin, and are usually due to too much of a kyphosis.

X-rays of a kyphotic spine frequently reveal Schmorl's nodes. These reflect discal herniation into the body of a vertebrae and are probably of no clinical significance.

Scheuermann's osteochondritis occurs as a source of pain in young athletes. Scheuermann's kyphosis in the upper or mid thoracic spine by definition consists of at least three vertebrae with wedging, vertebral end plate changes, and disc narrowing. Findings include a round back posture with forward shoulder thrust and a tight lumbar spine on bending. Treat with relative rest, analgesia, and dorsal parascapular muscle strengthening. Postural correction reduces excess lumbar lordosis by pelvic tilt and leads to extension of the thoracolumbar junction. Extension exercises to the dorsal spine are encouraged.

Bracing is rarely indicated for a scoliosis, and should be managed under the care of a specialist in spinal deformity.

Referred pain from the thoracic spine

Pain from the thoracic spine may be felt over the spine locally, but is more often to one side of the spine or radiating around the chest wall. Pain is

269

often worse lying, better sitting or standing. The patient may sleep in a chair rather than a bed. Chest wall or anterior chest pain without spinal pain may occur. Twisting to one side and breathing may hurt.

Thoracic disc injury

The dermatomal distribution of thoracic nerves extends from the upper chest and arm to the groin. The thoracic nerve T10 refers to the umbilicus, and those of the thoracolumbar junction to the groin via the ilioinguinal nerve. Thoracic disc injury is associated with pain on lateral bending or rotation. MRI scan confirms the diagnosis. There are two options in the management of pain severe enough to give radicular symptoms or cord compression: wait and see or early surgery. There are no clear guidelines but this should be the responsibility of an appropriate orthopaedic or neurosurgical specialist. Nor are there clear guidelines as to when to allow a person to return to sport.

Costovertebral joint injury

The diagnosis can be made by indirect pressure on the rib reproducing pain localised to the costovertebral junction. The pain may be aggravated by respiration. Treatment includes various mobilisation techniques. The upper ribs move in a bucket handle plane whilst the lower ribs move in a pump handle plane, and mobilisation techniques employ this variance. A local injection of corticosteroid employing an image intensifier for guidance can be curative.

Ribs

Rib fracture

A rib fracture following trauma to the chest wall is confirmed by pressure over the rib away from the fracture site causing pain. X-ray confirms the diagnosis. A concern in contact sport is pneumothorax and tension pneumothorax, therefore a player must be removed from the field of play. An intercostal nerve block gives excellent pain relief.

Stress fracture

Sports associated with stress fracture of the ribs include rowing, canoeing, and golf. A bone scan will confirm the presence of increased bone turnover; plain X-ray should show simple callus formation.

270

An unpleasant injury from contact sport is one to the rib tip. A separation of anterior costal cartilage from the rib is very slow to heal and easily re-injured. Allow 9–12 weeks for this to resolve.

Vertebral body fracture

These occur as a result of falls and direct trauma. They are usually stable, with the exception of high energy injuries such as those occurring in riding and motorsport. Expert assessment is required.

Thorax injury

Cardiac compression from direct trauma has been reported. Downhill cyclists wear body armour for protection from such injury. Injuries to the chest wall and thorax are very common in tae kwon do. Up to 20% depression of the original depth of the chest wall causes no injury and is fully reversible.

Acknowledgment

We are grateful to Mr John K Webb of the University of Nottingham, for comments on the original manuscript.

14   Head and neck injury

NEIL BUXTON AND JOHN FIRTH

Introduction: the craniospinal problem

The brain, spinal cord, head, and neck form a complex risk unit which represents the greatest single area of hazard in sport. Head injuries accounted for 14% of 1000 rugby injuries,[1] and 18.9% of equestrian injuries; with 50% of equestrian hospital admissions and over 70% of equestrian deaths being due to head and neck injuries.[2] Thirteen per cent of all head injury attendances at one emergency unit were sports-related[3] and up to 11% of all skiing injuries are to the head and spine.[4] Brain injury is more frequent than spinal cord injury, but both brain and cervical spine injury can be missed. The consequences of failed early detection can be devastating to victim, family, colleagues, and society alike. Sports authorities, doctors, first aiders, spectators, and players themselves have differing but complementary responsibilities. All must understand the basics of head and spinal injury. All have to be involved in their prevention and all need to know the first principles of head and spinal injury care.

Most sport is voluntary. Most sports injury, therefore, results from elective or planned activity. Most are therefore avoidable and, if avoidable, then unacceptable. Only the element of luck and the relatively low risk of accident renders tolerable the potential for brain and spinal cord injury which is the downside of the overall good that sport imparts. Within this balance of risk and benefit, deliberate or negligent injury is intolerable. This poses a challenge to the very ethos of some sports and to the regulation, conduct, and organisation of all others.

Head injury

Head injury results from the application of energy to the head. Common mechanisms are head impact or penetration, skull deformation and fracture, brain acceleration or laceration. So long as it is not lacerated, the brain within the head has a complex tolerance threshold to the many potential insults. Once that threshold is exceeded, the head injury is "significant";

significant in that brain injury has occurred; significant also in that once brain insult has reached this level, a secondary cascade of pathological factors can be set in train, any one or a combination of which can cause severe disability or death. Determining what is "significant" on the spot and in the heat of the moment is not easy. Hippocrates found as much 2500 years ago, noting that an apparently trivial head injury can lead to death; yet, the most hopeless situation, if tackled immediately, appropriately and with determination, may have a good outcome.

The only sure signs of "significance" in this context are head penetration, skull deformation, and the most important of all signs – an alteration of consciousness, however short. A disturbance of consciousness, even if not observed, may be inferred from an interruption of the player's memory. Loss or impairment of consciousness is a sure sign that enough energy has been transferred from the head to injure the brain and set in train the secondary complications of vasoparesis (loss of cerebrovascular autoregulation which can cause brain swelling) and intracranial haemorrhage (bleeding). Even if the initial injury was not severe, these two complications maim and kill if not promptly treated. As the head is mounted upon the neck, the same energy input is transferred on to the neck and may cause immediate spinal cord injury or spinal column instability, allowing subsequent spinal cord damage by inappropriate neck movement after the injury.

Progress is being made in head protection, but fashion and practice influence whether and what headgear is acceptable (see Appendix). Many designs are far from ideal. Much vital research still has to be done in this field.

Neck and cervical spine

Sport-related spinal injury is not uncommon. Sixteen per cent of all spinal injuries at one regional centre were suffered in sport.[5] Unlike the brain, in which conscious level is the key, spinal cord function may escape disturbance by the initial injury. Rather, the spinal column (vertebral bones) is destabilised or fractured by the initial injury, sparing the spinal cord only for it to destroyed later by injudicious movement of the victim's head, neck, or body. There may be no outward indication of a spinal injury. As a result, all head injuries must be presumed to have an unstable neck injury until proved otherwise.

If conscious, the victim may warn of spinal cord injury by transient symptoms in legs, trunk, and arms, together with neck pain, muscle spasm, or impaired neck movement. Children are at particular risk. They may complain of no more than momentary, often bizarre bodily and limb sensations, without objective signs and often appearing entirely

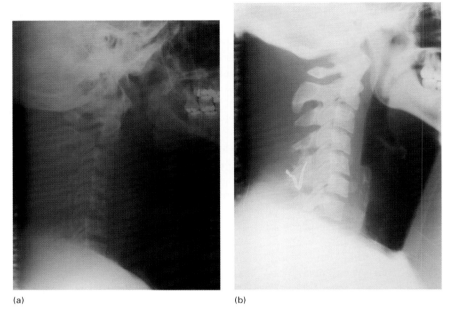

(a)   (b)

Figure 14.1   (a) Rugby injury of the cervical spine: C5–6 subluxation; (b) the injury following
operation

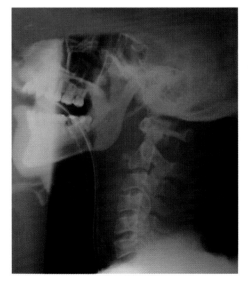

Figure 14.2   Hangman's fracture

normal on initial assessment. The symptoms themselves are enough to indicate that a sufficient spinal cord insult has occurred to disturb cord function, to induce local cord vasoparesis (spinal cord blood flow autoregulatory failure) and sympathoparesis (disturbance of the central grey reticulum of the spinal cord, impairing sympathetic nervous system function upon which the maintenance of systemic blood pressure depends). The combination of these two pathological mechanisms results in later, irreversible spinal cord infarction unless the significance of the situation is appreciated and the child or individual is kept flat. Cautious and careful examination may demonstrate neurological signs, head or neck deformity, and bruising or tenderness, but the pliability of the young spine and the spontaneous reduction of spinal fractures, once victims are placed supine, means that physical examination and spinal X-rays cannot be relied upon to identify or exclude cervical spine injury, a phenomenon known as spinal cord injury without radiological abnormality (SCIWORA).

This difficulty persists in hospital where suspicion, care and expertise are necessary to establish the diagnosis, and investigate and manage all neck injuries. In the spine, the history and a detailed description of the circumstances of the injury are the keys to successful management.

Neck injury is a particular hazard in some contact sports (notably rugby and American football) and some non-contact activities (horse riding and diving). Game development, rule changes, fashion, and increasing awareness among participants, referees, and governing bodies have reduced the incidence but not removed the hazard.[6]

Mechanisms of injury

Though strengthened by bony hoops and ridges, in impact terms the skull is little better than an eggshell containing the brain, within which the nerve cells and their processes (the axons and dendrites upon which connection and function depend) are supported in the jelly-like glia. Skull impact, deformation, and penetration not only disrupt this fragile arrangement but can tear blood vessels inside the head, so causing:

- Intracerebral bleeding within the brain which affects consciousness virtually instantaneously
- Subdural bleeding over the brain's surface, which impairs consciousness over seconds or minutes
- Extradural bleeding which results in loss of consciousness in minutes to hours as the clot expands between the brain's tough dural covering and the overlying skull.

275

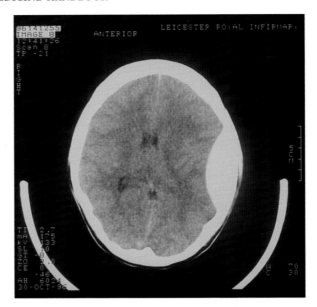

Figure 14.3   Extradural bleeding as seen on CT scan

These events compress and further disturb the brain and its vasculature, increasing any brain swelling that may already be present from the initial injury. Swelling alone or in combination with haemorrhage kills the victim unless this accelerating vicious circle of raised intracranial pressure is reversed by prompt, appropriate intervention.

The human spine (down the central canal of which the spinal cord runs from the brain) was developed by evolution for a horizontal, quadrupedal posture – "on all fours". Its static stability, flexibility, and dynamic integrity depend on the forward bowing (lordosis) of the cervical (neck) and the lumbar (lower back) spine. Its load-bearing ability depends on the anatomy and mechanical properties of vertebrae (the bones), the intervertebral discs, articulations, and ligaments, but above all in the impact situation on lordosis which enables the spine to act as a complex spring. The spine's protective performance is affected by the pre-impact shock-absorbing status of the viscoelastic intervertebral discs, paraspinal tonic muscle tone, and the performance of the segmental spinal reflex innervation. The voluntary, clonic, aerobic muscular system's response is too slow to react protectively in near-instantaneous impact pulses and acute injury loading. As viscoelastic structures, the intervertebral discs are only capable of elastic deformation and recoil from a pre-impact condition of distraction for which they were evolved. Pre-impact cervical kyphosis (slouching forward) causes intervertebral disc compression and the subsequent undamped transmission of impact and deforming forces to maximally pre-stressed disc annuli,

276

adjacent end plates, vertebral bodies, neurocentral and posterior articulations. The situation is compounded further in children. The younger the individual, the larger the comparative size of the head and the more horizontal the planes of the posterior facet joints, further reducing their resistance to transverse dislocation without bony fracture and enhancing their potential for spinal cord injury.

The spinal cord is protected by the bony and soft tissue elements of the spinal column surrounding the spinal canal, within which the spinal cord is further protected by suspension from the dentate ligaments within the dural sac which contains the impact-damping cerebrospinal fluid. But even such complex and efficient protective systems have their limits. Once exceeded, the integrity of the spinal column is compromised and the cord is exposed to potential damage.

Worse, anchorage by its dentate ligaments now focuses distorting forces ensuring that the cord's margin of tolerance to further spinal deformity is minimal. This gives spinal cord injury potentially an "all-or-nothing" character, so making the management of those with spinal column disruption with retained cord function even more critical. If some cord function persists after the initial neck insult, then with careful management a useful recovery can be made. But thoughtless handling can convert potential recovery into permanent disaster. The spinal cord is susceptible to distortion, compression, and vasoparesis. In the immediate management of spinal injury the keys to success are suspicion, recognition, spinal stabilisation, maintenance of normal cord anatomy, and control of spinal blood flow.

Avoidance of brain and spinal cord injury

The first principle and best solution is not to have a brain or spinal cord injury at all. Prevention is better than cure. If accident prevention fails, then protection is the second line of defence. A major improvement in the brain's tolerance of head injury is provided by modern helmets. Most helmets pose a greater challenge to skull base and cervical spine, to which the dampened but prolonged impact pulse is transferred. Neck impact tolerance and performance is compromised by pre-impact kyphosis (slouching), disc compression, and degenerative change. Focal degenerative disease impairs the overall bowspring behaviour of the cervical (and lumbar) spine and focuses imposed force. Both are compounded by poor muscle tone and fast, direct as well as segmental muscle reflex response. Posture, training, practice, habit, and integrated helmet design are the keys to brain and cervical cord protection. Injury avoidance is best achieved by training in infancy and childhood. Falling safely, rolling with facility, and escape without harm are abilities that are poorly learnt, rarely practised, and difficult to maintain in adult life. Yet the safety of many adult sportsmen or sportswomen depends upon just that.

Accident management

Once accident prevention, avoidance, and protection have failed, the objectives of injury management are the prevention of secondary complications, avoidance of further injury, and the promotion of recovery. The first person to the victim's side is usually neither a doctor nor a first aider. Simple basic procedures are therefore essential, which all can learn and apply. They are the foundations of successful treatment.

Immediate management in the field falls into several stages:

Stage 1   Assessment.
Stage 2   Primary care.
Stage 3   Control, transfer to hospital or return to sport.

Stage 1 Assessment: "ABC"

On reaching an injured individual, presume all to have head, brain, and unstable neck injuries. Do not move them until you have to.

Check what is most important, remembering "ABC":

- **Airway**: if not clear then clear it. Immobilise the head, neck, and body as one.
- **Breathing**: if not breathing for themselves, be prepared to undertake mouth-to-mouth ventilation immediately. If spontaneous breathing returns, periodically re-check breathing.
- **Circulation**: check for carotid pulse, and if not present, carry out cardiac massage. If spontaneous carotid pulse returns periodically re-check that the heart is still beating. Identify any bleeding points and stop them by direct pressure.

These are the first priorities. If you cannot clear the airway or the victim is not breathing and the position is preventing your mouth-to-mouth ventilation, stabilise the head on the neck using your hands and forearms and with the coordinated assistance of others "log roll" the victim on to their back. This usually requires at least three people to do safely. Continue to stabilise head-on-neck-on-shoulders, clear the airway and commence mouth-to-mouth ventilation.

If ABC are satisfactory, continue with your assessment.

278

Table 14.1 Glasgow Coma Scale

Score	Motor (M)	Conversation (V)	Eye-opening (E)
6	Obeys commands	—	—
5	Localises pain	Orientated	—
4	Withdraws from pain	Confused	Spontaneous
3	Abnormal flexion	Inappropriate	To speech
2	Extends	Sounds only	To pain
1	Nil	Nil	Nil
Total =			

- **D (Disability)**: conscious level (the key to the state of the brain). This is best assessed using the Glasgow Coma Score (GCS) (Table 14.1). Does the victim move (score 1–6)? Speak (score 1–5)? Open his/her eyes (score 1–4)?

If in any doubt about the victim's conscious level summon an ambulance immediately. Never leave an unconscious casualty alone. The airway will obstruct and any chance of a good recovery will be lost.

Spinal cord function?

1. Can the victim move arms, hands, fingers, legs, feet, and toes? Motor power recorded on the Medical Research Council (MRC) motor power scale (Table 14.2) is invaluable for later comparison, management, and

Table 14.2 Medical Research Council motor power (muscle strength) scale

Score	Movement at joint
5	Normal
4	Strong but not normal
3	Weak but can overcome gravity
2	Movement but not against gravity
1	Movement detected
0	No movement

audit. MRC 0 is no movement; MRC 3 is movement against gravity; MRC 5 is normal. So MRC 1 is a trace of movement, MRC 2 is obvious movement but not strong enough to overcome gravity, and MRC 4 is strong but not normal.

2. Can the victim feel his/her arms, hands, body, and legs? Local painful stimulation (pinch or pinprick) should be applied if there is any doubt and the individual is conscious enough to cooperate.

Other injuries? A, B, C (all three) will keep you busy enough. If they are normal, beware; check for:

1. Bruising (e.g. behind the ears in skull base fractures, **Battle's sign**).
2. Deformity and swelling.

3. Wounds.
4. Head and spinal tenderness (if the victim is awake, moving all limbs, and conscious enough to tell you; otherwise do not move until you can move with head, neck, body, and limbs as one "log", onto a spinal stretcher).

Assessment outcome

The above will establish whether the victim is conscious or not and provide a baseline on which further management will depend. The use of a standard head and spinal injury form recording timed observations from the moment of injury is invaluable to the hospital team to achieve optimum patient care and to sports authorities to document injury experience (see Figure 14.4).

Stage 2 Primary care: "ABCD"

The keys remain:

A The airway, always, with cervical spine immobilisation.
B Breathing, the victim's or yours doing it for them, mouth-to-mouth.
C Circulation.
D Conscious level (GCS) and cord function.

Your assessment will have established the victim's overall status. This can be categorised as one of the following.

1 No disturbance of consciousness

You can now establish whether there are or have been any neurological symptoms (momentary loss of memory, pain, "pins and needles" (paraesthesiae), numbness, clumsiness or weakness, incontinence), head or neck pain, or impaired movement. If in any doubt, treat as brain normal but potential spinal cord injury. Immobilise, log roll when moving, stabilising head-on-neck-on-shoulders, continue recorded observations, and evacuate to the nearest Accident and Emergency department for expert review.

2 Consciousness was disturbed but is now normal

The victim has been exposed to sufficient trauma to have caused vasoparesis, extradural or subdural bleeding. Establish the timing and duration of the disturbed consciousness. Even if no neck or neurological symptoms or signs are present, treat as an unstable neck injury and transfer with head and spine stabilised to the nearest Accident and Emergency department for an expert review. Stabilise the head and neck,

280

Name			Time											
Address	Airway	open Y/N												
	Breathing	Y/N												
Male Female	Circulation	Blood pressure												
DOB														
Injury site		Pulse rate												
	Glasgow	Coma Scale												
	Eye opening	Spontaneous	4											
		To speech	3											
		To pain	2											
		None	1											
	Motor response	Obeys commands	5											
		Localises	4											
		Flexion to pain	3											
		Extension to pain	2											
		None	1											
	Verbal response	Orientated	5											
		Confused	4											
		Innappropriate	3											
		Incomprehensible	2											
		None	1											
			Total											
	Pupils	Left	reacts Y/N											
		Right												
	Limb	Movements												
	Arms	Full power	5											
		Reduced power	4											
		Against gravity	3											
		Slight movement	2											
		No response	1											
	Legs	Full power	5											
		Reduced power	4											
Compressed ▲ Wound ○		Against gravity	3											
Fracture # Burn ◉		Slight movement	2											
		No response	1											
Drugs given?	Bloods taken?	Cannulation	Y/N	Where?										
Drug	Dose and time													
Other comments														

Figure 14.4   Head and spinal injury observation form

continue observation and recording of airway, breathing, conscious level, and spinal cord function (limb movements) whilst controlling any bleeding (circulation).

281

3 Consciousness impaired but improving

This may be the "lucid interval" when the brain is recovering; extradural bleeding is in progress but the clot is not yet big enough to distort the brain sufficiently to cause secondary deterioration of consciousness. Treat the patient as neurologically unstable and transfer as quickly as possible to the nearest Accident and Emergency department before clot expansion is compounded by vasoparetic brain swelling and rapid deterioration to death. You may have less than 30 minutes to play with and do not even depend on that. Continued serial recorded observation and maintenance of the airway remain vital.

4 Unconscious, not improving

Assume the victim has an acute subdural haematoma (blood), brain swelling, or both until proved otherwise. The only hope of a useful recovery

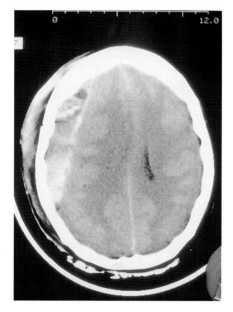

Figure 14.5   Acute subdural haematoma as seen on CT scan

is urgent clot evacuation with immediate intubation, ventilation to a $P\text{aco}_2$ of 3.5 kPa and dehydration (mannitol 1 g/kg IV) to counteract vasoparetic brain swelling on the way to the operating theatre. The time available here to prevent irreversible brain injury is measured in minutes. Maintain the airway and mouth-to-mouth ventilation if the tongue and lips are not pink until intubation and mechanical or hand ventilation is established.

5 Had improved, now deteriorating

This patient's status is now the same as (4) above: brain swelling, extradural haematoma, or both. Action as in (4). Speed to the operating theatre is the priority.

Stage 3 (A): field control of those not evacuated

Those with actual or potential brain and spinal cord injury require prompt hospitalisation. This leaves group (1) above, those who were not knocked out and had no disturbance of consciousness but were subject to gross head and neck impact/acceleration. Their care now centres on two decisions:

1. Do they need treatment for other injuries and if so can they be managed on the spot?
2. Can they return immediately to the game or competition?

Scalp injuries are a matter of debate. If they can be cleaned, sutured, stabilised, and protected, in the absence of other contraindications, a return to a competition or match has been considered both brave and reasonable. However, heat of the moment decisions are often later regretted and there are other potential public health matters of blood contact with, or contamination of the wounds of, others. Sporting bravery, enthusiasm, and loyalty are to be applauded, but such a return is best subject to medical advice.

The neurological hazards in this situation are, first, that brain and/or spinal cord are rendered vasoparetic by the force of the head impact and brain acceleration imposed by the accident. If so, with the enhanced cardiac output and raised blood pressure of renewed exercise, areas of vasoparetic brain or cord will swell, distorting surrounding brain or cord, rendering them in their turn vasoparetic and resulting in acceleration of secondary neurological deterioration. If a deterioration of consciousness occurs causing airway compromise then the treatment is mouth-to-mouth ventilation until intubation can be effected, hyperventilation established, and an intracranial clot excluded. These steps require urgent admission to hospital, as described above. The spinal cord hazard is greater in children.

The second hazard to be considered is the additive effect of a further head or neck impact, the "Second Impact Syndrome" (SIS). That second impact may be minor and not apparently sufficient by itself to disturb the brain and spinal cord. But with the brain still disturbed by the first insult, the two impacts have an added effect with very rapid vasoparetic brain swelling and early death unless arrested by immediate intervention with intubation, hyperventilation, dehydration, steroids, cerebral protection, and blood pressure control in a neurosurgical intensive care unit.

If the initial head and neck insult were sufficient to cause concern, then bed rest under the care of a responsible adult and referral to the individual's family doctor for review is prudent. Alcohol and agitation should be avoided and an advice card (Figure 14.6) for the carer is advised.

CARE AT HOME OF PATIENTS WHO HAVE SUSTAINED HEAD INJURIES

He/she should rest quietly at home for..day (s)

Bring him/her back to hospital IMMEDIATELY under the following circumstances:

If he/she:
- (a) Has a convulsion or fit
- (b) Complains of severe headache
- (c) Vomits repeatedly
- (d) Becomes increasingly drowsy and difficult to rouse. (Children should be woken every two hours during the first twelve hours after the injury to make sure that they are still rousable)

If you are worried about the patient's condition at any time

Figure 14.6   Advice card for home carers following a head injury

Stage 3 (B): transport of the victim

Treat all victims as having unstable spines. This requires managing them horizontal, supine on a flat surface with the head, neck, body, and limbs stabilised. This in turn means that they are more likely to obstruct their airway, swell their brains, and die. Continuous, uninterrupted, recorded observation is mandatory.

Therefore:

1. Manage the ABC. Continue to maintain cervical spine immobilisation. This is the task of the first person to arrive at the accident site.
2. Make the second person to arrive responsible for getting help and then stabilising the victim's head-on-neck-on-shoulders, maintaining constant alignment with their own hands, arms, and elbows. This must continue through movement and transfer until responsibility is taken over by ambulance crew, paramedics, or doctors in the Accident and Emergency department.
3. Slide, roll, or lift the victim as one, as if lifting a log, not allowing the head, spine, or neck to move on each other. This is best done using a spinal transfer board or scoop. Without aids, a minimum of four people are needed for this, depending on the size of the victim.
4. Transportation in any position other than horizontal and supine with the head stabilised invites a potential disaster, but this in turn hazards the airway, which must be constantly kept clear and breathing maintained.

Stage 3 (C): return to sport after injury

Subsequent return to sport requires careful review and a deliberate decision in each and every case. This will depend upon the injury, the extent of

284

recovery, the individual, the sport and the risk of a further brain or spinal cord injury compounding this accident.

The neuro-clinician has the following considerations in mind:

The second impact syndrome (SIS, above)   However, persisting vasoparesis is unlikely after 14 days if the individual is well and without symptoms.

Brain scarring   Causing focal abnormal brain stressing under later head impact or acceleration, particularly so if a post-traumatic epileptiform seizure occurred after the first accident.

Late bleeding   Into an area of brain contusion caused by the head injury. This is most likely at 10 days from injury, with a decreasing probability thereafter, to be unlikely after 3 weeks in someone who is otherwise well.

Impaired intellectual performance   Caused by the head injury. This can be cumulative (the "lame brain" syndrome of punch-drunk boxers and once common among jockeys), but also occurs in a "second impact" manner in those who return to sport before their recovery is complete. A return to sport before a full recovery has been achieved also ensures sub-standard performance and an enhanced risk of another head and/or spinal injury.

Frontal lobe and brain stem injuries   These are largely acceleration-induced and therefore more common in high speed road vehicle accidents than in sports. It is important to appreciate that it is the magnitude of brain acceleration/deceleration rather than initial velocity which injures. Low velocity but high acceleration/deceleration impact brain injury is a hazard in most sports. Recovery from such injuries can take 2 or more years with headache, dizziness, altered behaviour, and intolerance. Such symptoms were formerly labelled "post-concussional". They preclude a return to sport until they have cleared.

Potential spinal instability   Without internal fixation, neck fractures take at least 6 weeks to unite. Most spinal surgeons advise 3 months before union is considered stable. Focal reduction in spinal mobility places greater stress on neighbouring motion segments which may be further complicated by pre-existing spondylotic distortion (associated with the normal disc degeneration we all suffer).

Residual neurological deficit   May or may not compromise the safety of the individual or their colleagues.

285

Return to sport after specific injuries

Structural brain injury

Return should be subject to the advice of the victim's neurological adviser, but is unlikely to be recommended within 3 months.

Uncomplicated skull fracture (that is, without brain disturbance)

Return after 6 weeks, subject to written expert medical advice.

Uncomplicated brain swelling or cord vasoparesis

Return at 3 weeks from cessation of symptoms (including headache), on written expert advice.

Uncomplicated traumatic alteration of consciousness, "concussed"

"Concussed" is a term which has defied medical definition. It is not used neurologically, as it suggests that brain insult can be sufficient to "stun" yet insufficient to cause actual brain injury. Sadly this is not so. The player should have 3 weeks off and return only following medical review and written advice.

Spinal cord injury

Return should be only after written advice from the individual's neurological adviser, and with written confirmation from the spinal surgeon involved that it is reasonable to return to the specified discipline.

Current practice in various sporting disciplines

With the many forms sport takes, it is not surprising that many different attitudes and positions have been adopted. Examples of sporting authorities' guidelines follow. They are not exhaustive, and each relevant authority should be approached for definitive advice.

British Boxing Board of Control (BBBC)

- Boxers knocked out or stopped suspended for 45 days. No boxer stopped or knocked out to spar for 28 days.
- Any boxer knocked unconscious or who in the view of the doctor has taken excessive punishment should go to hospital. The board would

exercise its right to suspend any boxer ignoring medical advice either at the venue or at hospital.

Football Association (FA)

● A player who has left a match or training session with a head injury should only return following clearance by a qualified medical practitioner.

Jockey Club

● All competing under Jockey Club Rules are required to carry a personal injury "Red Book" which is inspected at each meeting by the racecourse medical officer (RMO) before each individual may race. Head injuries attract an entry and advice in red ink. These reflect the following:

1. "Concussion of a minor nature"	The RMO may suspend the rider from riding that day and for the next 2 days, a minimum of 2 full days.
2. Where the rider has: (a) suffered a short period of unconsciousness, or (b) any degree of post-traumatic amnesia, or (c) been sent to hospital in this connection	He/she is medically suspended for a minimum period of 6 full days.
3. If the rider has suffered a significant period of unconsciousness (>60 seconds)	He/she is to be sent to hospital and medically suspended for a minimum period of 20 full days.

Medical Equestrian Association (MEA)

1. Concussion of a minor nature	The competitor should not ride or drive a vehicle again on the same day or until completely recovered.
2. An episode of unconsciousness or post-traumatic amnesia.	The competitor should not ride or compete for a minimum of 7 days.
3. Prolonged unconsciousness	The competitor should not ride or compete for a minimum of 3 weeks.

Rugby Football Union (RFU)

1. Loss of consciousness	Requires review by a doctor who may recommend hospitalisation.

2. Definite concussion   No match or training session for 3 weeks and only then following proper neurological examination.

Rugby Football League (RFL)

1. Following head injury a player should be taken to hospital for medical review if there is anything unusual or he:

- develops new or increasing head pain
- has a fit (epileptic seizure)
- vomits
- is dizzy, drowsy, restless, irritable, or unrousable.

2. Recommended time off from the game depending on the severity of head injury as assessed by a doctor:

- "Mild"

Definition 1: no loss of consciousness (LOC) or memory loss	Can usually continue playing after being checked
Definition 2: memory loss	Leave field. No playing or training until passed by the club doctor

- "Moderate"

Definition: LOC <2 minutes	Leave field. No playing or training for 15 days and then only after check by club doctor

- "Severe"

Definition: LOC <3 minutes	Leave field. No playing or training for 22 days and then only after check by club doctor
Definition: LOC >3 minutes	Admit to hospital. No playing or training for 29 days and then only after check by club doctor

- "Severe concussion" (not defined)   Warrants X-rays of skull and cervical spine.

Parachuting

- Military   Medical Officer (MO) review of all head injuries. Return only when MO satisfied there are no post-traumatic sequelae.
- Sport   No parachuting following severe head injury, brain, or nervous system disease, including epilepsy.
  Tandem jumping more relaxed, but medical assessment required for specified illnesses.

Recommendations

1. Sport is to be enjoyed, not regretted. Brain and spinal cord injuries often recover incompletely, unlike the rest of the body. They are the principle cause of regret in sport. Prevention is better than cure.

2. As sport is not compulsory, such injury is by its very nature avoidable. It is part of the risk:benefit relationship inherent in the voluntary decision whether to engage in sport or not.

3. Because they are avoidable (by non-participation), the potential for head and neck injuries and their elimination or reduction is a challenge to each sporting discipline, its leaders, regulators, authorities, and participants.

4. The present incidence of brain and spinal cord injury can only be defended if appropriate steps are taken to identify and avoid the avoidable accident, define the injuries, promote prevention and protection, and introduce, improve, and practise arrangements for the prompt and appropriate management of casualties.

5. Accidents reflect past practice, posture and training, present circumstance, and the performance and physique of the individuals involved. Injury mechanism, scenario, victim, and post-traumatic management all contribute to the outcome. Although it is only the victim who suffers, all should learn from past experience and develop safe practice in all sports. This does not mean that the sports have to be any less competitive and enjoyable. Rather, as Professor Richard Schneider's influence on American football showed, the outcome can and should be to increase the fun, the fury, and the excitement whilst reducing the hazard.

6. The reduction, or better, exclusion of brain and spinal cord injury is a priority for the authorities of each and every sports discipline. That medical assistance to this end is on offer is exemplified by this book. Many disciplines require a major shift in attitudes, but few need to be inhibited and the overall contribution of sport to the general population's wellbeing will be enhanced. This responsibility cannot be ducked. Expert help and enthusiasm is available. Progress has, is, and must continue to be made to enhance enjoyment and cut casualties.

7. Once head and neck injury has occurred, the guidelines set out in Table 14.3 apply to all sports.

Table 14.3 Recommendations for a safe return to sport

Post-accident situation	Response	Return to sporting activity
1 No loss of consciousness or memory; no symptoms, however minor or bizarre	Check: conscious level and memory; voluntary head, neck, spine, arms, fingers, legs and feet movement; exclude muscle spasm, neck deformity, and head or neck penetration	Return when comfortable and able to participate effectively and fully
2 Transient alteration of consciousness or loss of memory	Significant head injury has occurred. Manage flat with ABC. Commence timed neurological observations, on the form provided. Be prepared for rapid evacuation to nearest A&E department if conscious level declines	No play same day, nor later until cleared by written medical advice
3 Any neurological symptom in the limbs, however transient or bizarre	Indicate spinal cord insult and an unstable spine until proved otherwise (in hospital). ABC, nurse horizontal, head and neck stabilised flat in neutral position without a pillow. Commence neurological observations on form provided. Transfer to A&E department for expert review. Beware respiratory failure due to cervical cord injury. Ventilate if in doubt	No return until spinal cord integrity and spinal stability established by expert, written review
4 Impaired or altered consciousness	Significant head injury, potentially unstable spine. ABC. Record timed observations. Urgent transfer as head and spinal injury	Minimum of 7 days; 21 more appropriate and then only following expert, written clearance
5 Seizure or epileptic fit	Manage as (4) above	Return only with written advice of usual neurological attendant
6 Unconscious or obvious severe head injury	Treat as (4) above	Unlikely within 3 months; then only on written advice of the responsible consultant
7 Unstable spinal/cord injury	Manage as (3) above. ABC. Urgent evacuation to hospital, head and neck stabilised. Beware: chance of recovery may be denied by careless handling	Minimum of 6 weeks, probably 3 months and only on the written advice of the victim's spinal and neurological surgeons

References

1 Adams ID. Rugby football injuries. *Br J Sports Med* 1977;**11**(1):4–6.
2 Nelson DE, Rivara FP, Condie C. Helmets and horseback riders. *Am J Prevent Med* 1994;**10**:15–19.
3 Young WW, Gunter MJ. *A study of the head injured population in Pennsylvania.* Pittsburgh. The Pittsburgh Research Institute, 1991, pp. 58–9.
4 Myles ST, Mohtadi NGH, Schnittker J. Injuries to the nervous system and spine in downhill skiing. *Canad J Surg* 1992;**35**(6):643–8.
5 Grundy D, Swain A. *ABC of spinal cord injury,* 2nd edn. London: BMJ Publishing Group, 1993.
6 Cantu RC. Head and spine injuries in youth sports. *Clin Sports Med* 1995;**14**: 517–32.

Appendix

Helmets and head protection in sport

Head protection has concerned man since the Stone Age. Without the aid of bronze or iron, Polynesians constructed helmets of wicker, fibre, and bone. The obvious need was and is to prevent head injury, but comfort ensured that low levels of acceleration were attenuated even if their significant mechanisms were not understood. Today lightweight materials have allowed a revolution in helmet design and fabrication that may yet rival the protective performance achieved by armourers of the Middle Ages (designing and bespoking helmets and suits for competitive jousting at the international level) but without the penalties in weight.

Head protection may be "active" (preventing the accident, avoiding the impact, or cushioning the head, as in the womb or by air bags within a crash shell) or "passive", the latter most commonly by the wearing of a helmet. In many accident circumstances any helmet is better than none, but each helmet is a compromise between conflicting requirements which include:

1. Cost.
2. Appearance, i.e. fashion.
3. Comfort, which includes fit, ventilation, centre of gravity.
4. Weight.
5. Protective performance:
   Acceleration
   Deformation
   Penetration.
6. Centre of mass, dynamic and aerodynamic behaviour, retention (head: helmet stability) in real world conditions.

7. Surface properties (ability to slide along road surfaces, not catch and acutely rotate the head).
8. Sensory impairment, avoiding restriction of sight, vision, and hearing.
9. Need for associated equipment: eye and face protection, visor, earphones, microphones, visual displays.
10. Scaling, to provide appropriate protection for all age groups.
11. Potential for induced or helmet-enhanced injury, particularly to neck or face.
12. Medicolegal threats.

The traditional rugby scrum cap is as simple as they come, but is better for the ears and morale than any impact attenuation provided. Formed polystyrene cycle caps have provided both attractive shapes and impressive test acceleration attenuation, only to be found wanting in practice when impacting the angled objects and edges with which children collide. An enclosing shell addresses this, although to provide penetration and deformation resistance the shell weight has to be considerable.

Present helmet systems comprise several defined component parts.[1]

1. Protection for the brain itself, susceptible to insult from any direction.
2. The skull and head with which the helmet has to form a single, stable, brain-protective unit which does not secondarily hazard the neck or face.
3. The suspension system. Maintaining head–helmet configuration, comfortably for most of the time, but accurately under one or more impacts from several directions during an accident, requires 3- or 4-point fixation to achieve this in practice. The suspension system has also to allow a comfortable, accurate fit to each and every head (no two ever being exactly alike) and the ventilation necessary to keep the wearer comfortable (and thus wearing the helmet).
4. Acceleration attenuation. This has variously been achieved in the past by plaiting the hair, the wearing of soft "inner" "arming" caps and above all by the suspension system allowing an air gap between the outer helmet shell (the helm of the armoured knight) and the head. This system is mimicked by industrial hard hats and by the 1915-pattern British Infantry Steel Helmet. Today the air gap has been replaced in many designs by a crushable liner which attenuates the acceleration as it is destroyed. The drawback is the high level of initial impact energy required to initiate the degrading process (which may be initially transmitted on to the brain) and the need to replace the helmet after each significant impact. Liner collapse may not be obvious to the casual observer and the very success of the helmet's performance detracts from the realisation of the protection provided. In the future it is likely that a return to the air gap will be made in most designs.

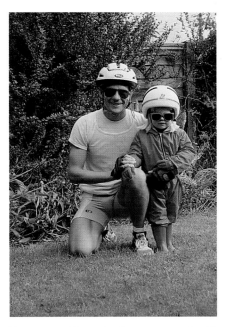

Figure 14.7   No two heads are ever exactly alike

5. Penetration and deformation prevention. Military helmets have moved on from steel to kevlar and exotic materials to achieve sufficient missile penetration protection with acceptable weight.[2] The financial cost is considerable and beyond most sporting budgets. How much weight is acceptable to the sporting public limits the degree of deformation resistance afforded. Cunning design allows sufficient integration of the various subsystems so that one enhances the performance of the other, the aim being that the protection afforded by the helmet as a whole is more than the sum of its separate parts. Such ambition may, however, be tempered by the need to meet mandatory standards (see below).

Current controversies centre on:

1. The present programme of European "harmonisation" of helmet performance specifications and whether European standards should be the "lowest common denominator", or better.
2. How much of the head to protect, without causing more accidents by limiting vision and hearing and by introducing the additional hazard of neck fracture by too low a helmet brim behind the head. The cut-out of American football and early aviation helmets prevents the latter.

293

3. Low lateral (temporal) and horizontal blow protection applied to the helmet brim. The motor cycling "full-face" helmet addresses this but is incompatible with some activities.

4. Helmet retention under high onset rate acceleration. Full face helmets with a single, 2-point under-chin fixation are still "flipping-off" in accidents, leaving the wearer unprotected. Equestrian experience has shown that 3-point fixation which encompassed the mastoid processes (the bony bulges behind the ears) largely avoids this and is as effective as and more comfortable than traditional 4-point fixation systems.

5. The "holy grail" helmet for all occasions. Although an ideal, and if achievable a great convenience, the present head protection scene is very much that of "horses for courses". This is supported by the British Standards Institute (BSI) and similar national and international bodies world-wide. In the BSI case each discipline is or can be supported by a BSI advisory committee experienced in that particular field and reflecting the many interests involved – sports authorities, participants, industry, medicine, research. They draw up a performance specification, rather than design constraints. The objective is to stimulate innovation whilst ensuring that any item which earns the BSI's "kite mark" provides state of the art protection. Minimum statutory 5-yearly review of the published standards is maintained, although active criticism and debate continues in each committee between each review, providing continuous surveillance of experience in practice.

6. Reporting and investigation of actual helmet performance in practice. This is the weakness of the present situation. Accurate data is essential for informed improvement, but either the helmet works so well that the incident is discounted as insignificant (as head injury did not occur) or the helmet is forgotten in the heat of the moment, often lost and its part in the accident not considered in detail by accident departments, medical teams, neuropathologist, and coroners. The situation is changing. Sports injuries now contribute significantly to overall national disability. Reporting of sporting injuries is being promoted. At the same time, individual sporting disciplines are improving their own surveillance systems. Those of the British Horse Society and the Jockey Club in the UK are examples in which multidisciplinary review is already in place. The principal problems are initial referral to the discipline's system and secondly, the fact that these systems are run by volunteers. Bureaucratic alternatives, however, would be extremely expensive and possibly ineffective. Once again the privilege of the freedom to engage in sport carries with it the obligation to address its consequences. In the mid-term the combination of an increasing awareness of the importance of accurate information coupled with individual enthusiasm and altruism, backed by the various authorities and the BSI, is the most likely

combination to produce results.[3] How soon these appear depends on voluntary, financial, and industrial support.

7. Design details. The "soft-outers" (soft outer layer over the shell) versus "sandwich" (outer and inner shell, intervening liner) versus air gap versus compound helmet controversies continue, ensuring healthy competition between designers, manufacturers, and research. So far support by the latter has been limited. Slow basic science progress in defining the human brain's acceleration toleration envelope and absence of funding for animal research itself means that the medical research community is having to pull itself, and all others, up by their "own boot straps", relying on the painfully slow and labour-intensive methods of real life accident research. Fortunately, collaborative enthusiasm may now be engaging the interest of research funding bodies. Stimulated by each accident, and supported by and disseminated through the various sports and standards authorities, this "proper study of man is man" approach will ensure the most rapid provision of real world data to improve successive generations of helmet designs.

Present advice to sports participants

1. The head was not designed to be hit. If this is a feature of the sport of your or your child's choice, think hard before *not* wearing a helmet.
2. The "universal helmet" is still an ambition. Very good protective headwear is already available for most sports where head protection is appropriate. Hats are now "in". They demonstrate intelligence and maturity and are no longer "sissy".
3. It is very difficult, at point of purchase, to compare the impact performance of one hat against another. For this reason only buy an up-to-date BSI "kite"-marked helmet.
4. To be worn enjoyably a helmet has to look good and be comfortable. You are the best judge of fashion and only you can feel if the hat fits both tight and right: sufficiently tight that it is part of your head should you fall; "right" so that the helmet conforms to all your head, spreading its weight, without "pressure points" and becoming as or more comfortable than your hair, which it should retain.
5. If you should suffer head strike and are unaffected, be grateful, but check the liner and if in doubt consult the retailer. If you change it, make sure that the hat and a short report of the incident goes to your sport's governing body for their information and surveillance. If you do not change the hat, let them know the circumstances just the same. Details of helmet success and "non-injuries" are just as important.
6. Buy your helmet from a trained retailer. Manufacturers now ensure that their outlets understand the importance of comfort, fit, and product

support. It is in their and their employees' financial interest. Take advice. Make sure that the helmet is properly fitted, adjusted, and fastened for you and write the name of the fitter within the label.

7. A helmet that is not on the head cannot work. A helmet that is not fastened will fall off before you hit anything. The equivalent of the equestrian advice "Don't go within 10 m of horse without your hard hat, fastened" holds for all sports.

References

1 Firth JL. Equestrian injuries. In: Fu Hu, Stone DA (eds). *Sports injuries. Mechanisms, prevention, treatment.* Baltimore: Williams & Wilkins, 1994, pp. 315–31.

2 Carey ME. Analysis of wounds incurred by US Army Seventh Corps personnel during Operation Desert Storm, February 20 to March 10, 1991. *J Trauma* 1996;**30**(3 Suppl):S165–169.

3 Simpson D. Helmets in surgical history. *Aust NZ Surg* 1996;**66**:314–24.

296

15   Injuries of the hand and wrist

NICHOLAS BARTON

In a modern Western country, most injuries to the hand are sustained at home or work, but a significant number happen in sport. The hand is obviously at risk in sports such as basketball, volleyball, and netball,[1] but may be damaged in any sport. The most common mechanisms of injury are the impact of a ball or a fall. Less common causes are running into the wall or fence around the playing area or being hit (accidentally or deliberately) by an opponent or a bat, racquet, or other sporting implement.

The injuries which may occur to the hand or wrist during sport are, on the whole, the same injuries as occur in any other activity. There are some which are especially common and some largely confined to sport.

In a group of patients studied in Sunderland, UK, in 1985,[2] the most common sport causing hand injuries was association football (soccer), probably because it is the game most played. The goalkeeper is the only player allowed to handle the ball, but other players often fall onto an outstretched hand and injure it (see Table 15.1).

Some injuries to the hand or wrist are obviously serious. Many are minor. The danger area is those which appear minor but are, in fact, major. The

Table 15.1   Sports causing hand injuries in a large town in northern England in 1985

Sport/activity	No. of cases
Soccer (association football)	14
Rugger (rugby football)	6
Cricket	5
Skiing	4
Karate	3
Boxing	3
Horse riding	2
Training	2
Boating	1
Skating	1
Rounders	1

From Campbell (1985).[2]

first priority is to make a full diagnosis. I use the word "full" because there may be more to the injury than meets the eye: an obvious dislocation of a finger, which is relatively easy to treat, may in fact be a fracture–dislocation which is a serious injury requiring urgent specialist treatment. Figure 15.1 shows a useful classification of injuries of the hand and wrist.

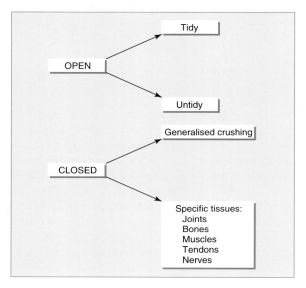

Figure 15.1 Classification of hand injuries

Open injuries

Any cut on the hand or wrist must be assumed to have damaged tendons and/or nerves until proved otherwise. Carefully examine the distal parts. Each digit has two digital nerves, and each must be tested by comparison with a corresponding area on the uninjured hand. Ask "Does this feel exactly the same as that?" (the uninjured area).

Each finger has two flexor tendons and one extensor tendon with a complicated plexus-like arrangement. The thumb has one long flexor tendon and three extensor tendons (if one includes abductor pollicis longus, which is really the extensor of the carpometacarpal joint). Each tendon must be tested.

Table of tendon tests

1. Observe hand posture and compare with uninjured side.
2. Active and passive extension of proximal and distal interphalangeal joints.

  (a) Mallet finger or thumb (avulsion of the insertion of the long extensor). The distal joint will not actively extend, but can be passively extended in the early stages.

  (b) Boutonnière deformity (tearing of the extensor hood over the proximal interphalangeal joint). The joint will not actively extend, but can be passively extended in the early stages.

3. Active flexion of terminal phalanx with middle phalanx held by examiner.

  (a) Jersey finger (flexor digitorum profundus avulsion). The joint will not actively flex, but can be passively flexed in the early stages.

4. Tests for flexor digitorum superficialis: the proximal interphalangeal (PIP) joint must be seen to flex fully, while the other fingers are restrained by the examiner in full extension.

5. Pain against resisted movement may indicate a partial rupture.

Tidy injuries are those produced by a sharp knife or blade. The best results will follow immediate repair of tendons or nerves. Late repair or reconstruction is unlikely to be as good.

Untidy injuries are jagged and dirty, the sort of damage inflicted by a circular saw. Clean the wound, stabilise the skeleton if necessary and obtain skin cover (by skin grafting if necessary). Repair or grafting of tendons and nerves must wait until the skin is fully healed, the soft tissues are supple, and physiotherapy has restored a good range of passive movements.

Ice skating commonly produces open injuries. The skater falls onto the outstretched hand which is then skated over by another skater following too closely behind. The blade produces a laceration which may divide extensor tendons and cause fracture, joint injury, or partial amputation. These are usually fairly tidy injuries[3].

Closed injuries

These are more common in sport. They are less dramatic but can be equally troublesome.

Crushing of a fingertip, even if it is accompanied by a fracture, usually only needs cleaning and the passage of time. The fingernail should be retained if possible as it affords some protection to tender tissues.

The hand

Joint injuries

A normal X-ray does not mean everything is normal. Injuries to ligament and capsule may occur without a fracture.

299

Dislocations

Not all fingers which look a funny shape are dislocated (Figure 15.2). Reduction is kinder under local anaesthetic (Figure 15.3). Difficulty in

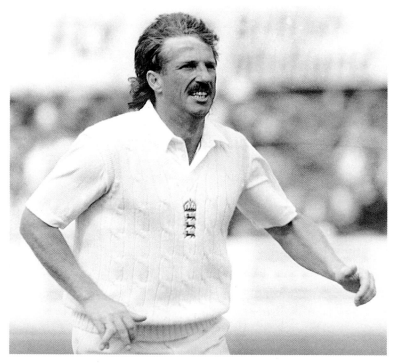

Figure 15.2   This international cricketer, while fielding in a Test Match, was struck by the ball and is seen here leaving the field with a torn radial collateral ligament of the PIP joint of the right ring finger. (Photograph courtesy of IT Botham and of the Nottingham Evening Post*)*

reduction may mean there is soft tissue interposed and surgical exploration is necessary.

Reducing the dislocation (Figure 15.4) does not mean that a normal joint is restored. The ligaments which normally prevent dislocation were torn, and they remain torn after reduction. Assess the lateral and AP stability at the joint. In the thumb it is necessary to immobilise the joint for a while to allow the ligament to heal; in the fingers this does not apply. If the joint re-dislocates immediately after reduction, the dislocation is probably accompanied by a fracture. An "on the field relocation" requires *X-ray within 24 hours* to exclude a fracture–dislocation. A note should be made of the direction of the dislocation to guide subsequent treatment.

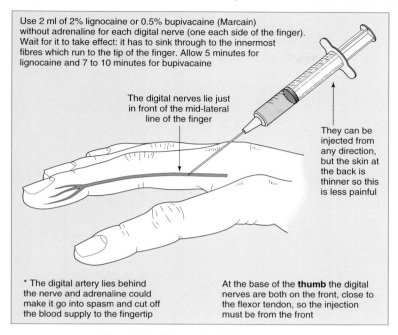

Use 2 ml of 2% lignocaine or 0.5% bupivacaine (Marcain) without adrenaline for each digital nerve (one each side of the finger). Wait for it to take effect: it has to sink through to the innermost fibres which run to the tip of the finger. Allow 5 minutes for lignocaine and 7 to 10 minutes for bupivacaine

The digital nerves lie just in front of the mid-lateral line of the finger

They can be injected from any direction, but the skin at the back is thinner so this is less painful

* The digital artery lies behind the nerve and adrenaline could make it go into spasm and cut off the blood supply to the fingertip

At the base of the **thumb** the digital nerves are both on the front, close to the flexor tendon, so the injection must be from the front

Figure 15.3   How to do a digital nerve block

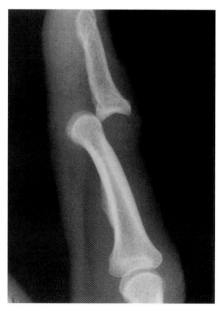

Figure 15.4   Dorsal dislocation of the DIP joint. Sometimes the skin is torn too, making it an open dislocation with the risk of the joint becoming infected

301

Management of dislocations

1 Reduce under local anaesthetic
2 Test stability
3 Arrange an early X-ray

Torn ligaments

Ligaments may tear without dislocation. Collateral ligaments support the side of the metacarpophalangeal and interphalangeal joints. They tear at one end rather than the middle and may bring a tiny flake of bone, technically a fracture but in practice a ligamentous injury. Usually the digit has less angulation than in Figure 15.2, but it is swollen, tender, and unstable.

Ulnar collateral ligament of the thumb: "skier's thumb" Common in skiers, not only on snow but also artificial ski slopes where there is the additional hazard of holes in the skiing surface. It is usually the cord attached to the handle of the ski stick which causes the damage.

Anatomically, it is a unique injury[4] because the ulnar side of the metacarpophalangeal joint of the thumb is overlain by the proximal end of the aponeurosis of the adductor pollicis muscle. Following the tear, the torn ligament returns to overlie the aponeurosis, preventing healing.

The diagnosis is essentially clinical; swelling, tenderness, and bruising on the ulnar side of the joint and obvious laxity when stressing it sideways. This must always be compared with the other thumb as some patients have considerable natural laxity. An X-ray must be taken to exclude a fracture.

My practice is to take stress X-rays of both thumbs under general anaesthetic. This usually reveals gross laxity and I reattach the ligament. The repair is protected for 3 weeks in a "scaphoid" plaster. The aponeurosis is not repaired.

Abrahamsson *et al*[5] state that if the ligament is displaced superficial to the aponeurosis, it can be palpated during clinical examination, but I find this difficult. Numerous methods of investigation have been employed, including arthrography, ultrasound scanning, MRI, and arthroscopy. MRI appears to be the most reliable non-invasive method. I have explored all of these injuries which I have seen over the past 30 years and only once have I failed to find the torn ligament displaced as described above.

Late repair cannot be undertaken. Various ingenious methods of reconstructing the ligament have been described, but none is entirely satisfactory. If joint laxity is causing real difficulty, arthrodesis of the

302

metacarpophalangeal joint is an excellent operation, producing surprisingly little disability provided the other joints are normal.

The radial collateral ligament of the thumb This ligament is less often damaged. There is no aponeurosis on the radial side. The capsule may also be torn, allowing some anterior or posterior subluxation of the joint on X-ray, requiring repair. With no subluxation, immobilization in a "scaphoid" plaster cast for 3 weeks is adequate. A strapping spica will not protect the joint adequately.

Torn collateral ligaments of the fingers These much less common injuries usually occur at the PIP joint. Tears at the metacarpophalangeal joint are rare.

At the PIP joint the torn end of the collateral ligament can get hooked into the joint. A true PA X-ray centred on that joint ensures that the surfaces are absolutely parallel: if not, interposition is diagnosed and the joint explored. If the surfaces are parallel but the joint was unstable (Figure 15.5), then conservative treatment is usually satisfactory (except perhaps

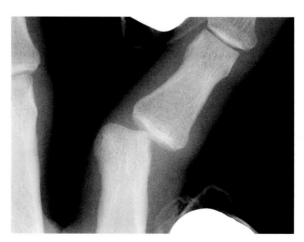

Figure 15.5 Stress X-ray of another international cricketer who tore the collateral ligament of the PIP joint. He was successfully treated by straightening the finger and strapping it to the neighbouring finger on the radial side. (Reproduced with permission from Sports Injuries, *2nd edn, ed. MA Hutson, Oxford University Press, 1996)*

on the radial side of the index finger) in the form of neighbour strapping to the injured finger. Narrow strapping should be used, not covering the joints, permitting mobilisation to avoid stiffness while still protecting the ligament (Figure 15.6).

303

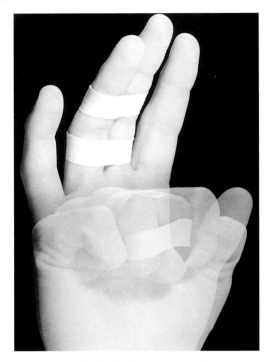

Figure 15.6 Neighbour strapping, allowing flexion and extension but preventing sideways movement. The joints themselves are not covered. There is no need to put anything between the fingers, but if you do, it should be thin and flexible: an empty length of tubigrip is satisfactory

Sprains

A sprain is a partial tear of a ligament and is often more painful than if the ligament is completely torn.

These injuries may remain painful for a year and swollen for 2 years. In the early stages, protective neighbour strapping is wise but later treatment is the passage of time. They do get better in the end.

Volar plate injuries

Forced extension of the finger may injure the thick anterior capsule known as the volar plate.

In most cases the volar plate itself remains intact but pulls off one or both of the little bony tubercles to which it is attached distally. This is most often seen at the PIP joint and is discussed below under fractures.

The joint must be X-rayed, but when the volar plate itself is torn, the X-ray is normal.

304

The joint should be splinted in 10 degrees of flexion for 3 weeks, after which it is mobilised and kept under close review. The ensuing scar tissue tends to draw the joint down into a flexion contracture. Progression is prevented by resuming splintage in a straight position for another 3 weeks, then using a dynamic splint. Occasionally the reverse phenomenon is seen, especially in adolescent girls with lax joints. There is no healing of the volar plate and the joint keeps hyperextending and a swan neck deformity develops. There are operations which can be done for this if necessary. Alternatively, a mild swan neck deformity may develop secondary to a chronic mallet finger (see below), but the PIP joint can be flexed actively and does not need treatment.

Tendon disorders

In sport, tendons are most often damaged in a closed injury, i.e. torn not cut. Healing may occur, but treatment is needed to make sure it heals at the correct length and not in a lengthened position.

Mallet finger

This common injury is caused by forcible flexion of the fingertip. The extensor tendon is torn over the DIP joint and the end of the finger droops, but passively it can be extended fully (Figure 15.7). PA and lateral X-rays

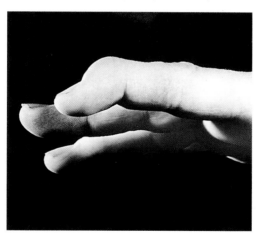

Figure 15.7   Typical mallet finger deformity. There is swelling over the torn tendon. (Reproduced with permission from Sports Injuries, *2nd edn, ed. MA Hutson, Oxford University Press, 1996)*

are taken centred on that joint, as management is different if there is a fracture (see below). If it is a pure tendon injury,[6] then a decision must be taken with the patient as to whether to treat it or not. Treatment is

305

continuous and uninterrupted splintage of the DIP joint in a straight position for 6–8 weeks. The best type of splint is the Stack moulded plastic splint* (Figure 15.8). Apply the splint carefully as the splint may press on

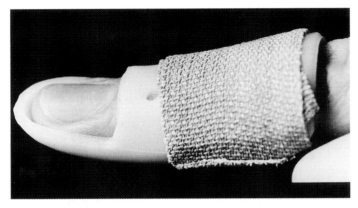

Figure 15.8   Mallet finger treated in Stack splint. The straight edge proximal to the nail can be trimmed with a scalpel if it is pressing on the skin. The DIP joint must be kept straight continuously throughout the period of treatment. (Reproduced with permission from Watson Jones' Fractures and Joint Injuries, *6th edn, ed. JN Wilson, Churchill Livingstone, 1982)*

the skin near the base of the nail. If necessary the splint can be trimmed with a scalpel to prevent this. The patient *must not* remove the splint to wash or to see how the finger is getting on because the injured part needs to be immobilised continuously if it is to heal correctly. If it is not, a permanent mallet finger results. However, the deformity causes no real disability and most patients soon forget about it.

Boutonnière injury

Injury to the slip of extensor tendon which extends the proximal interphalangeal joint is less common and often overlooked.[7] This is because the intact lateral bands of the extensor tendon, which more distally join to form the tendon which extends the DIP joint (that tendon which is damaged in mallet finger), are at first still able to extend the PIP joint. However, the injury has torn not only the central slip but its attachments to the lateral bands on either side and, over the next few weeks, the lateral bands slip progressively forwards so that they cease to extend the PIP joint and, if they go forwards far enough, may even flex it. Secondarily, there develops

---

* Available from Promedics Ltd, Clarendon Road, Blackburn, Lancs, BB1 9TA. They come in six sizes and you have to buy boxes of ten, each size costing £25 per box. Most A&E departments have a stock of various sizes. Stack's splints have also been pirated by an American company which, with extraordinary cynicism, sells them under the name of Stax splints.

306

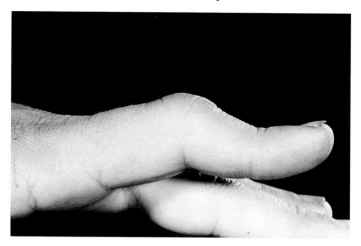

Figure 15.9 Boutonnière deformity: flexion at the PIP joint and hyperextension at the DIP joint. In the early stages these may be passively correctable; later they become fixed. (Reproduced with permission from Sports Injuries, *2nd edn, ed. MA Hutson, Oxford University Press, 1996)*

hyperextension at the DIP joint (Figure 15.9), resulting in the full-blown boutonnière deformity (known in French as "le buttonhole", because the joint comes through between the two lateral bands like a button through its buttonhole).

Tenderness and swelling, with no fracture, over the centre of the back of the PIP joint should suggest this injury and the joint should be splinted in extension for 3 weeks and reassessed. After that, a lively splint should be used to permit some flexion but automatically return the joint to extension for another 3 weeks. The patient must be kept under review until it is clear that all is well.

In practice, the injury is often overlooked and the patient not seen until later when a flexion contraction has developed so that the PIP joint can no longer be extended fully, even passively. In this situation, serial splintage or some form of dynamic splint must be used to get the joint straight and hold it straight for at least 6 weeks. Surgery has little to offer: it can get the joint straight, but often at the cost of loss of flexion, which is worse than the original problem.

Avulsion of the flexor digitorum profundus tendon ("jersey finger")

This is an injury almost confined to rugby football and American and Australian-rules football.[8] Typically, a player is tackling another and grasps his opponent's shorts waistband or pocket, flexing strongly while the other player, trying to escape, forcibly extends the finger. For some reason, it is almost always the ring finger which is injured. A piece of bone may be

307

avulsed from the base of the distal phalanx, which makes repair and fixation easier, but usually an X-ray is normal and the diagnosis is not made until weeks or months later.

Anybody treating sportspeople should be aware of this injury and players should be advised that their shorts should have no pockets. The damage is detected by holding the PIP joint straight and asking the patient to flex the end of the finger at the DIP joint. Do it first on an uninjured finger so the player gets the idea.

If diagnosed at the time, the tendon can be reattached by a hand surgeon. If seen later, the choice lies between a tendon graft (with an uncertain prognosis and the risk of compromising the hitherto normal PIP joint), fusion of the DIP joint in slight flexion, and accepting the slight disability: most patients choose to accept it.

Tendon sheath disorders

I doubt if tendinitis can ever occur: there are so few cells inside tendons that it would be hard to raise an inflammatory reaction. The disorders which do occur arise on the surface of the tendon and involve its various ensheathing layers.

Tenosynovitis

This diagnosis is frequently made, but usually without a shred of justification. Where tendons pass under fibrous retinacula, as at the wrist and on the front of the fingers, they are protected by a **synovial** sheath which separates the tendon from the retinaculum. Inflammation of this tendon sheath, or tenosynovitis, occurs in an acute form in tendon sheath infections and chronically in rheumatoid disease and tuberculosis. Perhaps it occasionally occurs from overuse, although I doubt it, believing such patients to be really suffering from one of the conditions described below.

Stenosing tenovaginitis

Thickening of the **fibrous** sheath, whose cause is usually unknown, causes two common conditions. In *de Ouervain's* disease there is pain, tenderness, and swelling on the radial side of the wrist, over the tendons of abductor pollicis longus and extensor pollicis brevis. The pain is felt when using the thumb or ulnar-deviating the wrist. Finkelstein's test involves making a fist with the thumb under the fingers, then ulnar-deviating the wrist to reproduce the pain. Treatment consists of rest, followed by gentle stretching and strengthening exercises, and a gradual return to function. Local anaesthetic and steroid may resolve the pain; if that fails then surgical release is usually curative. In *trigger digits*, the fibrous sheath is thickened at the base of a finger or thumb, usually causing the typical triggering but sometimes just pain or difficulty in bending the digit. Treat with steroid injection followed by surgical release if that fails. [Editor's note: Rock climbers have reported to me that massage of the area may allow the triggering to resolve. RGH]

Rupture of the fibrous flexor sheath in the fingers

Rock climbers, hanging by their fingertips from tiny ledges of rock, apply enormous strain not only to the flexor tendons, which are designed to withstand this, but to their fibrous sheaths which are not. This produces a condition, well known in the climbing fraternity but not among doctors, where the fibrous sheath is torn or stretched and the flexor tendon can therefore bowstring across the front of the flexed finger. Bollen[9] examined the hands of 67 climbers taking part in the British Open Climbing Competition and found evidence of this in 18 (25%), usually in the ring finger of the dominant hand. Climbers often deal with it by wrapping tape round the finger. It seems unlikely that any surgical repair would withstand forces strong enough to damage a previously healthy sheath in a fit young person.

Extensor indicis proprius syndrome

Ritter and Inglis[10] described two athletes with pain and swelling on the back of the wrist over the tendon of extensor indicis proprius. At operation it was found that the muscle belly extended further distally than usual, into the fibrous tunnel on the back of the wrist. This is, therefore, a slightly different condition to stenosing tenovaginitis: it is not the walls of the tunnel which are thickened but its contents which are larger than normal. It is almost a form of compartment syndrome. Surgical decompression relieved the symptoms.

Peritendinitis crepitans

In this condition there is pain, swelling, and a characteristic crepitus on movement, occurring about 2 inches above the wrist, towards the radial side of the extensor aspect, where the extensor pollicis longus tendon crosses obliquely over the tendons of extensor carpi radialis longus and brevis; for this reason it is known in America as the intersection syndrome. It is not tenosynovitis as there is no tenosynovium at this level.

The condition is undoubtedly brought on by repeated and rapid flexion and extension of the wrist. It was originally described in industry and invariably settles with rest, but Williams[11] described seven cases in top-level oarsmen and one in a canoeist who were unwilling to rest and were cured almost immediately by surgical decompression. The condition in oarsmen is caused by gripping the oar more tightly as fatigue sets in. This prevents the oar from sliding through the hand, leading to exaggerated dorsiflexion of the wrist at the end of the stroke. Peritendinitis crepitans also occurs in skiers and weight-lifters.

Fractures of the hand

"Hand fractures can be complicated by deformity from no treatment, stiffness from over-treatment or both deformity and stiffness from poor treatment".[12]

What is required, therefore, is to distinguish between those hand fractures needing little or no treatment (and which are better without treatment) and those which need reduction, splintage, or operative fixation. Of the latter, it has been rightly said that "too often these fractures are treated as minor injuries, and major disability results".[13] These are summarised in Table 15.2 and discussed in more detail below.

Table 15.2 Treatment of some common fractures of the hand

Mobilisation in strapping or bandage	Reduction and splintage	Operation
Fractures of the fingertip Tiny flake fractures without subluxation Fractures of the neck of the fifth metacarpal Undisplaced fractures of the shaft of a metacarpal Fractures of the base of the proximal phalanx Epiphyseal fractures	Fractures of shafts of phalanges Mallet finger fractures without subluxation Fractures of the base of the first metacarpal, distal to the trapezio-metacarpal joint	Fractures of shafts of phalanges which cannot be held by splintage Fractures with subluxation of a joint Fractures carrying a large part of a joint surface Multiple fractures in the hand

In all cases, X-rays must be taken in two planes at right-angles to each other: PA and lateral. These will yield much more information if they are centred on the injury. Many X-ray departments only take PA and oblique films, but you should insist on a lateral film to assess angulation and displacement and to see small fragments which may otherwise be obscured.

However, there may be more than one fracture in the hand or even in one part of one finger, and a dislocation may be accompanied by a fracture. Do not stop looking when you have seen one abnormality.

The variety of fractures in the hand is great: those listed below are the more common or important ones. I have given more detailed accounts elsewhere.[14,15] Broadly speaking, those which are likely to cause permanent problems are ones involving the PIP joint and the shafts of the bones on either side of that joint: the proximal and middle phalanx.

Fractures needing little or no treatment

Fractures of the fingertip Crushing injuries often produce fractures of the tuft of the distal phalanx. These always heal and can be ignored: it is the soft tissue injury which needs to be treated. A painful sub-ungual haematoma should be released by using the red-hot end of a paperclip to burn through the nail or drilling through it with the pointed end of a scalpel blade.

Tiny flake fractures without subluxation These are common, especially on the front of the PIP joint (Figure 15.10). The flake of bone has been pulled

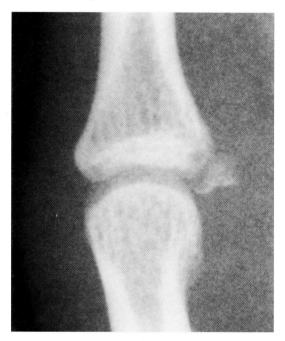

Figure 15.10 A virtually undisplaced pull-off fracture from the base of the middle phalanx. The joint is not subluxed. Mobilisation in strapping is the best treatment, but the finger will be painful and tender for several weeks

off by the ligament or capsule attached to it. It is best not to call them "chip" fractures, because that implies that they have been knocked off. They should be regarded and treated as ligamentous injuries, i.e. mobilised in neighbour strapping. It has been shown that this gives better results than splintage.[16]

However, it is very important to *ensure that there is no subluxation*: the joint surfaces must be absolutely concentric and normally lined up. If they are not, this is a serious injury (see below).

311

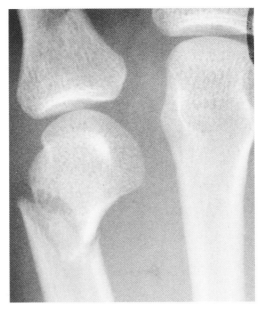

Figure 15.11   Fracture of the neck of the fifth metacarpal: a common injury needing minimal treatment

Fractures of the neck of the fifth metacarpal (Figure 15.11)   Though often called boxer's fractures, these are seldom sustained in proper boxing but commonly in informal fights, often by a drunk who misses his less inebriated opponent and hits a wall instead. Other people punch the wall deliberately as an expression of anger or frustration, presumably copying actors in American films.

Ford *et al.*[17] showed that excellent functional results are obtained by early mobilisation. I usually recommend a crepe bandage to remind the patient and other people that the hand has been injured, but this is not really treatment for the fracture. Cotton wool under the bandage is neither necessary nor desirable, as it restricts movement. These fractures will unite unless somebody interferes with them, but often with some deformity. In this case the deformity is only visible if the patient makes a fist, when the head of the fifth metacarpal is less prominent than normally, and very few patients are bothered by this. There is often a lag in extension of the little finger for a few months, but this almost always recovers fully. The fact that the fracture has united in flexion (fractures of the metacarpals invariably go into flexion) does not cause a bony prominence in the palm because there is enough movement at the fifth carpometacarpal joint to allow the fifth metacarpal to extend so that its head is still in line with the others.

312

The only bad results I have seen after this type of fracture have been following attempts at operative treatment.

Fractures which run into the *head* of the metacarpal (and thus enter the metacarpophalangeal (MP) joint) require more careful consideration; although some can be treated by simple mobilisation, others may require surgery.

Undisplaced fractures of the shafts of a metacarpal In most cases, these are adequately splinted by the adjoining intact metacarpal, though a protective bandage is used. Remember to check the finger end-on for rotational deformity (which may not be apparent on the X-ray), especially with spiral fractures.

Displaced or multiple metacarpal fractures may require splintage or surgery.

Ensure there is no dislocation between carpal and metacarpal bones by palpation and X-ray.

Fractures of the base of the proximal phalanx Although these involve the MP joint, it is not always necessary to achieve anatomical reduction and internal fixation. If the joint is mobilised after a few days, when the pain has settled down, the fractured base of the proximal phalanx will be moulded into roughly the right shape by the curved head of the metacarpal. A surprisingly good range of movement will result (Figure 15.12).

Epiphyseal fractures The epiphyses in the hand fuse – and growth stops – at the age of 13–14 in girls and 14–17 in boys. The one in the first metacarpal (which is proximal) fuses before those in the other metacarpals (which are distal). In the phalanges they are all proximal, but those in the distal phalanges fuse before the middle and proximal phalanges.

If there is gross deformity, it should be reduced but residual or minor deformity will be completely corrected by growth, provided the deformity is in the plane of movement of the adjacent joint. However, rotational deformity will *not* correct itself.

After care With these types of fracture, the limiting factor in the patient resuming their sport is pain. Usually 2 or 3 weeks off sport will be needed. Neighbour strapping (see Figure 15.6), or a bandage should be worn during this period and perhaps when first playing again, as a warning sign.

Fractures needing reduction and splintage

It makes no sense to reduce a fracture and not splint it, or it will slip out of place again. External splintage is satisfactory for some fractures and should usually be maintained for 3 weeks.

313

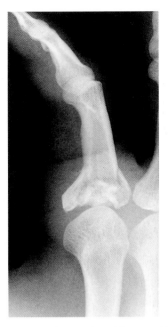

Figure 15.12   Oblique view showing severely comminuted fracture of the base of the proximal phalanx in a professional cricketer. He was treated by mobilisation in neighbour strapping and was playing county cricket again in 6 weeks

When a hand is injured, it tends to get stiff with the MP joints straight, the interphalangeal (IP) joints flexed and the thumb (if involved) adducted. This is the position of failure; it is often incurable and there is no excuse for it. If a hand needs splinting, it should be done in the opposite position to that above: the MP joints should be flexed as much as possible and the IP joints straight. If the thumb has not been injured, it should be left free but, if it has to be immobilised, it should be in a position of palmar (anterior) abduction. This is called the safe position or the position of immobilisation: the position from which it is easiest to regain a full range of movements.

Note that neither of these is the position of rest, that assumed by the hand when not in use or when its owner is asleep. The position of rest is nearer to the position of failure than to the safe position and the injured hand should not be allowed to remain in this position.

If only one finger is broken, it can be satisfactorily immobilised on a padded aluminium splint, such as those made by Zimmer, applied as shown in Figure 15.13, *not* as shown on the picture on the box containing the splint. The splint should only be on the *palmar* surface of the finger, leaving the end of the finger uncovered so that it can be examined end-on to make sure that any rotational deformity has been corrected. The splint should

314

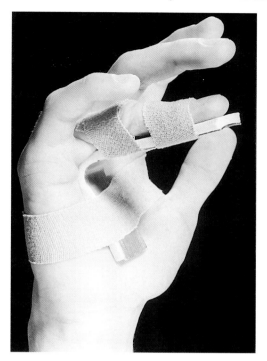

Figure 15.13 The correct way in which to splint a finger (see text). The right-angle bend in the splint should be at the palmar crease, not *at the base of the finger, and the tip of the finger should be visible so you can check rotation. (Reproduced with permission from* Sports Injuries, *2nd edn, ed. MA Hutson, Oxford University Press, 1996)*

be flexed to 90 degrees *at the palmar creases* because these, not the creases at the base of the finger, are the creases for the MP joint. The splint should not cross the wrist, or it will be joggled when the wrist is flexed and this force transmitted to the finger which is supposed to be immobilised.

If more than one finger is involved, volar and dorsal plaster slabs may be used, with the ends of the fingers exposed. The thumb can be satisfactorily immobilised in a plaster cast: in fact the only indication for a so-called "scaphoid plaster" is, in my opinion, an injury to the thumb or first metacarpal. If the fracture is in the distal half of the thumb, the plaster will need to be extended to the tip of the thumb.

Fractures of the shafts of the phalanges   In the phalanges, in contrast to the metacarpals, the angulation is always concave dorsally (Figure 15.14). This must be corrected, not only to realign the finger but to restore a smooth unstepped surface to the front of the phalanx, which is the floor of the tunnel in which the flexor tendon moves. If the tendon cannot glide smoothly, the finger will certainly stiffen.

315

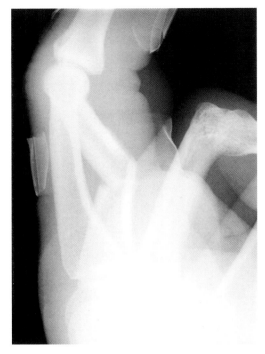

Figure 15.14   Fracture of the proximal phalanx of the ring finger with about 40 degrees of angulation concave dorsally. This must be corrected and held in the corrected position by a splint, as shown in Figure 15.13

Lateral X-rays are essential to assess the angulation and, after splinting, to check that it has been reduced. Severe rotational deformity is visible on the X-rays but milder forms can only be detected clinically (Figure 15.15a). If the finger is allowed to unite with a rotational deformity the deformed finger crosses over one of its neighbours in flexion. This is easy to correct at the time of the fracture, but difficult afterwards. That is why it is so important, with every fractured finger, to look at it end-on and compare the alignment of the fingernail with that of the other fingers. Do so again after manipulation to make sure that it remains correctly aligned.

Mallet finger fractures without subluxation   Bony involvement paradoxically permits you to immobilise the finger for a *shorter* period than if there is no fracture. Bone heals better than tendon and immobilisation of the DIP joint in a straight position on a suitable splint, such as a plastic Stack splint, need only be for 3 weeks. However, the joint must be X-rayed in the splint immediately after it has been applied to make sure that it has not caused subluxation. Subluxation or greater than 30% involvement of the joint surface requires operative treatment.

316

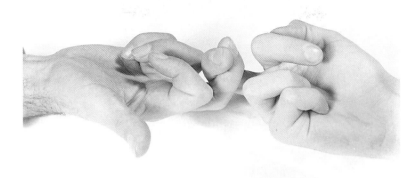

(a)

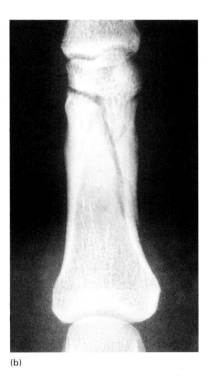

(b)

Figure 15.15 (a) Finger wrestling applies a twisting force to the finger which (b) caused this spiral fracture of the proximal phalanx. Any rotational deformity must be corrected

317

Fractures of the base of the first metacarpal, not involving the carpometacarpal joint These angulate into flexion so that the thumb is adducted across the palm and the span diminished. This should be corrected and held in a "scaphoid" plaster.

After care Fractures of the shaft of the proximal phalanx should be immobilised for 3 weeks, and then gently mobilised with the injured finger strapped to an adjoining intact finger. Contact sports and ball games should be avoided for 6 weeks.

Metacarpal fractures needing splintage should also be immobilised for 3 weeks.

Fractures of the shaft of the middle phalanx are uncommon but prone to non-union, so they may need longer splintage. They should be treated by an expert.

Fractures requiring open reduction and internal fixation

1. Fractures of the shafts of the proximal or middle phalanx in which splintage has failed to maintain satisfactory position.
2. Fractures into a joint with either:
   (a) a large fragment, carrying a third or more of the joint surface; or
   (b) subluxation, especially at the PIP joint as shown in Figure 15.16 (in the DIP joint, stiffness does not matter so much, but I think one should still correct subluxation) or the carpometacarpal joint of the thumb (i.e. Bennett's fractures).
3. Multiple fractures in the hand.

All these should be referred to an expert immediately. It is no good waiting 4 or 5 days; the fracture will already be uniting in the wrong position and the operation will be more difficult with less chance of a good result.

After care Internal fixation is to hold the fracture together until it heals. It is not strong enough to withstand similar forces to that which caused the injury.

The sportsperson has had an operation because, if this had not been done, the injury was likely to have resulted in permanent stiffness or deformity or both. If sport is resumed too soon, the fracture will come apart and nothing will have been gained from the operation. A player's career is more likely to be at risk from being left with a permanently crooked or stiff finger than from missing another few games.

318

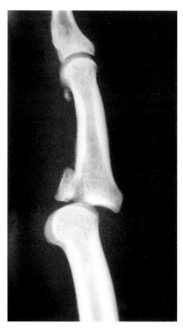

Figure 15.16   This injury is quite different from that shown in Figure 15.10 as there is not only a volar fracture but there is subluxation. The base of the middle phalanx is displaced dorsally in relation to the head of the proximal phalanx. This is a serious injury and difficult to treat; it needs an expert. (Reproduced with permission from Watson Jones' Fractures and Joint Injuries, *6th edn, ed. JN Wilson, Churchill Livingstone, 1982)*

Light training could begin after 4 weeks, but serious sport should be deferred until 6 weeks.

Nerve compression

The commonest type of nerve compression, carpal tunnel syndrome, is not particularly associated with sport but, because it is so common, may be seen in sportsmen or sportswomen. It is most common in women between the ages of 35 and 55. In men, symptoms are often atypical.

Cyclists may bear up to one third of their body weight on the handlebars and this compresses the ulnar nerve at the base of the hypothenar eminence, causing handlebar palsy. Sometimes only the deep motor branch of the ulnar nerve is affected and the sensory branch is spared.[18]

Dedicated ten pin bowlers, who play five or more times a week, may develop fibrous tissue around the ulnar digital nerve of the thumb where it is inserted into the hole in the bowl.[19] This can be relieved by changing the grip or stopping bowling.

319

The wrist

Fractures

Fractures of the wrist always need treatment and should always be assessed by an orthopaedic or hand surgeon within a day or two of the injury. To dismiss them as "just a crack" is to invite trouble in the future. An X-ray is essential but first you must examine the wrist with care. Each carpal bone can be fractured. Fractures of the scaphoid are the most common and most important. The distal end of the radius is very commonly fractured in the elderly. In younger people this injury is serious. The bone is stronger and therefore a more violent impact is necessary to fracture it.

Wrist fractures usually result from a fall on the outstretched hand. The soccer goalkeeper may have his wrist forcibly extended by the impact of the ball on his hand. Fracture of the scaphoid is quite a common injury in goalkeepers.

A normal X-ray does not exclude a ligamentous injury. These will be discussed in the next section.

Examination

The purpose of clinical examination is to localize tenderness. Press carefully all round the wrist at the level of the distal radius and ulna, then again over the proximal row of carpus and finally around the distal row of carpus to discover the *most tender spot*. The reason for this is to enable you to order the appropriate X-rays. If you ask just for X-rays of the wrist, you will get X-rays of the wrist, and this will serve you right. These may not show a fracture of the scaphoid and almost certainly will not show a fracture of the hook of the hamate: those require special views and, on the basis of clinical suspicion as to which bone is fractured, you must order the X-ray views which are necessary to show that fracture. Alternatively, the tenderness may be at the joint between two bones (e.g. the scapholunate joint), indicating a ligamentous injury.

Fractures of the scaphoid

Abnormal tenderness in the anatomical snuff-box indicates a fracture of the scaphoid, but some tenderness there is normal, as you are pressing on the terminal branches of the radial nerve; you must compare it with the other wrist. X-rays should be taken with the wrist in ulnar deviation. The fracture may not be obvious on the X-rays and the medicolegal consequences of failing to X-ray or diagnose a fracture of the scaphoid are all too often seen in the law courts. It is better to be on the safe side. Even without a fracture, there has been an injury which is causing pain and it will be more

320

comfortable and more likely to settle down quickly if it is immobilised completely for 2 weeks.

Small fractures of the tuberosity at the distal end of the scaphoid (Figure 15.17) are not very important and only need 3–4 weeks in plaster, but any

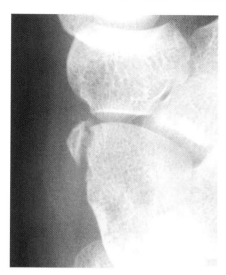

Figure 15.17   Fracture of tuberosity of scaphoid, either comminuted or a few weeks old. This only needs 4 weeks in plaster

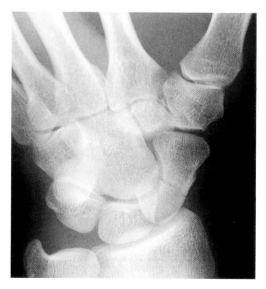

Figure 15.18   Fractures across the scaphoid sometimes lead to non-union even if treated, and probably always fail to unite if not treated. The fracture is not always as obvious as this one

321

fracture which goes right across the scaphoid (Figure 15.18) should sound warning bells.

There is clear evidence that delay in starting immobilisation of a fractured scaphoid leads to an increased likelihood of non-union. The longer the delay, the greater the likelihood. Sportspeople will try to dismiss the injury because they want to play next week. They do not understand the potential problems: insist on proper treatment. It is not worth risking the development of non-union and arthritis which may put an end to the player's sporting career.

Any painful injured wrist should be immobilised in plaster-of-Paris for 2 weeks and then reassessed, with further X-rays, by an experienced orthopaedic or hand surgeon. If the wrist is still painful and the X-rays remain doubtful, a technetium bone scan should be done without any further delay. A normal scan rules out a fracture, although not a ligamentous injury. If the scan is hot, it will show you which part of the wrist is injured.

Traditionally, the treatment of fractures of the wrist of the scaphoid in the UK has been in a below-elbow plaster cast including the first metacarpal and proximal phalanx of the thumb. In America and continental Europe it is usual to employ an above-elbow cast for the first 6 weeks followed by a below-elbow cast for another 6 weeks. There is no conclusive evidence that this is any better.[20] Our own research showed that there is no advantage in immobilising the thumb. I believe that the best treatment is a below-elbow plaster, with the wrist slightly extended and the thumb free, making it easier for the patient to use his hand. The important thing is that the wrist is effectively immobilised and the plaster is not allowed to become loose, soft or broken.

Treatment should be supervised by an orthopaedic or hand surgeon. Unfortunately, it is difficult to determine when union has occurred. The tenderness usually disappears quickly and X-rays, even after 8 weeks, are often ambiguous. In my opinion, all fractures across the scaphoid should be completely immobilised for 8 weeks. If there is still doubt, clinically or radiologically, a further 4 weeks in plaster is recommended.

Even after proper treatment, about 12% will fail to unite; more if the fracture is near the proximal pole. However, without treatment, they probably all fail to unite, so treatment is important.

Non-union will lead to osteoarthritis in 10 years in 90% of patients, and most of these will develop symptoms. The only cure is an operation of bone grafting, with or without internal fixation, possibly followed by another period of immobilisation. Only about 75% are successful in achieving bone union so, if the patient has no symptoms at all, it may be best to accept the situation. One famous English soccer goalkeeper played successfully in the World Cup with a longstanding non-united scaphoid fracture which was causing little trouble.

Fractures of the triquetrum

The second most common carpal fracture is a dorsal flake fracture of the triquetrum.[21] It is visible on the lateral X-ray, where it may look as though it came off the lunate. The flake of bone has been pulled off by the ligament to which it is attached and this can be regarded and treated as a ligamentous injury. Three weeks in a plaster cast with the wrist straight is enough.

Fractures of the hook of the hamate

This rare injury is almost confined to sport.[22,23] It is caused by the impact of the end of a golf club, cricket bat, tennis or badminton racket, or similar implement on the hook of the hamate (Figure 15.19). This is situated

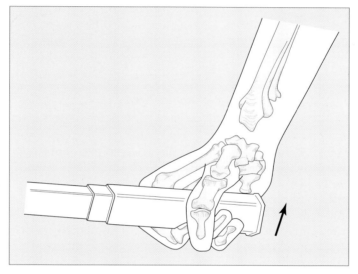

Figure 15.19   Mechanism of a fracture of the hook of the hamate. (Reproduced from Stark et al,[23] *with permission)*

about one centimetre distal and slightly radial to the pisiform, although covered by fat and not so easy to palpate. In sports like golf and cricket, it affects the top hand and is usually caused by an impact such as the golf club hitting the ground instead of the ball. The clues to diagnosis are the history and the precise site of the tenderness over the hamate. As the flexor tendons to the ring and little fingers run alongside the hook, there may be pain on moving these fingers. There may also be sensory changes in those fingers, as branches of the ulnar nerve pass over the hook. Ordinary X-rays will not show this fracture. It requires an oblique view (in about 30 degrees of supination) or a "carpal tunnel view" in which the beam runs along the

323

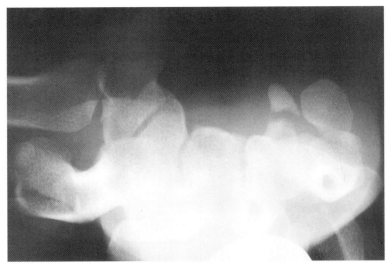

Figure 15.20   Carpal tunnel view of wrist. The main carpal bones and the metacarpals (some seen end-on) are below. Above, from right to left: pisiform, fractured hook of hamate, scaphoid and trapezium. (Reproduced with permission from Sports Injuries, *2nd edn, ed. MA Hutson, Oxford University Press, 1996)*

carpal tunnel (Figure 15.20). For this the wrist has to be dorsiflexed, which may be prevented by pain, in which case a CT scan will be needed to show the fracture.

This injury is not well known and is therefore usually missed. The patient is often not seen until later, by which time he has painful non-union of the fracture, cured by excision of the hook. This should be done by an experienced hand surgeon, as the ulnar nerve is only millimetres away.

When I have seen recent injuries, I have treated them in the same way, as immobilisation seems unlikely to succeed and internal fixation of the hook (although possible) would be very fiddly and might not produce rigid fixation.

Fractures of the trapezial ridge

The trapezium has a ridge on its palmar surface which may be fractured by a fall on the outstretched hand.[24] This is another fracture that cannot be seen on ordinary X-rays. It is diagnosed by the history and by finding tenderness localised to the front of the trapezium (just distal to the scaphoid tuberosity but proximal to the base of the first metacarpal). It can be confirmed by carpal tunnel view X-rays, as in Figure 15.20, although the trapezium is rather dark and its ridge is hard to see.

This injury seems to be uncommon, but I suspect it is often missed. Fresh cases should be immobilised in plaster for about 4 weeks: in late cases excision of the fractured fragment has been recommended.

Joint injuries of the wrist

Dislocations

It takes a violent force to dislocate the wrist and these uncommon injuries seldom occur in sport. Depending on the nature of the dislocation, there may or may not be obvious deformity. You should *not* attempt to reduce the dislocation. An X-ray must be taken first to define the exact nature of the injury because:

- Reduction is difficult and requires full anaesthesia: unskilled attempts may do harm
- There may be an associated fracture
- The future stability of the wrist depends on the exact pattern of injury and displacement. The orthopaedic surgeon treating the patient needs to see X-rays with the wrist in the dislocated position.

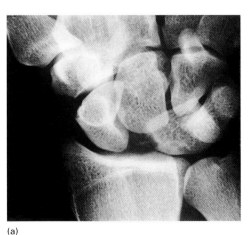 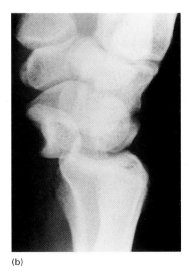

(a)   (b)

Figure 15.21   Anterior dislocation of the lunate, into the carpal tunnel. This is more obvious on the lateral view, where the lunate is not only dislocated forwards but dislocated and rotated through 90 degrees so that its distal concavity is now facing forwards. However, it should also be obvious from the PA view that something is badly wrong: the normal smooth arc of the mid-carpal joint is broken and there is a gap between the scaphoid and lunate (with a tiny flake of bone detached from the latter)

325

Almost any pattern is possible, but the three least uncommon are:

1. *Perilunar dislocation*. The lunate stays in its correct relationship to the radius but the rest of the carpus dislocates dorsally around it.
2. *Dislocation of the lunate* (Figure 15.21). This is believed to be a second stage of perilunar dislocation. The carpus returns to its normal position, pushing the lunate forwards into the carpal tunnel, where it may compress the median nerve. Open reduction may be needed. Surprisingly, the lunate seldom goes avascular afterwards, because it retains a soft tissue pedicle which presumably carries an adequate blood supply.
3. *Trans-scaphoid perilunar dislocation*. The dislocation is accompanied by a fracture through the waist of the scaphoid. These are very unstable injuries and the scaphoid fracture is particularly prone to non-union. Operation is required.

If any of these injuries is suspected or indeed possible, the patient must be taken to hospital and X-rayed immediately. Although the abnormality on the X-ray should be obvious, it is unfortunately sometimes overlooked by inexperienced casualty officers who are not used to looking at lateral X-rays of the wrist. A senior opinion should be obtained.

Torn ligaments

A normal X-ray does not mean a normal wrist. Individual ligaments can be torn, but these are sometimes hard to diagnose accurately, even by

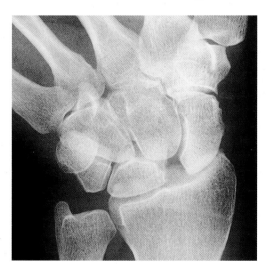

Figure 15.22 The ligaments joining the scaphoid and lunate have been torn, allowing a gap to develop between these bones. This is sometimes called the Terry-Thomas sign because of its resemblance to the gap between that actor's front teeth. The injury also allows the scaphoid to flex in relation to the other carpal bones. This is one form of carpal instability

experts. The best clue is tenderness localised to one of the intercarpal joints. An X-ray may show a gap between the scaphoid and lunate (Figure 15.22), or the lunate tilted back into dorsiflexion, but the changes may be subtle and difficult to detect.

If the injury is missed, the patient will probably present later with carpal instability (see below).

Sprained wrist

There is an old adage that "sprained wrist does not exist". This is not strictly true but should always be borne in mind, because it is a diagnosis which can only be made in retrospect. To diagnose a sprained wrist without getting an X-ray is irresponsible, foolish, negligent, and unforgivable.

Chronic pain in the wrist

In these cases there is often a history of an apparently minor injury. Many people, especially sportspeople, frequently suffer minor injuries and may wrongly attribute their pain to some small injury.

The path to a correct diagnosis follows a proper history, a thorough examination, and appropriate investigation. Obtain as much detail as possible about the mechanism of the injury and its relationship to the onset of pain: did the pain come on at once or not until weeks or months later? Painful clicking is usually significant but some people just have clicky wrists. Localised tenderness is the most useful physical sign. Clinically detectable instability of the wrist (i.e. abnormal AP movement on stress) is uncommon but testing for it may cause pain, which is significant. Examine the inferior radio-ulnar joint and observe full pronation and supination of the forearm. X-rays must be of good quality. A series of views of the wrist in various positions, including an AP (standard views of the wrist are PA) with the patient gripping tightly, may reveal an abnormal gap between the carpal bones or abnormal alignment of one of them. X-ray screening of the wrists is more useful. Various directions of stress can be applied. Both wrists should be screened, for comparison. Ideally, this should be done with (not by) the radiologist and should be recorded on videotape so that it can be studied over and over again to pick up some change in the rhythm of movement. Typically, some bones lag behind during movement and then catch up suddenly with a painful click. Best of all, while screening, get the patient to reproduce the movement or position which produces their symptoms.

Ligamentous injuries may also be visible on arthroscopy and MRI can be invaluable, for example in the early stages of avascular necrosis of the lunate before radiologically visible changes have occurred.

327

Kienboch's disease

Avacular necrosis of the lunate or Kienbok's disease is reported to be more common in those who participate in martial arts. Symptoms include loss of grip strength, pain, and reduced range of motion. X-rays will show the progression of the disease. Treatment is dependent upon the X-ray findings and should be managed by a hand surgeon.

Carpal instability

This is a particularly difficult subject.[25] Essentially, there are two main types: dissociative, in which there is a gap between two bones in the same row of the carpus (Figure 15.20), and non-dissociative, in which part or all of one carpal row (usually the proximal row) is malaligned in relationship to the other row and adjoining bones. The proximal row is fitted in between, or "intercalated" between, the fixed distal end of the radius and ulnar and the distal row of carpal bones which is fairly rigidly fixed to the bases of the metacarpals. This proximal row, or intercalated segment, is freely mobile and controlled only by ligaments, so that if those are damaged it can tilt into dorsiflexion (dorsal intercalated segment instability, or DISI) or, less often, into palmar – or volar – flexion (volar intercalated segment instability, or VISI). These gaps or malignments may be present all the time ("static" carpal instability) but – which can make diagnosis so difficult – they may be intermittent and only occur in certain positions or activities ("dynamic" carpal instability). Intermittent instabilities may be hard to demonstrate and diagnose. X-ray screening is useful, as the patient can attempt to reproduce the phenomenon while you are observing the movements of the carpal bones. Patients should be treated by a specialist hand surgeon.

Conclusion

Many hand injuries are minor but some, although appearing to be minor, can cause lasting and important disability. Do not jump to conclusions and accept an apparently obvious diagnosis, because there may be other injuries too: for example, a dislocation may be accompanied by a significant fracture. It is always wise to obtain an X-ray, especially in injuries of the wrist; in the hand, the X-ray should be centred on that part which is injured if it is to yield useful information.

Wrist injuries should always be assessed by an expert. Injured fingers can be treated according to the scheme shown in Figure 15.23.

The reason for treating the potentially serious injuries is to prevent permanent disability. This will delay a return to sport but, even for

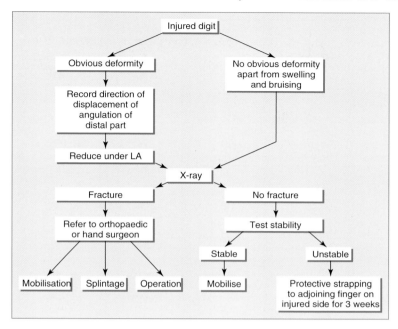

Figure 15.23   Scheme of management of a closed injury to a finger or thumb. LA, local anaesthetic

professional sportspeople, this is less likely to jeopardise their sporting future – and indeed their lives after sport – than being left with a permanently painful wrist or stiff crooked finger. Serious treatment and an adequate period of recovery after these more serious injuries is in the player's best interest.

References

1 Amadio PC. Epidemiology of hand and wrist injuries in sports. *Hand Clinics* 1990;**6**:379–81.
2 Campbell AS. Hand injuries at leisure. *J Hand Surg* 1985;**10B**:300–2.
3 Murphy NM, Riley P, Keys C. Ice-skating injuries to the hand. *J Hand Surg* 1990;**15B**:349–51.
4 Stener B. Displacement of the ruptured ulnar collateral ligament of the metacarpophalangeal joint of the thumb. *J Bone Joint Surg* 1962;**44B**:869–79.
5 Abrahamsson S-O, Sollerman C, Lundborg G, Larsson J, Egund N. Diagnosis of displaced ulnar collateral ligament of the metacarpophalangeal joint of the thumb. *J Hand Surg* 1990;**15A**:457–60.
6 Burke F. Mallet finger. *J Hand Surg* 1988;**13B**:115–17.
7 Souter WA. The boutonnière deformity. *J Bone Joint Surg* 1967;**49B**:710–21.
8 Lunn PG, Lamb DW. "Rugby finger" – avulsion of profundus of ring finger. *J Hand Surg* 1984;**9B**:69–71.

9 Bollen S. Injury to the A2 pulley in rock climbers. *J Hand Surg* 1990;**15B**: 268–70.
10 Ritter MA, Inglis AE. The extensor indicis proprius syndrome. *J Bone Joint Surg* 1969;**51A**:1645–8.
11 Williams JGP. Surgical management of traumatic non-infective tenosynovitis of the wrist extensors. *J Bone Joint Surg* 1977;**59B**:408–10.
12 Swanson AB. Fractures involving the digits of the hand. *Orthop Clin North Am* 1970;**1**:261.
13 Lipscomb PR. Management of fractures of the hand. *The American Surgeon* 1963;**29**:277.
14 Barton NJ. Fractures of the hand. *J Bone Joint Surg* 1984;**66B**:159–67.
15 Barton NJ. Fractures and joint injuries of the hand. In: Wilson JN (ed.). *Watson Jones' fractures and joint injuries*, 6th edn. Edinburgh: Churchill Livingstone, 1982, pp. 739–88.
16 Phair IC, Quinton DN, Allen MJ. The conservative management of volar avulsion fractures of the PIP joint. *J Hand Surg* 1989;**14B**:168–70.
17 Ford DJ, Ali MS, Steel WM. Fractures of the fifth metacarpal neck: is reduction or immobilization necessary?. *J Hand Surg* 1989;**14B**:165–7.
18 Richmond DR. Handlebar problems in bicycling. *Clin Sports Med* 1994;**13**: 165–73.
19 Dobyns JH, O'Brien ET, Linscheid RL, Farrow GM. Bowler's thumb: diagnosis and treatment. A review of seventeen cases. *J Bone Joint Surg* 1972;**54A**:751–5.
20 Barton NJ. Twenty questions about scaphoid fractures. *J Hand Surg* 1992;**17B**: 289–310.
21 Bartone NF, Grieco RV. Fractures of the triquetrum. *J Bone Joint Surg* 1956; **38A**:353–6.
22 Bishop AT, Beckenbaugh RD. Fracture of the hamate hook. *J Hand Surg* 1988; **13A**:135–9.
23 Stark HH, Jobe FW, Boyes JH, Ashworth CR. Fracture of the hook of the hamate in athletes. *J Bone Joint Surg* 1977;**59A**:575–82.
24 Palmer AK. Trapezial ridge fractures. *J Hand Surg* 1981;**6**:561–4.
25 Taleisnik J. Carpal instability. *J Bone Joint Surg* 1988;**70A**:1262–8.

Appendix Additional conditions affecting the hand and wrist by Roger G Hackney

Impaction syndromes

Ulnar impaction syndrome occurs in gymnastics with weight-bearing activities with the wrist in a position of dorsiflexion, pronation, and ulnar deviation. Pain and swelling are found over the wrist on the ulnar side at the distal radio-ulnar joint, aggravated by ulnar deviation. In young gymnasts, the distal radial epiphysis may be damaged leading to a positive ulnar variance (a longer ulna). The triangular fibrocartilage complex (TFCC) is at greater risk of injury from the impaction and torsion on the pommel horse and vault in particular.

Examination shows weakness of grip with pain and clicking on the ulnar side of the wrist, made worse by ulnar deviation. Differential diagnosis includes stress fractures, dorsiflexion, and dorsal wrist capsulitis. Pain on impaction with dorsiflexion is worse over the scapholunate ligament.

Diagnosis is by clinical examination aided by MRI scanning and arthroscopy of the wrist.

Treatment is along standard lines with rest from aggravating activities, especially important in the young. Adjusting the gymnast's technique is important in avoiding a recurrence.

Nerve entrapments in chronic pain in the wrist and forearm

Pronator syndrome is compression of the median nerve in the elbow or forearm. It is found in sports using repeated forceful pronation and gripping, for example throwing. Athletes complain of forearm pain and hand pain which is worse on activity. Sensory deficit is less common than with carpal tunnel syndrome. The three sites of compression include under pronator teres either at a high origin or between the two heads, under flexor digitorum superficialis, or under the ligament of Struthers if this is above a supracondylar process. Test for the syndrome by deep palpation over the area of entrapment to reproduce the symptoms and Tinel's sign. Treatment is by rest from any aggravating activities, analgesia, and splinting if severe. Surgery is reserved for those who have not settled after 5 months.

Distal posterior interosseous nerve syndrome

There is compression of the deep terminal branch as it passes over the distal radius. The condition presents with a dull ache in the wrist worse on hyperextension. It is a diagnosis of exclusion.

Anterior interosseous nerve syndrome

The motor branch of the median nerve may be compressed in the forearm. The athlete may present after a single episode of activity with pain and an inability to pinch the fingertips of index finger and thumb together. This usually settles with rest and non-steroidal anti-inflammatory drugs (NSAIDs).

Infection

Infections of the hand may develop rapidly with apparently few clinical signs. Paronychia, infections of the nail bed, and infections of the distal finger pulp once established are best treated with surgical drainage.

331

Antibiotics alone will not adequately deal with the pus. There are several tissue planes or potential spaces along which infection may spread. The degree of swelling and other clinical signs may be much less than expected given the amount of pain. Pain on palpation together with some warmth and swelling should ring alarm bells. Infection speading along a tendon sheath gives rise to intense pain on moving the affected finger. The treatment is urgent surgical drainage.

16 Injuries of the elbow and forearm

ROGER G HACKNEY

Anatomy

The elbow joint consists of two types of articulation and hence two types of motion. There is a hinge joint between the ulna and humerus which allows flexion and extension. The radiohumeral and radioulnar joint allows rotation in an axial plane as well as a hinge movement. The elbow sits in a varying amount of valgus, the so-called carrying angle. The joint is stabilised by collateral ligaments. The annular ligament permits rotation of the radial head. The forearm musculature is attached to bony prominences of the humerus. There are complex relationships between muscular attachments and the three major nerves which cross the elbow.

Epidemiology

Studies of the incidence of a history of elbow, forearm, and wrist injuries in tennis players have shown that roughly half have experienced lateral elbow pain; 47% of recreational and 45% of world class players. A similar incidence of 50% was found among players over 30 years old in three clubs. Medial pain is 20% as common. Elbow injuries occur in other sports that involve gripping, such as fencing, as well as throwing, and in swimming. Occupational activities that require use of the forearm also give rise to elbow pain.

Classification

Overuse injuries are divided into their anatomical site and will be described as such in this chapter. Lateral, medial, and posterior injuries occur of both soft tissue and bone.

Lateral injuries to the elbow

Lateral epicondylitis

Tennis elbow was originally reported as lawn tennis elbow in 1883 by Runge. The pain is located at the common extensor origin in tennis players aged 35–50 years. The incidence increases the more tennis is played. The risk relates to activities that tension the wrist and hence the extensors and supinator muscles. The pain and pathology are located around the extensor origin specifically at extensor carpi radialis brevis (ECRB), but also at the other extensor muscles of the common origin. The onset is usually insidious and gradual.

Pathology

The cause is repetitive microtrauma, resulting in microtears, fibrosis, granulation, and mucoid degeneration, with partial failure of the tendon

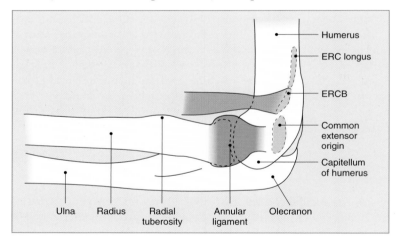

Figure 16.1 Origin of extensor carpi radialis brevis (ERCB)

of ERCB. At surgical inspection, there is oedema with friable grey tendon which has lost the parallel alignment of resilient properly tensioned fibres. There is a vascular fibroblastic invasion, i.e. degeneration, a tendinosis similar to that seen in other overused tendons.

History

The pain is located at the lateral epicondyle, and is worse on playing the aggravating sport. There is morning stiffness, an aching pain, and wrist extension is painful anterior to or over the lateral epicondyle. The pain

334

may radiate into the forearm. In the sporting context, the stroke which produces the pain should be identified.

Examination

The site of pain is the lateral epicondyle. Pain is also felt over the radio-ulnar joint and the extensor muscle mass. Resisted extension of the wrist reproduces pain. More specifically, forced flexion of the extended index and middle fingers is painful. Range of movement (ROM) is restricted in severe cases.

Investigation

X-rays exclude calcific deposits and degeneration of the radiocapitellar joint.

Treatment

Conservative   Control of pain with rest, ice, and NSAIDs, is important. When the forearm is strong enough to shake a hand then rehabilitation can begin in earnest. Activity modification and exercises together with modification of technique and equipment form the basics of treatment. Initially, racquet sports are avoided depending upon the degree and severity of symptoms. Those with chronic symptoms are usually less compliant and ice is less effective. NSAIDs may be needed for several weeks.

Gentle passive and active range of movement exercises to preserve and improve ROM are performed 3–6 times daily. Symptoms should not be reproduced.

The Mills manoeuvre, a sudden forced flexion of the wrist, is said to break down scar and give relief, but is painful and should only be attempted by those with experience in manipulation.

Bracing with a 20 degree wrist splint may be helpful. The forearm counterforce braces seem to reduce pain, but probably work by reducing muscle expansion, reducing muscle contractile tension and hence work done by the forearm muscles. The brace should be worn during the day and whenever racquet sports are played.

When full elbow and wrist ROM are achieved, the rehabilitation programme can become more aggressive. Active wrist exercises without external resistance are introduced, including extension, flexion, and circumduction. Forearm supination and pronation work with isometric contractions leads to repetitions with light weights or rubber tubing with progression over weeks. This strengthening regimen is to reduce the risk of re-injury.

335

Local anaesthetic and steroid should be used only rarely, and then for non-competitive athletes with acute pain which makes normal life difficult. Prednisolone (40 mg) with local anaesthetic are injected locally, into the point of maximum tenderness, the sub-aponeurotic space of ERCB. The practitioner must beware of subdermal atrophy from leakage back under the skin. No more than three steroid injections should be given in a year. Injections should not continue if there has been only a temporary response.

The most important means of avoiding recurrence is to improve stroke play and racquet technique (see Appendix).

Surgery The indications for surgery are a year's symptoms, calcification at the extensor origin, multiple cortisone injections, constant pain, and poor modification of the patient's activity. High performance athletes may require earlier surgery. There are many surgical options, but debridement of granulation tissue at the site of insertion of ERCB addresses the pathology. Other authors decorticate the epicondyle.

Postoperatively, 7 days immobilisation are followed by ROM exercises when painless, at around 3 weeks. A strengthening programme for 3–6 months with maintenance of flexibility and correction of technical errors will allow a return to full competition. A counterforce brace can be used during rehabilitation.

Differential diagnosis

The differential diagnosis of lateral elbow pain includes radiocapitellar osteoarthritis. There is pain on axial loading on supination and pronation, which is not painful with lateral epicondylitis.

Lateral injuries to the elbow in children

- **Acute**
  Osteochondritis dissecans of the capitellum, including separation
  Osteochondrosis of the capitellum
  Avulsion fractures of the lateral humeral condyle
  Fracture of the capitellum and distal humerus
  Anterior subluxation of the humeral head
  Fracture of the proximal radius

- **Chronic**
  Lateral humeral epicondylitis
  Radial head hypertrophy
  Loose bodies
  Osteochondritis of the capitellum and radial head

Entrapment of the radial nerve produces similar symptoms with pain around the extensor–supinator mass at the lateral elbow. The pain radiates into the forearm but the character of the pain is different, more vague and aching in nature, and the most tender spot is distal. The nerve can be entrapped anywhere along its course from radial head to supinator. Electromyelography is not usually helpful in making the diagnosis, which is largely clinical. Pain from nerve root entrapment more proximally in the neck can mimic lateral elbow pain, but there are usually adequate signs of a problem in the neck.

Throwing injuries

The throwing mechanism is fully described in Chapter 17. The valgus stresses on the elbow during the acceleration phase of throwing produce

Throwing injuries to the elbow

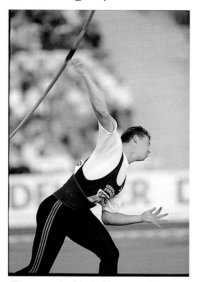

(Photograph: Mark Shearman)

The acceleration phase of throwing produces a very rapid movement of the elbow with angular velocities of 5000 degrees per second and accelerations of 500 000 degrees per second. Repetitive throwing causes injury to the elbow. Throwing places a valgus strain on the elbow, particularly in the acceleration phase. The term valgus overload is used to describe the spectrum of injuries that results in all compartments of the elbow. In the position of abduction and external rotation the weight of the forearm and implement is borne by the anterior band of the ulnar collateral ligament. The forces involved may exceed the tensile strength of the ulnar collateral ligament. Continued traction on this ligament results in weakening and stretching. This permits an increase in valgus deformity with traction on medial structures and compression laterally. Excess compressive loads laterally damage the radiocapitellar articulation. Valgus stress in children damages the growing medial epicondylar epiphysis. Posteriorly, impingement of the medial tip of the olecranon in the olecranon fossa results in osteophyte and loose body formation.

Valgus stress can be reduced by limiting the number of throws performed by a child and by coaching the use of a high elbow in the acceleration phase.

compression injuries on the lateral elbow. The elbow of the growing child is most at risk.

Osteochondritis dissecans

The repetitive valgus forces in throwing injure the articular surface and underlying bone. This trauma leads to osteochondrosis and osteochondritis

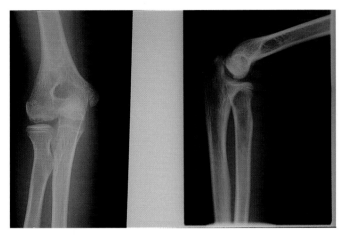

Figure 16.2   Osteochondritis dissecans of the capitellum

dissecans (OCD). The youngest and least experienced baseball pitchers are most at risk. The cause of osteochondritis dissecans is a vascular insufficiency which is aggravated by valgus compressive forces. The condition is different from Panner's disease, a fragmentation of the entire capitellar ossification centre in children aged 7–12. OCD occurs in older children aged 13–16. OCD produces joint surface deformity, collapse, and loose body formation. The long term consequences are joint irregularity and arthrosis.

These phenomena are seen in young baseball pitchers, in whom the condition is called Little Leaguer's Elbow. Little Leaguer's Elbow presents with elbow pain, radial head overgrowth, loss of supination, and extension. Similar injuries are seen in gymnasts, where the carrying angle produces the valgus stress with weight-bearing on handstands. The lesions can be treated arthroscopically with removal of the loose bodies, and drilling the subchondral bone to encourage regrowth of articular surface.

338

Panner's disease

Panner's disease is an osteochondrosis avascular necrosis of the capitellar epiphysis during initial ossification. It occurs in baseball pitchers and gymnasts, from repeated compression forces to the lateral side. Sufferers complain of tenderness, loss of range of motion, swelling, crepitus, and pain on valgus loading. X-ray shows sclerosis, fissuring, and irregular margins of the capitellum.

Treatment is by rest, maintaining ROM, rehabilitation, and re-education in technique. If diagnosed early then Panner's disease can heal. If it continues, then growth arrest and collapse occur.

The radial head overgrowth is caused by a hyperaemic response during the healing phase. Loss of joint congruity leads to secondary osteoarthritis. An arthroscopic debridement can be done.

Osteochondritis dissecans looks very similar and the condition of Panner's disease may be a continuum. X-ray of OCD shows subarticular rarefaction, cyst formation, and cortical fragmentation or flattening with loose bodies.

Posterior injuries to the elbow

Posterior injuries

- **Acute**
  Olecranon fractures, apophysitis and spurs
  Triceps strain
  Olecranon bursitis

- **Chronic**
  Olecranon traction apophysitis, spurs
  Loose bodies in the posterior compartment
  Synovitis
  Posteromedial spurs

Triceps overload: tendinitis and apophysitis

The elbow undergoes a very rapid extension from flexion in the acceleration phase of throwing. The pull of the triceps can lead to injury to the muscle tendon or the bone itself as an avulsion injury or stress fracture. In children the growth plate is injured.

339

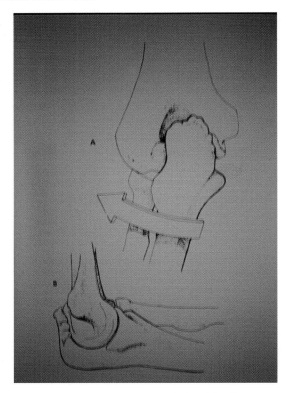

Figure 16.3   Posterolateral injuries of the elbow

Examination

The triceps tendon or bony insertion are tender. A reduction in range of movement should be taken seriously.

Investigation

Plain X-ray is used to exclude loose bodies and avulsion injuries.

Treatment

The overuse usually settles with adequate rest and pain relief. Chronic lesions give rise to spur formation, impingement, and loose bodies. Avulsion of the olecranon is rare, and may be undisplaced when rest will permit union. If displaced, then fixation will prevent non-union and continuing disability.

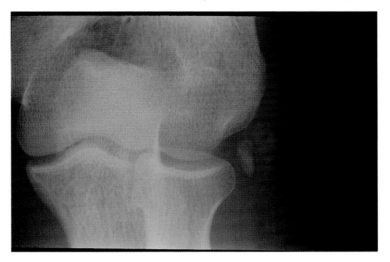

Figure 16.4   Loose bodies in the elbow

Hyperextension overload

Valgus stress, especially with a degree of medial laxity, leads to repeated hyperextension stress and impingement of the medial tip of the olecranon into the olecranon fossa. This causes osteophyte formation and, when they break off, loose bodies in the posterior fossa. There may be an area of damage to the posterior trochlea in the olecranon fossa. This articular surface degeneration corresponds to the lesions on the olecranon, so-called kissing lesions.

History

The history is of sudden pain in the elbow on throwing at the follow-through phase. The syndrome is associated with other damage in the elbow and a general aching is common.

Examination

There is a block to extension compared with the normal side and reproduction of pain on forced extension.

341

Investigation

Plain X-ray does not show the osteophytes as well as a CT scan.

Treatment

The osteophytes and loose bodies can be removed arthroscopically or by open operation. This may permit full extension and is the best hope for a return to sport, although this is not guaranteed.

Olecranon fractures

These may occur as a result of repetitive trauma causing a physeal stress fracture, from baseball pitching in the acceleration and follow-through phases. A bone scan confirms the diagnosis. Treatment is by rest or surgical fixation for displaced fractures. Fractures as a result of traumatic events require surgery.

Olecranon bursitis

This bursa lies beneath the olecranon at the point of the elbow. This is often injured in a fall or blow resulting in bleeding and a painful swelling. Elbow guards should be used where possible. Infection may occur when spontaneous pain, swelling, and redness are obvious. Treatment is drainage and treating any infection appropriately. Chronic inflammation may leave an elbow which is very painful to rest on. Surgery usually cures this.

Medial injuries to the elbow

Valgus stress can lead to medial pain from:

● Medial epicondylitis
● Medial epicondylar fractures
● Medial collateral ligament (MCL) injury or insufficiency
● Ulnar nerve tension neuropraxia
● Medial elbow intra-articular pathology.

Medial epicondylitis

Medial elbow pain requires a careful assessment because of the many possible causes. The incidence is 20% of that of lateral epicondylitis. Medial epicondylitis is related to wrist flexor activity and pronation, as in throwing and the pull-through stroke in swimming.

History

The athlete complains of pain and tenderness in the medial side of the elbow around the flexor and pronator origins. The tennis serve and overhead strokes are more responsible for producing medial pain, by repeated valgus stresses to the soft tissues of the medial elbow with wrist flexion and pronation. Forehand strokes can also lead to valgus overload. This is more common in tennis players who use a lot of top spin. The forced pronation aggravates symptoms at the pronator muscle.

Examination

Resisted flexion and pronation reproduces symptoms. The differentiation between medial epicondylitis and injury to the ulnar collateral ligament (UCL) can be difficult, indeed they may co-exist. Medial epicondylitis is distinguished from chronic UCL sprain by applying a valgus stress to an elbow that is slightly flexed, while the forearm is pronated and the wrist flexed. This position eliminates the effects of medial epicondylitis and results in a painless valgus stress test in the absence of an injury to the UCL. Injury to the ulnar nerve often occurs with medial epicondylitis pain. An incidence of 60% of ulnar nerve neuropraxia in those undergoing surgery for medial epicondylitis has been reported.

Pathology

Degeneration similar to that found in lateral epicondylitis is found at the interface between pronator teres and the other muscles of the common flexor origin. Major ruptures are uncommon.

Investigation

X-ray or bone scan will identify intra-articular pathology.

Treatment

Overall management is similar to the epicondylitis of the lateral side. Control of pain is followed by flexibility and gentle resistance exercises, emphasising pronation and wrist flexion. Suggestions include 3–6 sets of 10 reps 2–3 times daily, using the other hand or Theraband with progression as tolerated.

Surgical treatment for medial epicondylitis is less effective than for lateral epicondylitis. For persistent symptoms which fail to respond to conservative measures a return to racquet sports can be expected by 3 months. The flexor origin is freed from bone to remove granulation tissue. The surgeon

343

must reattach the flexor origin, if necessary with a suture anchor. The common flexor origin is a major stabiliser for the medial elbow. Over-aggressive surgery may cause instability.

Medial epicondylar fractures

An acute stress from a fall or throwing may result in a fracture through the epiphyseal plate. The elbow has a block to extension. The growth plate may become displaced into the joint and its position must be confirmed on X-ray. Surgical repair is then indicated.

Ulnar collateral ligament (UCL) injury (adults)

Overhead throwing or serving in tennis places valgus stresses upon the elbow. The anterior bundle of the UCL is the primary restraint to valgus

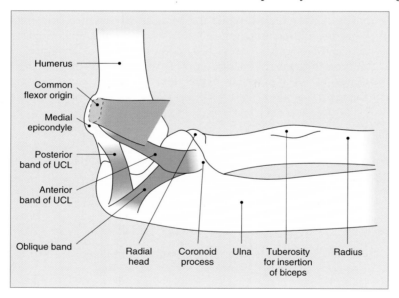

Figure 16.5 Anatomy of the ulnar collateral ligament (UCL)

stress in the acceleration phase of throwing. In this position the shoulder is abducted and externally rotated. Repeated valgus overload can produce ligamentous injury, pain, and instability, and a sense of loss of control of the throw. The pain is felt in the acceleration phase. Acute rupture of the UCL is uncommon in racquet sports but does happen in throwers, especially as an end result of chronic strain. This leads to valgus instability.

UCL pain is difficult to distinguish from medial epicondylitis. Co-existing injury to the ulnar nerve from traction is common. Ulnar nerve traction injury is found in 40% of those who undergo surgery for UCL insufficiency.

The articular configuration of the elbow joint is a secondary stabiliser. Abnormal stresses on the joint surfaces lead to degenerative changes with osteophytes that can lead to medial pain. The valgus overload also gives rise to lateral pain because of radiocapitellar joint compression and asynchronous firing of the forearm muscles. There is increased activity of ECRB in those with an injured UCL compared with the uninjured. This will lead to further joint compression laterally.

History

Elbow pain is felt in the tennis service stroke, and cocking and acceleration phases of throwing. There is a gradual increase in symptoms and pain on palpation of the UCL. Excessive use of top spin in racquet sports is implicated. Pain is felt as the forearm pronates.

Examination

Pain is palpable over the medial epicondyle and aggravated by pronating the forearm. Check for UCL stability (see below). There should be a detectable end point on stressing the ligament. Check for ulnar nerve function.

Investigation

Minor UCL sprain shows little change on X-ray, but films should be taken to identify medial traction spurs, bony avulsion, bony hypertrophy in the ulnar groove and loose bodies. Bone scan can reveal bony pathology. MRI scan shows the soft tissue injury.

Treatment

If the UCL is not unstable, treatment is along conventional lines with rest and a strengthening and stretching programme. An active rest from throwing of 6 weeks for mild and 3–4 months for moderate tears is recommended. No local steroid should be used in order to avoid inducing a rupture. Valgus stress is avoided, whilst strengthening and stretching exercises for the wrist flexors and extensors are performed. Shoulder and trunk conditioning is important or there may be problems with technique on return to throwing. Treatment of a UCL which fails to settle or is unstable is discussed below.

Ruptures of the ulnar collateral ligament

The anterior band of the UCL is the primary stabiliser against valgus stress to the elbow joint. Throwing imposes great demands upon this ligament, and poor technique by dropping the elbow in the acceleration phase increases the loads applied. The ligament is injured by overuse with micro- and macrotrauma.

History

There is usually a history of repetitive overload through throwing activities. There may be a history of a gradual onset of aching in the medial elbow. The athlete then experiences a sudden pain or pop following which he is unable to throw far without reproducing a sharp pain. The length of preceding history is very variable. The athlete will complain of pain, loss of distance, accuracy, or control, together with a sensation of instability and local swelling. The pain is felt in the late cocking and acceleration phases.

The UCL can rupture as an acute traumatic event in a contact sport with a direct blow and valgus force, but this is very uncommon. Few of those cases complain of instability.

Ulnar nerve symptoms are frequently associated with a rupture of the UCL.

Examination

Valgus stress is applied to the elbow in 30 degrees of flexion with the athlete seated. The examiner must be careful not to apply flexion to the elbow or confusion will arise. It is suggested that the examiner stands behind the patient with the forearm in the patient's axilla and the examiner's finger over the UCL. The elbow can be in a position of nearly full extension. It is not necessary to fully unlock the joint. There is some movement on the normal side. The end point or rather lack of it together with any local pain with increasing displacement are important features; 5 mm displacement is significant.

Investigation

Plain X-rays identify heterotopic ossification in the medial ligament, loose bodies, and osteochondritic lesions. The *gravity stress test* is used to identify the degree of laxity. The patient lies supine on the table with the shoulder in full external rotation and the elbow over the edge of the table. The weight of the forearm is borne by the anterior band of the UCL. More

346

than 2–3 mm of opening of the medial side of the elbow is significant. MRI can detect the partial thickness undersurface tears.

Treatment

The elbow will function sufficiently well to cope with day-to-day activities with a rupture of the UCL. The elbow will settle even after complete rupture if a functional brace is worn. Conservative treatment is followed even for full thickness tears for 3–6 months, although racquet sports place less stress on the ligament than does overhead throwing.

If a return to overhead or throwing sports is desired, then surgery is frequently required. The duration of symptoms prior to surgery does not affect the outcome. A more immediate surgical repair may be needed if there are significant ulnar nerve symptoms. Surgical reconstruction using a tendon graft works better than repair.

Postoperative rehabilitation

Grip strength work for 10 days during elbow immobilisation is followed by active shoulder and elbow range of motion exercises. Strengthening work begins at 4–6 weeks. When normal strength is achieved gentle backhand strokes or gentle throwing are permitted. At 6 months racquet sports players may begin to serve and smash, but throwers should still be only throwing 20 m with an easy wind-up. It will take a year or more to return to competitive sport.

Ulnar nerve

Anatomy

The ulnar nerve is susceptible to injury as it crosses the elbow joint. The nerve may be tethered at the arcade of Struther's, 8 cm above the medial epicondyle, and in the cubital tunnel. The cubital tunnel narrows as the elbow is flexed, the roof stretches 5 mm in 90 degrees flexion, and the proximal edge becomes taut. Distally, the UCL bulges, and together these reduce the volume in the tunnel. The intraneural pressure rises sixfold with elbow flexion. The nerve is required to be quite mobile, elongating 4.7 mm in flexion, and moving 7 mm medially during motion.

Pathophysiology

In throwing there are very rapid angular velocities and forces generated about the elbow as it passes from 90 to 0 degrees with full pronation. The ulnar nerve is injured as part of the complex of injuries of valgus stress. In addition, the harder the ball is thrown the further the forearm lags behind the upper arm, and the greater the valgus stresses. The elbow of a pitcher's throwing arm when compared with the other one shows bony hypertrophy of the humerus, an enlarged olecranon and fossa, fixed flexion contractures and muscle hypertrophy, and an increased valgus carrying angle. Injury to the UCL causes medial instability which causes traction on the nerve. There are both physiological and pathological causes of ulnar nerve injury. As a result of the medial injuries the nerve may additionally become tethered by scars, traction spurs, and calcific deposits, irritated by the irregular ulnar groove from a previous injury, or entrapped beneath the thickened retinaculum, or hypertrophy of the forearm or triceps muscles. Recurrent dislocation also occurs in throwers. Forty per cent of those undergoing surgery for UCL instability have ulnar nerve symptoms.

Symptoms

Symptoms as a result of throwing are generally fairly mild. Clumsiness or heaviness may be the major complaint. Athletes complain of numbness and tingling in the distribution of the 4th and 5th fingers. This precedes muscle weakness which is uncommon. The muscles flexor carpi ulnaris and flexor digitorum profundus are often spared because the fibres are sited deep in the nerve. Symptoms are worse with exercise and better with rest. There may be pain in the elbow which runs down the ulnar aspect of the arm.

Investigation

Electromyelography is often unable to demonstrate damage to the nerve at the elbow, but the report is helpful if positive.

The nerve should be carefully palpated; it may feel thick or doughy. Observe for subluxation in flexion/extension. Tinel's sign, tapping the nerve to reproduce the tingling, may be positive.

On X-ray, the cubital tunnel view may show osteophytes or loose bodies.

Treatment

Conservative treatment consists of rest, pain control, and immobilisation if symptoms are severe. Any underlying cause such as UCL instability must be treated. Conservative treatment of a longstanding neuropathy usually fails. Surgical release and decompression of the nerve is followed by anterior transposition. Osteotomy of the epicondyle is not desirable in the competitive athlete.

Prevention

Strengthening, flexibility, and a warm-up are essential. Coaching assistance must be sought to ensure proper throwing mechanics. A conditioning programme for shoulder and trunk stability reduces stress upon the elbow. Overload and fatigue are predisposing factors.

Differential diagnosis

The differential diagnosis includes cervical rib, scalenus anterior syndrome, superior sulcus tumour, cervical prolapsed disc, and more distal compression in the forearm.

Elbow dislocations

These result from a fall onto the outstretched hand with the elbow extended and forearm pronated. There may be associated fractures, growth plate injuries in children, nerve injuries, and ischaemic contractures as a result of extensive bleeding and compartment syndrome. Associated fractures include those of the coronoid, radial head, and capitellum.

Neurovascular assessment must precede reduction, and X-rays will be required.

Reduction usually needs a general anaesthetic. Occasionally, operative reduction is necessary where the head of the radius buttonholes the capsule. The elbow is usually stable immobilised at 90 degrees of flexion. Displaced fragments of growth plates should be reduced.

After reduction the elbow is immobilised for 3–10 days depending upon the concomitant injuries. A cast brace may be needed for up to 3 weeks. Early range of motion exercises usually ensure no residual deficit.

Distal biceps rupture

Avulsion of the distal end of the biceps occurs as a result of tensile overload. The injury is reported in body-builders and weight-lifters, and is linked with abuse of anabolic steroids. The history is of a sudden pop or tear in the elbow followed by weakness of elbow flexion and supination of the forearm and cosmetic deformity. Treatment is surgical repair using two incisions to avoid injuring the post-interosseous nerve. Good results are expected. A missed rupture causes weakness of elbow flexion; delayed repair will give improved function.

Forearm

Ulna stress fracture

This rare injury presents with pain in the forearm, worse with activity, in the middle third of the forearm. They tend to be transverse fractures with a periosteal reaction indicating healing, which will occur with rest.

Median nerve

The median nerve runs over the front of the elbow and forearm. There are several potential sites of compression, most commonly between two heads of pronator teres.

History/examination

Sensory symptoms are intermittent, in the thumb, palm, and forearm. Athletes are likely to suffer more in the forearm than wrist, for example, volleyball players who suffer repeated trauma to the front of the forearm. Careful palpation is required for the site of maximum tenderness. Entrapment at the lacertus fibrosus gives painful resisted elbow flexion at 120 degrees with forearm supination. Resisted pronation produces pain with pronator teres syndrome.

Investigation

X-ray is needed to exclude supracondylar bony process. Electromyelography is *no good*.

Treatment

Initially conservative with rest, NSAIDs, physiotherapy, and flexibility. Surgical release is rare in sport.

Anterior interosseous nerve

With an injury to the motor branch of the median nerve, the athlete cannot form the OK sign, and has a weakness of pinching. These usually settle with rest.

Radial nerve

The nerve passes in the radial tunnel between the radial head and the supinator muscle. There is tenderness over the supinator, pain on elbow extension, resisted forearm supination, or forearm pronation and wrist flexion. Motor loss is incomplete. The lateral epicondyle is non-tender except with compression of the radial recurrent nerve, which is nearby. Treatment is conservative, with surgical release if symptoms fail to settle.

Rehabilitation of the elbow: general principles

1. Control of inflammation and healing phases. Anti-inflammatory measures include NSAIDs prior to exercise, cold application with the cryocuff, and counterforce bracing.
2. Warm-up period. A general body warm-up is used rather than local heat to the elbow. Avoid strength and flexibility work whilst a lot of inflammation is present.
3. Strength training. This should be done in proper sequence, aimed at normal and injured tissue:
   - **Isometric**: the patient remains in control. Hold contraction of the elbow and wrist for 3–5 seconds and 50 reps per day. Alter the position of shoulder, wrist, and hand to affect different muscle groups.
   - **Isotonic**: both concentric and eccentric exercises. Avoid muscle soreness, which can lead to loss of motion. Use rubberised cord.
   - **Isokinetics**: useful for comparing strength of sides.
4. Flexibility. Premature attempts at regaining full range of movement (ROM) may cause harm by placing excess stretching forces upon vulnerable injured tissue. The elbow seems particularly susceptible to injury with early exaggerated passive attempts at stretching to a full ROM, therefore introduce this at a later stage of rehabilitation to ensure healing has occurred. Mechanical blocks must be overcome. Most resolve without surgery.
5. Avoid inflammation with careful exercise progression under supervision with patient education as to what is intended, together with written instructions.
6. Return to competition with SAID, Satisfactory Adaptation to Imposed Demands.

Appendix   The elbow and racquet sports

The causes of lateral epicondylitis for a racquet sport are deficiencies of force and flexibility in the forearm extensor muscles, together with a lack of accuracy in play and excessive grip tightness. All these factors must be addressed in managing a racquet player. The trauma is an overuse injury from impact forces between racquet and ball and vibrations transferred to the arm.

The work of wrist muscles contracting to hold the racquet is increased in unskilled players due to poor technique.

Vibration

Excessive vibration transmitted to the forearm is implicated. There is one impact location, the node of the fundamental bending which gives the least vibration. In most modern racquets this is found at the centre. The vibration dampens more quickly with a firmer grip. The greater the distance from this node that the ball strikes the racquet, the greater the amplitude of oscillations. Unskilled players suffer more vibration as they hit the "sweet spot" less frequently. The amplitude of vibration is increased by harder, faster balls whilst a stiffer frame deforms less and hence produces less oscillation. The intrinsic damping of the racquet is still much less than that of the hand. The effect of string dampeners is so small that these have very little effect.

Racquet weight

A heavy racquet exacerbates the requirement for the inexperienced player to grip too hard with inadequate control. Even if missing the ball, the action may give problems. Heavy heads increase torsion by shifting the moment away from the elbow. On the other hand, using a light racquet may induce the player to try to hit the ball harder, and hence the stroke may be less accurate increasing the twisting force on the racquet. The use of a Y configuration reduces air resistance; large heads reduce vibration.

Shock and jar

Contact at the centre of gravity, the balance point of a racquet, does not produce much force on the hand. There is greater shock the greater the distance the ball is hit from the centre of percussion. The further off axis the ball impacts the greater the rotation. One inch off centre is enough to twist the racquet, regardless of how hard the grip, although this may not be noticed by the player. Wider racquets are more stable. Softer strings, lower string tension, and thinner, more elastic strings with an open string pattern all increase dwell time on the racquet frame and reduce peak force, as will a flexible shaft and a softer grip. Old balls require greater power to hit as do wet balls and a fast surface. Cushion grips reduce vibration transfer to the forearm. Lowering string tension during the recovery phase by 3–5 lb reduces stress transfer.

352

Grip

A player's grip is simply not strong enough to resist completely the torsional forces. Fatigue leads to reduced control. Off centre top spin goes faster when hit with a hard grip but this means greater forces in the arm. Elite players have a tighter grip. Grip size is important; an alteration in the grip diameter may relieve symptoms. A guide for the correct size of grip is that the circumference of the grip should equal the distance between the mid palmar crease and the tip of the middle finger (Figure 16.6).

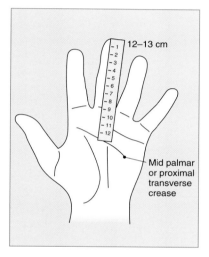

Figure 16.6   Distance between the mid palmar crease and tip of the middle finger equals circumference of grip of racquet handle

Positioning of the player for the shot is an important factor. A player off balance will not strike the ball correctly. General fitness, trunk strength, and the use of fast small steps for speed and balance contribute towards avoidance of injury.

Backhand

The correct stroke demands a long torque arm when reaching for the ball. The one-handed backhand requires greater strength and sequential movement of body parts to produce the shot. Step, hip, trunk, shoulder, elbow, wrist, and racquet follow in a smooth flow, although coordination may be a problem leading to an inaccurate stroke. For the two-handed stroke there is a greater reliance on trunk as opposed to upper limb strength. After the step, the trunk and arms rotate as one. Premature

353

trunk rotation leads to "opening up too early" and excess use of elbow and shoulder power. There is an increased incidence of tennis elbow in the one-handed stroke. A leading elbow in backhand causes tennis elbow.

The modern game demands spin. Excess top spin and lack of strength to control the shot in both back- and forehand may contribute to elbow pain.

17   Shoulder injuries

LARS NEUMANN, ROGER G HACKNEY AND
W ANGUS WALLACE

Introduction

The shoulder is the most mobile joint in the body. The anatomy and
biomechanics that permit this range of motion predispose the glenohumeral
joint to injury. Sport increases the risk. Trauma to the shoulder is frequent
in contact sports, whilst sports involving throwing and swimming demand
a large range of motion, risking instability and impingement.

Symptoms from many differing pathological conditions of the shoulder
are similar, so establishing an accurate diagnosis can be challenging.
However, athletes' shoulder problems can be managed effectively by
relatively simple treatment such as exercise therapy and injections. Only
in a relatively small number of cases is surgery necessary. The treatment
in most cases should not prevent the athlete from maintaining his fitness
and if properly planned not cause serious setbacks in his sporting prowess.

Anatomy

The glenohumeral (GH) joint has poor intrinsic bony stability, necessary
to achieve a great range of motion. Stability is reliant upon a number of
soft tissue structures.

The GH joint is one of five joints making up the shoulder joint complex.
All these components need to be assessed when dealing with problems of
the glenohumeral joint. Motion of the GH joint does not take place alone
but is accompanied by movement in the sternoclavicular (SC) joint, the
acromioclavicular (AC) joint and the thoracoscapular (TS) joint. The GH
joint rotates and glides; up to 4 mm of transverse or vertical movement is
normal. The subacromial space is a sliding joint under the roof of the
shoulder formed by the acromion, coracoacromial ligament, and distal
clavicle. The glenohumeral joint "floats" on the chest wall. Anteriorly the
clavicle acts as a strut preventing the shoulder complex moving anteriorly
around the chest. Scapular movement increases the mobility of the shoulder
complex.[1,2]

The glenohumeral joint

Static stabilisers

The ball-and-socket GH joint consists of a ball – the humeral head – of approximately 50 mm diameter seated in a shallow socket – the glenoid – the surface area of which is only about a quarter of that of the humeral head. The stability of the bony components of the shoulder joint has been compared with that of a ball balanced on the end of a seal's nose. Both sides are free to move independently; they are unconstrained. The cavity of the shallow glenoid is deepened by the glenoid labrum, a rim of fibrocartilage. There is a negative pressure of 30 mmHg within the joint. This creates a suction effect akin to the cup on the end of a child's arrow which contributes to joint stability.

The capsule of the GH joint is a static stabiliser of the shoulder with thickenings which function as ligaments (Figure 17.1).

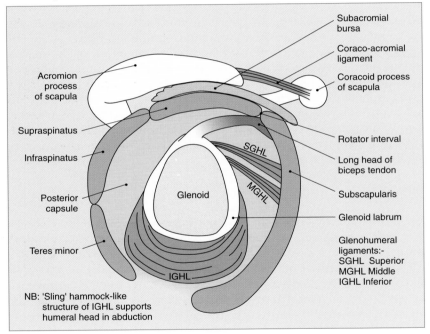

Figure 17.1 View of the glenoid and shoulder stabilisers with the humeral head removed. The muscles from back to front are: teres minor, infraspinatus, supraspinatus, and subscapularis. The glenohumeral ligaments (GHL) are seen as thickenings of the joint capsule

The superior glenohumeral ligament originates from the glenoid rim just anterior to the insertion of the long head of biceps tendon and inserts near the lesser tuberosity of the humerus. It prevents inferior subluxation of the GH joint when the arm is by the side.

356

The middle glenohumeral ligament originates from the anterosuperior labrum and the adjacent supraglenoid tubercle and inserts onto the lesser tuberosity, contributing to anterior stability.

The inferior glenohumeral ligament consists of the capsule attached to the middle and lower part of the glenoid extending posteriorly beyond to the 9 o'clock position. It inserts onto the humeral neck just inferior to the head. This is the ligament which becomes detached in the presence of a Bankart lesion and it is probably the most important anterior and inferior stabiliser of the GH joint with the arm in abduction and external rotation.

Dynamic stabilisers

Four muscles originate from the blade of the scapula and insert on to the greater and lesser tuberosity along the articular surface of the humeral head to form the rotator cuff. These play a vital role in stabilising the shoulder. These rotator cuff muscles from anterior to posterior are the subscapularis, supraspinatus, infraspinatus, and teres minor (Figure 17.1). The function of the rotator cuff muscles is to centre the humeral head in the glenoid and provide some tensioning of the capsular ligaments. They are essential in maintaining a normal movement pattern of the shoulder joint complex. Supraspinatus is especially important in depressing the head of the humerus against the superior pull of the deltoid. The long head of biceps (LHB) inserts into the superior rim of the glenoid labrum and also acts as a humeral head depressor. The rotator cuff and LHB run between the humeral head and the acromion with the acromioclavicular joint and the acromioclavicular ligaments.

The acromioclavicular joint

This small joint between the clavicle and the acromion transfers heavy loads during elevation. As the shoulder moves, the acromioclavicular (AC) joint rotates and glides. The joint contains a small meniscus and is partly stabilised by superior and inferior acromioclavicular ligaments which reinforce the capsule. The conoid and trapezoid ligaments form the coracoclavicular ligament which is the major lateral stabiliser of the clavicle.

Terms and definitions of instability

The terms used to describe shoulder instability are frequently confused. Appropriate treatment depends upon a clear understanding of the different types of instability. Instability may occur in one or more directions. Selecting the wrong management for an unstable shoulder may aggravate instability rather than curing it.

357

Joint laxity (hypermobility)

There is a normal range of motion for a given individual. Hypermobility is an excessive range of motion when compared with the average person. There are no apprehension signs on testing. This is often inherited and bilateral. This condition is not pathological as long as the athlete remains asymptomatic and is able to maintain stability, keeping the humeral head centred in the glenoid. Beighton's tests[3] for joint laxity will score higher than 5 for an adult, 6 for a child (Table 17.1).

Table 17.1 Beighton's 9-point scale for the evaluation of generalised joint laxity

Left/Right	
1/2	Thumbs to meet forearm by flexing wrist
3/4	Little finger passive 90° dorsiflexion
5/6	Elbow hyperextended >10°
7/8	Knee hyperextended >10°
9	Ability to place palms flat to floor by bending forwards from standing with knees straight

Instability

Instability occurs where laxity of the GH joint becomes symptomatic. Instability may take the form of complete dislocation or subluxation where the joint congruity is only partially lost. The patient usually has positive apprehension signs when tested at the extremes of movement.

Dislocation

A total loss of congruity of the two components of the GH joint.

Subluxation

A loss of congruity of the GH joint which is incomplete and which is usually a temporary phenomenon. Episodes of recurrent subluxations are involuntary, and patients have positive apprehension signs. Subluxation is a significant symptom and can be very disabling.

Multidirectional instability (MDI)

MDI is defined as instability in more than one direction.

Voluntary subluxation

The ability to sublux or dislocate the shoulder at will. The condition is painless and apprehension is absent.

Habitual

The humeral head dislocates or subluxes with a particular movement.

Aetiology

TUBS versus AMBRI

Thomas and Matsen[4] introduced these acronyms, which are useful as a rough guide to the understanding of patients with instability. TUBS stands for Traumatic, Unidirectional, with Bankart lesion treated with Surgery. AMBRI stands for Atraumatic, Multidirectional, Bilateral, treated by Rehabilitation with Inferior capsular shift surgically. These two populations represent two ends of a spectrum; the majority lies somewhere between the two.

Traumatic instability

Anterior instability is most commonly seen. During the initial dislocation or subluxation damage is inflicted on the capsular or bony structures of the joint leading to tearing, stretching, and permanent damage. Nearly 90% of acute dislocators have a tearing of the glenoid labrum from the glenoid. The tear of the glenoid labrum is known as a Bankart lesion. The labral tearing together with increasing stretching of the capsule with further episodes of instability form the basis for recurrence.

Atraumatic instability

Hypermobility of the shoulder may be converted into an unstable shoulder either with significant trauma or by repetitive capsular stretching.

Pathoanatomy of instability

The anterior **Bankart lesion** is almost always seen in the traumatic anterior instability. A posterior version is also found in posterior dislocation. At the time of the dislocation the capsule is torn or stretches. The labrum and the adjacent capsule with its ligamentous structures – including the most important, the inferior glenohumeral ligament – may be avulsed from the glenoid rim. Occasionally the periosteum is stripped from the scapular neck in continuity with the capsule. The pocket so created shows little or no tendency to heal back onto the bone. In some cases the glenoid rim is fractured during the dislocation – a bony Bankart lesion (Figure 17.2a). With repeated instability episodes, the capsule stretches still further, the

359

glenoid rim becomes worn and any remaining labrum is abraded, leading to recurrent instability.

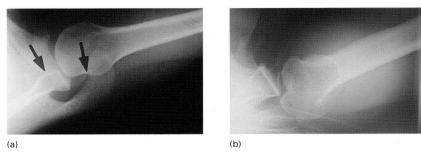

(a)   (b)

Figure 17.2   (a) Hill–Sachs lesion of humeral head caused by impaction on glenoid rim; (b) humerus head dislocated

The **Hill–Sachs lesion** is an impaction fracture of the humeral head when the head is pushed onto the glenoid rim during the dislocation (Figure 17.2a). In an anterior dislocation the lesion is in the back of the humeral head; in the posterior dislocation the lesion is in the front of the head – a reverse Hill–Sachs lesion (Figure 17.2b).

Following the initial dislocation, the presence of these intra-articular lesions makes recurrence more likely. A large Hill–Sachs lesion will cause a further dislocation to occur more easily and prevent spontaneous relocation.

Voluntary instability

Patients with hypermobile, lax shoulder joints sometimes get into the habit of dislocating and relocating their shoulder joint and often demonstrate this ability as a "trick movement". As long as this happens under control it rarely causes any problems to the patient. Unfortunately after a while the patient may no longer be able to control the dislocations which then happen in situations without intention. The instability has now changed from voluntary intentional into an involuntary unintentional. As the patient at this stage has lost his normal movement pattern, stabilising the shoulder is extremely difficult. Specialised physiotherapy with biofeedback is necessary. Surgery should be avoided if at all possible.

SLAP lesion

The term was introduced by Snyder and co-workers in 1990.[5] SLAP means Superior Labrum, Anterior and Posterior and consists of a tear of the labrum anterior and posterior to the biceps insertion.

Various grades of the lesion are seen. The frayed type 1 and 2 are probably chronic lesions whereas the more extensive type 3 and 4 involve

360

the biceps insertion and are acute lesions, usually caused by a fall on the outstretched arm.

Pathoanatomy of impingement

Subacromial impingement

Tendinitis, tendon tears, bursitis, and impingement are seen in the subacromial space. Subacromial impingement has been divided into several "stages" by Dr Charles Neer.[6] Dr Frank Jobe later modified this to include a fourth category.[7] The classification is open to misinterpretation in that the stages should not be regarded as being a path along which an athlete passes.

- **Stage 1** Age group under 25 years. Early changes of oedema and mild haemorrhage commonly caused by overuse from overhead activity in young athletes.
- **Stage 2** Age group 25–40 years. Recurrent episodes of impingement cause the supraspinatus tendon to become chronically inflamed.

 These stages usually respond well to reduced activity and conservative measures.

- **Stage 3** Age group over 40 years. This usually presents in older athletes who have a history of multiple episodes of pain and impingement. A small rotator cuff tear of less than 1 cm is often present, associated with a bony osteophyte of the acromion and clavicle inferolaterally. Conservative treatment at this stage may fail but should be attempted.
- **Stage 4** Any age group. Rotator cuff tears greater than 1 cm. Surgical management may be necessary, although there are reports of acceptable results using conservative treatment in professional pitchers with full thickness tears.

There is undoubtedly a strong connection in some athletes between impingement, instability, and rotator cuff tears. The group where this is most obvious is in throwing athletes, where instability or poorly controlled hypermobility leads to the acromion coming into contact with the rotator cuff causing mechanical wear of the tendons.

In young patients, especially in swimmers and overhead athletes, until otherwise proved, impingement is always related to instability and a loss of the rotator cuff muscles' ability to keep the humeral head centred in the glenoid fossa during movement.

Dr Jobe further describes a spectrum of impingement and instability divided into four groups:

- **Group 1 Pure impingement no instability.** This group will include older throwers of 35 years or more who have positive impingement but negative apprehension and relocation tests. Severe impingement will give rise to pain on apprehension testing but no pain relief on testing with the relocation test.

- **Group 2 Primary instability due to chronic labral microtrauma with secondary impingement.** This group consists of those overhead athletes who have developed a chronically unstable shoulder as a result of their sporting activity. Examination reveals impingement and pain but not apprehension until the relocation test is performed. Examination under anaesthesia (EUA) may not detect instability as the findings can be so subtle. There may be increased anterior movement of the humeral head. Arthroscopically findings are undersurface cuff tears, anterior labral damage, and attenuation of the inferior glenohumeral ligament. There may be minor posterior labral damage and posterior humeral head chondromalacia, the so-called kissing lesion, associated with internal impingement in the cocking and early acceleration phases of throwing.
- **Group 3 Instability due to generalised increased ligamentous hyperlaxity with subsequent impingement.** The findings on clinical examination are the same as group 2, with additional evidence of generalised laxity. Scapular pseudo-winging is common. These shoulders are hypermobile on EUA, frequently bilateral. Arthroscopically they may have fraying of the rotator cuff. The inferior glenohumeral ligament is loose on probing and it does not tighten on external rotation. The humeral head can be seen to be pushed over the edge of the glenoid labrum which is small but intact. The arthroscope can be passed easily between the humeral head and the anteroinferior glenoid, the drive-through sign.
- **Group 4 Pure instability without impingement.** These patients will usually have had a major traumatic episode with anterior subluxation or dislocation. There is a negative impingement test but pain with apprehension testing and relief of pain with the relocation test. EUA reveals anterior instability. Arthroscopy shows anterior labral damage due to subluxation, with corresponding humeral head defects and capsular injury. The rotator cuff is normal.

Long head of biceps

Rupture of the long head of the biceps tendon is a sequel to subacromial impingement or degenerative changes in the bicipital groove impingement. The tendon may sublux out of the bicipital groove. Bicipital tendinitis in isolation is extremely rare.

Pathology of the rotator cuff

Rotator cuff tears are uncommon in the younger athlete, the incidence and size increasing with age. Chronic tears are caused by either external impingement from the acromion or, in overhead athletes, from internal impingement of the supraspinatus tendon onto the posterosuperior glenoid rim during full elevation. They respond well to treatment of the underlying cause. After the age of 40 cuff tears become more frequent as the tendon tissue which in the young individual is extremely strong becomes relatively degenerate and weak. In the young athlete the tears are usually "sprains", i.e. partial thickness tears only, whereas in the older athlete, avulsions of the tendon from the insertion on the tuberosities become more common.

Calcific tendinitis is seen in athletes. The presence of a calcific deposit in the tendons of the rotator cuff is a sign of degeneration visible on X-ray. The calcium deposit only becomes symptomatic when resolution begins, when the shoulder suddenly becomes acutely inflamed and extremely painful. If left untreated, this inflammation usually leads to spontaneous discharge of the calcium with subsequent pain relief. A defect is left in the cuff.

Pathology of the acromioclavicular (AC) joint

Acromioclavicular joint subluxation or dislocation is a very common sports injury. The clavicle is bound by both coracoclavicular ligaments and acromioclavicular joint capsule and ligaments which are ruptured with complete dislocation. The patients are classified using the six grades of the Rockwood classification.

- **Grade 1** is a minor sprain with pain and swelling but less than 50% translation.
- **Grade 2** is a 50–100% translation of the clavicle against the acromion.
- **Grade 3** is a full dislocation with complete rupture of the restraining ligaments.
- **Grade 4** is an unreducible dislocation with the clavicle stuck into the trapezius.
- **Grade 5** is a full dislocation, which risks perforating the skin.
- **Grade 6** is an inferior dislocation under the coracoid.

Osteoarthritis of the acromioclavicular joint is common and increases with age. Even quite marked changes are often asymptomatic. Downwards directed AC joint osteophytes can add to a subacromial pain problem by impinging on the supraspinatus tendon.

Osteolysis, bone resorption, of the distal end of the clavicle is seen in some sports where the AC joint is particularly stressed, such as weight-lifting and gymnastics.

Adhesive capsulitis

Capsulitis or "**frozen shoulder**", although more common in the middle-aged, can be seen in athletes. It can be either primary, i.e. develops without any apparent cause, or secondary, i.e. develops after a shoulder trauma or shoulder surgery. The primary condition has a higher incidence in diabetics. The aetiology of the condition is still poorly understood, but the symptoms and clinical findings are typical: the shoulder is usually very painful. Movement is restricted both passively and actively, in particular in external and internal rotation. If an arthrogram or arthroscopy is carried out a very tight GH joint is found. Capsulitis is often confused with impingement pain or rotator cuff lesions. Shoulders with subacromial pathology usually have full passive movement but limited active movement due to pain.

History and examination

History

In over 50% of the cases the correct diagnosis can be made solely on a careful history. Table 17.2 details some important points to be brought out in the history.

Details of the onset of symptoms are important. When obtaining the history, remember that shoulder pain may originate from the neck. You should always question the patient about neck pain. Changes in sensation or power in the arm are important symptoms to elucidate. Neck pain is felt over the top of the shoulder around the trapezius. Acromioclavicular joint pain is well localised over the joint itself. GH joint pain is often referred down the upper arm near to the insertion of the deltoid on the humerus.

Where instability is suspected, it is important to assess the degree of force required to produce the initial injury and the direction of the dislocation.

Clinical examination

It is important to remember that many pathological conditions of the shoulder are painful. A relaxed and comfortable patient is essential to allow a careful and full examination of the shoulder. The examination must be carried out gently and at a speed that leaves the patient confident that he or she can stop a painful manoeuvre before it causes unnecessary pain. It is the examiner's duty to make sure that this trust is established before the examination takes place.

It is common for both shoulders to be "abnormal", even although only one is symptomatic. The examiner should **examine the asymptomatic shoulder first**. This will allow him to establish the "normal values" against which the findings in the symptomatic shoulder can be compared. The examiner should develop his own established routine for shoulder

Table 17.2 A detailed history of shoulder problems

General		
Complaints	Symptoms	Pain
		Functional limitations
		Treatment? If so, any benefit?
		Change in symptoms since onset
Onset	Trauma	Nature of trauma, how severe?
		Position of the arm at the time of incident
		Immediate/delayed symptoms, weakness of deltoid and loss of sensation over the tip of the shoulder = axillary nerve injury
	Non-trauma	Relation to specific activities or positions of the arm
		Provoking/relieving factors
Specific		
Pain	Nature	Burning, aching
	Intensity	
	Location	Neck, trapezius, AC joint, deltoid, forearm
	Duration	Night pain, following sport
	Onset	Relation to sport and shoulder position
	Radiation	Forearm, hand, deltoid insertion
	Aggravation	At rest, movement, sport
	Relief	Position, analgesia, treatment
Instability	Dead arm syndrome	
	Impingement-related	
	Subjective feeling of instability	
	Position of arm when symptomatic	
	"Do you trust the shoulder?"	
Stiffness	Associated pain	
	Diabetes	
	Posterior dislocation	
	Arthritis	
Other complaints	Weakness	
	Locking and/or clicking	
	Deformity	

examination. The following is the authors' preferred way of assessing and examining the shoulder. A logical sequence to the examination using the sequence of look, move, feel, and "special tests" is recommended.

Look

When inspecting the patient, both shoulders should be studied at the same time from both behind and in front. The arms should also be exposed, to allow unrestricted movement. The examiner looks for wasting of the muscles around the shoulder. Shoulder posture is important for comparison; holding the shoulder in an elevated position indicates an injury.

Localised muscle atrophy can be a sign of a rotator cuff lesion, a nerve injury, or disuse.

Swellings: look at the soft tissue and bony contours. The outline of the AC joint may show a step from a dislocation or a ganglion. An unreduced dislocation is not as obvious as might be anticipated and requires careful assessment. A muscle or tendon injury such as a rupture of the long head of biceps or pectoralis major is distinctive.

Move

The standard movements of forward flexion, abduction in the plane of the scapula (30 degrees anterior to the coronal plane), and extension are recorded. Internal and external rotational movements are tested with the elbow by the side. Internal rotation can also be measured by asking the patient to reach as far up their backs from below, as possible. In younger patients, passive external rotation in 90 degrees abduction should also be measured. A standardised nomenclature for shoulder movements has been recommended by the American Academy of Orthopaedic Surgeons.[8]

Examine the range of motion of the neck.

Ask the patient to tell you when any pain begins and ends. Observe the ratio of movement of the scapulothoracic and the glenohumeral joints. One of the joints may be relatively fixed, with all movement taking place in the other joint. It is possible to achieve nearly 90 degrees of abduction by moving the scapula alone without using the GH joint at all.

The movement of the humeral head should also be observed from the front. If it visibly rises upwards, even only a small amount, at the start of abduction or flexion, this indicates deficient rotator cuff function. The movement pattern can be distorted as a sequel to instability, as the patient may have developed compensatory movements of the scapula to keep the shoulder in joint during movement.

Observe any "trick" movements used to fully elevate the arm, suggesting a subacromial problem. The "trick" movement may be used to avoid the supraspinatus tendon impinging under the acromion.

The supraspinatus and the deltoid muscles both contribute to elevation.[9] If an imbalance exists between these muscles, the normal movement pattern is lost and the patient is no longer able to centre the humeral head during movement, usually leading to upward migration of the humeral head and impingement.

With instability, increasing elevation of the GH joint may lead to a subtle inferior subluxation, compromising the normal GH rhythm.

When testing the passive range of motion, the patient must be completely relaxed. The movement is then tested in the same planes as the active movement. The examiner notes the difference between the active and passive range of motion.

Causes of reduced passive and active movement

- Mechanical restriction
    tight capsule as in capsulitis
    displaced fracture, e.g. greater tuberosity
    degenerative disease
    persistent dislocation, e.g. posterior dislocation limits external rotation
- Joint is too painful to take through a full range of motion
    impingement
    calcific tendinitis
    recent injury

Causes of reduced active range, passive range is full

- Muscle injury
    rotator cuff tear
- Pain
    impingement syndrome
    recent injury

If the movement is restricted by pain, or if only a part of the motion is painful, the examiner notes the range of pain during the movement. Three typical painful arcs are found (Figure 17.3).

1. A capsulitis painful arc: pain from a point of elevation below shoulder level and total active elevation is limited to about 100–120 degrees. Passive elevation is limited to the same extent as active movement.
2. A subacromial painful arc: pain is felt from a point of abduction just below or at shoulder level and continued during movement but reduces 20–30 degrees before reaching full elevation. Subacromial impingement also occurs at the extreme of flexion.
3. An AC joint painful arc: pain is increased during the last 10–20 degrees of elevation. In addition, cross-arm adduction is painful.

Power

Muscle strength is assessed, comparing both sides. Important findings are reduced power and/or pain during resisted movement; combinations are commonly seen. Pain without loss of power indicates tendinitis; loss of power with pain indicates a cuff tear, although this is a guide and does not hold absolutely true.

367

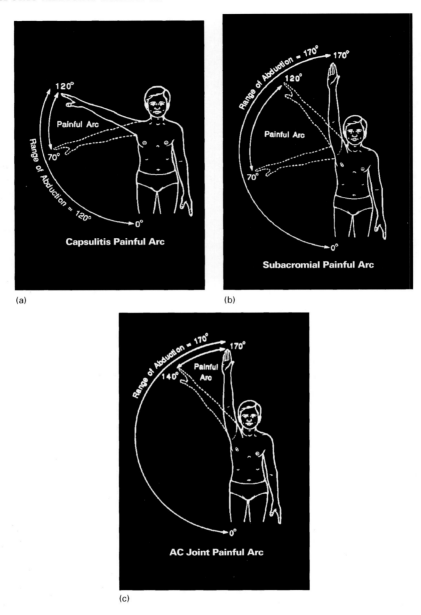

(a)   (b)

(c)

Figure 17.3   The three painful arcs. (a) The capsulitis painful arc. Both active and passive movement is reduced. Pain mainly at the end range of movement. (b) The impingement painful arc. Pain starts during elevation at shoulder level and disappears during the last 20–30 degrees of the range. (c) AC joint painful arc. Pain is felt at the end of the range in full elevation

368

Rotator cuff

Supraspinatus is tested by active resisted movement of the straight arm held at a position of around 45 degrees of abduction and 30 degrees of flexion – i.e. in the plane of the scapula with the arm in internal rotation, as if holding an upturned cup. This test – "the supraspinatus test" – is probably the most useful of the isometric tests.

Infraspinatus is tested with the elbow flexed to 90 degrees and stabilised at the patient's side by one hand of the examiner who then resists active external rotation.

Subscapularis is tested using the "lift-off" test which eliminates the influence of pectoralis major. The patient rests his arms, palms facing outwards, on the lower back and then attempts to lift the hands away from the body. Weakness indicates damage to subscapularis.

The three parts of the deltoid are tested separately, all with the arm hanging down. The anterior third is tested by resisted flexion, the lateral third by resisted abduction, and the posterior third by resisted extension. Deltoid should be specifically tested following anterior dislocation.

Impingement tests

Impingement may occur when bringing the arm actively up into full flexion. A more useful test is performed by raising the arm from a position of 90 degrees abduction and 30 degrees flexion. The humerus is then internally rotated by the examiner, causing impingement.

Feel

Palpation is performed at the end of the examination, as the previous procedures have now indicated the most likely location of the pathology.

Some areas are directly palpable, such as the AC joint and the clavicle, and others such as the anterior joint line and bicipital groove, depending upon muscle bulk and adiposity.

Palpate the tendinous part of the rotator cuff and its insertion to detect localised tender areas. The more experienced examiner can directly palpate a large defect in the rotator cuff. The anterosuperior part of the cuff is brought out from the subacromial space by extending and internally rotating the shoulder by placing the hand behind the back. The examiner palpates just anterior to the acromion, and gently moves the humeral head in rotation and flexion/extension to detect irregularities and tender areas in the cuff.

369

Special tests for instability

These tests, especially the stress tests, should be performed with care in patients who have had dislocations in the past as there is a risk of dislocating the shoulder.

Sulcus sign

Pull the arm directly downwards whilst preventing the torso from following with a gentle hand over the roof of the shoulder. The sulcus sign (Figure 17.4) is an indentation under the acromion as the head subluxes interiorly. This indicates inferior laxity.

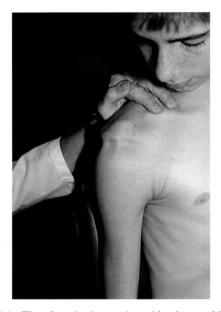

Figure 17.4   The sulcus sign in a patient with a hypermobile shoulder

Draw signs

With the patient's arm hanging down and relaxed, the examiner stands behind the patient and stabilises the shoulder girdle by holding the acromion with one hand, and the humeral head between index finger and thumb. The humeral head is pushed backwards and forwards on the glenoid. Some translation is found in normal shoulders. A translation up to or over the rim of the glenoid is helpful in assessing laxity and instability.

370

Apprehension test

The anterior apprehension test (Figure 17.5) can be performed either with the patient sitting or supine. The arm is abducted to 90 degrees and is

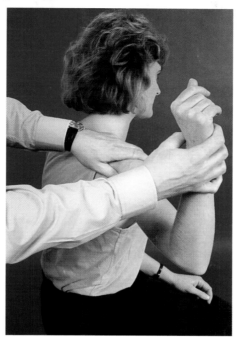

Figure 17.5   The apprehension test. The examiner supports the patient's shoulder with his left hand and takes the patient's symptomatic shoulder into external rotation in 90 degrees of abduction. In a shoulder with anterior instability this manoeuvre will cause apprehension

passively brought into external rotation. If this causes apprehension, or if muscle spasm prevents the same amount of external rotation as is seen on the asymptomatic side, this is strongly suggestive of anterior instability. By moving the shoulder from 60 to 140 degrees in abduction while maximal external rotation is maintained, the point where instability is at its maximum can be identified.

Stress tests

The stress tests require a relaxed, cooperative patient, and are often better assessed under general anaesthetic.

Anterior stress test   The patient is supine and the examiner fixes the scapula with his contralateral hand and the elbow with his ipsilateral hand. With the shoulder in 90 degrees of abduction and maximal extension the examiner

371

applies an axial load to the humerus while gently rotating the arm, trying to anteriorly sublux the head. While maintaining the axial load, the arm is taken to a flexed/adducted position across the chest. If the humeral head was subluxed initially, it will relocate during this manoeuvre with a palpable and often audible clunk.

Posterior stress test   With the arm in 90 degrees of flexion, the examiner stabilises the scapula by placing his contralateral hand behind the scapula. By pushing the humerus backwards, the examiner tries to sublux the humeral head posteriorly. Sometimes the subluxation can be felt by the hand holding the scapula. The axial load on the humerus is maintained, and the arm is now brought into abduction. If the humeral head has been subluxed the head of the humerus will suddenly relocate with a clunk or click.

Jobe relocation test

This is a very sensitive test for assessing symptomatic anterior instability. The patient lies supine with the symptomatic shoulder over the edge of the couch. With the arm in 90 degrees of abduction, the humerus is externally rotated to the point of pain and apprehension. Maintaining this position, firm downwards pressure is applied to the upper arm at the level of the humeral neck. This pressure is continued and further external rotation applied until pain recurs. The pressure on the humeral neck is suddenly removed. A positive test is produced by a sudden increase of pain. This pain is similar to the pain felt when symptoms from the shoulder are experienced. If this test is positive, symptomatic anterior instability is present.

The term "relocation test" is used because the original theory was that the humeral head anteriorly subluxed with the initial external rotation and then reduced by bringing the humeral head back into its correct position in the glenoid by direct pressure. The sudden pain on release was said to be due to a sudden anterior subluxation. Dr Jobe now believes that the pain is due to internal impingement of the posterior superior labrum onto the rotator cuff. Arthroscopically, performing the equivalent to the relocation test, this can be demonstrated to occur.

The stress tests may be difficult to perform in the apprehensive patient and may have to be deferred until an examination under general anaesthesia can be performed. The EUA must include the anterior and posterior stress tests.

Diagnostic local anaesthetic injections

Neer's test[6] helps establish the origin of shoulder pain and makes it possible to distinguish between bursal inflammation and rotator cuff tears. After examination of the shoulder, the subacromial space is injected with 10 ml of bupivacaine. Twenty minutes later the examination is repeated and the findings compared. If the pain is eliminated and strength and range of motion is restored, impingement and subacromial bursitis is the most likely diagnosis. If a limited range of movement and weakness persist, a rotator cuff lesion is likely.

The AC joint can be injected with 1–2 ml of local anaesthetic (with or without corticosteroid) to establish the source of pain from that joint. Care must be taken to ensure that the needle does not pass through into the subacromial space.

Investigation

X-rays

Most shoulder pathology in the athlete arises from the soft tissues, and only secondary changes are visible with conventional radiography. For example, the depth of the subacromial space can be measured (this should be at least 7 mm). Subchondral sclerosis of the acromion with corresponding changes on the humeral head confirms a clinical suspicion of impingement.

Usually, an AP and an axillary view are sufficient, although further views may be used with trauma.

X-ray findings

- Calcification in the rotator cuff tendons indicating degenerative changes
- Superior translation of the humeral head on the glenoid indicating a deficient rotator cuff
- Subacromial sclerosed bone and osteophytes
- AC joint changes, e.g. AC joint arthritis, osteophytes
- Old trauma
- Defects of the glenoid

Arthrograms

Evaluation of the rotator cuff can be carried out using double-contrast arthrograms. This examination is only useful for diagnosing joint side partial thickness tears and full thickness tears, and gives no information on the bursal side of the cuff. This is an invasive procedure and has been superseded by the MRI scan where available.

373

Computerised axial tomography (CAT) scan

The CT scan is the investigation of choice if there is suspicion of pathological bony relations, such as glenoid dysplasia, or to assess in detail the extent of a Hill–Sachs lesion or glenoid rim damage. If combined with intra-articular contrast – a CT arthrogram – detailed information on the condition of the capsule and labrum can be obtained.

Magnetic resonance imaging (MRI) scan

The MRI scan provides a detailed picture of the soft tissues of the shoulder and is now the procedure of choice to identify rotator cuff tears or tendinitis. The scan is extremely sensitive, and has even been shown to demonstrate pathological changes in asymptomatic shoulders. MRI is used in the investigation of instability where it can easily show defects of the glenoid labrum and capsule. The use of contrast medium enhances this feature. Occasional unexpected findings such as a ganglion impinging upon the suprascapular nerve leading to rotator cuff atrophy mean that the use of MRI scanning for shoulder problems will increase in the future. The scans are not very sensitive in assessing SLAP lesions. MRI scanning is unfortunately expensive.

Ultrasound

Recently, the use of ultrasonography in assessing the cuff has been advocated. This is a low cost non-invasive procedure. The accuracy is highly dependent upon the skill of the examiner and the equipment used. It has been found to be very useful, in particular in specialised centres where many examinations are carried out.

Arthroscopy

Examination under anaesthetic and diagnostic arthroscopy is useful in assessing instability and the associated intra-articular lesions.

Electromyelogram

Nerve conduction studies may be required when a nerve lesion is suspected. The most common nerves studies are the suprascapular nerve which supplies the spinati, the musculocutaneous nerve which supplies biceps, and the axillary nerve which supplies deltoid.

The shoulder in throwing sports

To have a concept of the stresses placed on the shoulder during throwing, it is important to understand the movement of the humerus and its relations while the throw takes place.

The throwing movement has been fully analysed and very carefully described by Perry[10] in baseball players during pitching, and has been divided into six phases. Only 30% of the velocity of the throw is produced by the shoulder, the majority comes from the legs, pelvis, and trunk. Throwing a javelin has a slightly different technique. The bowling movement in cricket is somewhat different due to the rules demanding that the elbow is kept straight. The movements associated with the overhead smash in racquet sports or the crawl or butterfly stroke in swimming are similar to the throwing movement.

The wind-up phase

With the ball in the throwing hand, the thrower stands on his ipsilateral leg and then puts his contralateral leg forwards. The shoulder is in a neutral position. The body is rotated towards the throwing arm with the opposite shoulder pushed forwards in the direction of the throw.

Early cocking phase

The thrower puts his foot forwards and at the same time the shoulder starts external rotation and abduction. The pitcher still has his opposite shoulder pointing towards the direction of the throw.

Late cocking phase

External rotation of the shoulder (often as much as 180 degrees in pitchers) and abduction is now taken to its maximum, putting a great stress on the anterior GH joint capsule by stretching it. The greater tuberosity moves medially and posteriorly under the coracoacromial arch. Subscapularis and supraspinatus are at the peak of activity as the shoulder is at most risk of anterior subluxation. The pelvis and trunk are forcefully rotated bringing them square onto the direction of throw.

Acceleration phase

The arm follows the trunk into internal rotation and horizontal flexion about the shoulder in an extremely rapid and forceful movement.

Contraction of the latissimus dorsi, the pectoralis major, and deltoid provide the power for the throw. Professional athletes demonstrate selective use of the individual cuff muscles, and are able to use subscapularis exclusively during this phase. Amateurs tend to use all the cuff muscles and biceps. Proper coordination of the trunk renders the supraspinatus, infraspinatus, teres minor, and biceps unnecessary for acceleration.

Deceleration (release) phase

After release, a force nearly equivalent to body weight must be counteracted to avoid damage to the shoulder. The upper arm internally rotates and adducts across the front of the body. Deceleration reduces the angular velocity to zero, with deceleration values of 500 000 degrees per second. The external rotators (infraspinatus and teres minor) contract eccentrically.

Follow-through

The body continues to move forwards as the shoulder adducts, movement being stopped by landing on the contralateral foot. In this position the greater tuberosity is taken under the acromion.

To obtain the maximum effect from the throwing movement, the thrower must make use of the entire range of motion of the shoulder, bringing the shoulder's static stabilisers to the limit of their range of movement. The laxity of the anterior capsule, and in particular the inferior GH ligament, permits an increased translation of the humeral head which must be controlled by the rotator cuff. If the dynamic stabilisers become fatigued the humeral head is allowed to sublux anteriorly, leading to abrasion of the labrum and further trauma to the capsule. This sets up a vicious circle where the increased translation requires greater effort from the already fatigued cuff, leading to further damage. Damage to the undersurface of the rotator cuff is more common than intrasubstance tears, and is probably due to internal impingement aggravated by a tight posterior capsule.

Treatment of shoulder injuries

Rehabilitation

The return of the athlete to competition can largely be achieved via a well balanced rehabilitation programme. The general principles which apply pre or post any surgery are as follows:

1. Rest from the sport or upper body training that produces symptoms. Note: As with any athlete, there should be encouragement to train non-injured parts and maintain cardiovascular fitness.
2. Reduce inflammation and pain with NSAIDs, up to three corticosteroid injections and cryotherapy.
3. Maintain range of motion. Begin with passive movements using pulleys, hydrotherapy, and improve stretching and progress to active movements then strengthening techniques for power and endurance. The emphasis is on movements in the scapular plane. Useful techniques include exercises with rubberised cord, for example Cliniband or Theraband. Proprioceptive feedback techniques are an important addition to conventional programmes.
4. Progression to free weights, emphasising scapular stabilisation and muscle strengthening. The use of isokinetic apparatus helps provide a baseline and comparison between sides.
5. Finally, progression to functional, sports-orientated work, including plyometrics and specific drills with coaches to correct any fault in technique. Low effort drills are gradually increased in intensity towards a return to competition.

Rehabilitation must also address the technical errors found in athletes with injuries; liaison with the coach is essential.

Rehabilitation

Muscle groups to be considered, and trained in that order!

- **The protectors:** Four rotator cuff muscles, concentric and eccentric exercises, in the plane of the scapula, with emphasis on scapula control, when exercising the cuff
- **The pivoters:** Scapula stabilisers, shoulder shrugs, rowing, pro- and retraction of the shoulder, progress through to press-ups with wider hands and then sideways walking
- **The positioner:** Deltoid, working all three parts of the muscle, with progressively longer lever arms
- **The propellors:** Power muscles, pectoralis major, latissimus dorsi, biceps, exercises such as pull-downs, biceps curls, internal rotation work

---

Treatment of shoulder instability

Dislocation

A first time anterior dislocation of the shoulder is traditionally managed by resting in a sling for a 6 week period. The evidence that 6 weeks' immobilisation reduces that risk is poor. Many studies have demonstrated

377

that a young sportsperson below the age of 30 years and involved in contact sports has a high chance of suffering not just a recurrent dislocation but significant symptoms from subluxation episodes. The Bankart lesion does not repair.[11]

Our current practice is to prescribe one week's rest in a sling to allow pain and discomfort to subside, followed by a rehabilitation programme. This programme should focus on rotator cuff strengthening exercises, exercises for the scapular stabilisers and deltoid. Shoulders with traumatic instability still risk a recurrence of symptoms while shoulders tending towards the atraumatic instability end of the spectrum have better results.[12]

Serious consideration is now being given to acute repair of the first time dislocator with no preceding symptoms and no evidence of joint laxity. Initial results have been highly encouraging. Arthroscopic repair in the hands of a specialist is being investigated as potentially the best option for young sportspeople in the future.

Subluxation

Where symptoms are of vague instability, subluxation, secondary impingement pain, or dead arm syndrome, a conservative rehabilitation programme should be pursued. The majority will respond to an appropriate regimen. Throwing athletes develop a tightness of the posterior capsule which contributes to anterior instability symptoms and responds well to a stretching programme.

Surgery for shoulder dislocation

The indications for surgery are a failure of conservative management, although the case for acute repair in certain circumstances can be made.

The surgeon must ensure that he is confident of the exact nature of the instability using appropriate stress tests. The presence of any additional capsular laxity determines which surgical procedure is most appropriate.

Shoulder arthroscopy and an examination under anaesthesia before proceeding provide useful extra information.

In the presence of a Bankart lesion, a Bankart repair is carried out.[13] If instability is present in more than just the anterior direction then a capsular shift procedure[14] is added to the Bankart repair. For this, the joint capsule is double-breasted from superior to inferior, tightening the joint without restricting external rotation movement significantly.

After repair the arm is kept in a sling with blocked external rotation for 2 weeks. A self-controlled rehabilitation programme is then begun, leaving the patient to mobilise at his own pace. No formal exercises or physiotherapy are given to avoid stretching the repair before solid scar tissue has formed. If at 6 weeks active elevation is less than 130 degrees and external rotation lag is more than 30 degrees, physiotherapy is given with gentle stretching exercises. If movement is satisfactory the patient can concentrate on building up strength, with a return to light sports such as swimming with careful breaststrokes and jogging at 10 weeks, and to full unrestricted activities at 4 months, including contact sports. At this stage, with a well timed rehabilitation programme the athlete should be fit to return to his sport at the previous level with a normal or near normal range of movement.

Dead arm syndrome

Dead arm syndrome includes a spectrum of complaints. At the mildest level, symptoms are of pins and needles in the throwing arm following a throw. At the other extreme, a sudden paralysing pain shoots down the arm which hangs useless by the side. The syndrome is always associated with instability, which may be occult. If undiagnosed these patients give up throwing or other forceful overhead activities. Treatment is initially conservative with rehabilitation and modification of throwing technique. Rehabilitation focuses upon scapular and rotator cuff muscle control, proprioception, stretching of the posterior capsule, and avoidance of the extremes of abduction and external rotation. If that fails, then surgery to address the instability is required.

Subacromial impingement

Following a diagnosis of impingement in a sportsperson, and in particular for an athlete whose sport involves overhead activity, a careful investigation programme should be carried out. The presence of instability must be excluded. In the presence of a painful arc and impingement signs, use of local anaesthetic helps confirm the diagnosis. If positive, the cause of the impingement must be found. AP and axial radiographs and a supraspinatus outlet view (to visualise the subacromial space) are necessary to assess the relations between the bony components of the shoulder. Often an AC joint view is also useful.

Steroid injections in the subacromial bursa work very well in relieving local inflammation but do not address the cause of the impingement. Corticosteroid injections should be given into the subacromial bursa. *Never* push steroid into tendon tissue. An abnormal movement pattern should be corrected by intensive physiotherapy during which up to three steroid injections into the bursa may be helpful in controlling the pain. Physiotherapy includes muscle strengthening and proprioceptive work to improve control of motion.

In cases of resistant impingement, if bony changes are found on the acromion or in cases where no primary cause for the impingement has been found, a subacromial decompression can be carried out. Today most athletes will have an arthroscopic decompression. Postoperative pain and the rehabilitation period is reduced for arthroscopic procedures, with success rates approaching that of open repair. Following any surgery to the subacromial space, rehabilitation is crucial. If mobilisation is not started immediately, i.e. from day one after surgery, scarring and adhesions form and can lead to stiffness and chronic inflammatory pain. In our practice all our patients have passive and active mobilisation using pulleys and physiotherapy-assisted exercises.

A calcific deposit can be released arthroscopically, usually with very good pain relief.

It cannot be overemphasised that subacromial decompression should *not* be carried out before the underlying cause has been fully addressed.

Rotator cuff tears

In younger patients the aetiology of the cuff tear must be sought. Osteophytes, and other causes of reduced subacromial space may be seen on plain X-ray. Internal impingement is recognised as the cause of undersurface tears in the throwing athlete. Tension overload from chronic fatigue and overuse of the cuff tendon produces a central degeneration.

The rotator cuff tendon can usually heal quite well once the causative factor and the inflammatory reaction has been addressed. A rehabilitation programme should be used as the first line of management. Some authors have reported success in treating full thickness tears in this way. Larger full thickness tears of the tendon should be treated with a formal repair to restore strength and function. Full restoration may be difficult to achieve, even with a technically successful repair. Patients with a full-thickness rotator cuff tear are kept in an abduction splint for 6 weeks to take the tension off the repair. Only passive exercises are used during this time. Active exercises above shoulder level are only begun when muscle strength has been restored so that elevation can take place using a near normal movement pattern.

A defect in the form of a partial or a full thickness tear may remain in the tendon following release of a calcific deposit or after trauma. Those of a limited size and involving partial thickness of the tendon only may be treated with decompression only followed by rehabilitation.

Acromioclavicular joint subluxations and dislocations

The initial approach after trauma is conservative for grades 1–3. There is no evidence that surgery improves the outcome. An early return to sport does seem to aggravate symptoms, and some efforts at rehabilitation in the form of mobilisation and cuff work seem beneficial. However, there is evidence in favour of operating for the rare grade 4, 5 and 6 cases. There should also be a lower threshold for surgery if the clavicle is significantly displaced in a posterior direction.

Subluxations may be more symptomatic than complete separations of the two joint surfaces. This is probably because in the subluxed joint symptomatic secondary arthritis and inflammation is more likely to occur. Pain and reduced function may develop over the following months or years. In these cases, an excision of the lateral end of the clavicle of no more than 1 cm with a slightly medially directed cut is a useful treatment.

If the coracoclavicular ligaments are found to be stretched or torn, they can be reconstructed using the acromioclavicular ligament. The acromial end of the ligament is detached and fixed onto the cut distal end of the clavicle – the Weaver–Dunn procedure.[15] It has been thought that resecting the distal end of the clavicle causes weakness of the arm, but a recent paper has shown that this is rarely the case. The Weaver–Dunn procedure is our preferred method for treating complete symptomatic dislocations of the AC joint.

Following excisions of the distal end of the clavicle the arm is kept in a broad arm sling for 2 weeks, but pendulum exercises are carried out as early as possible after surgery. If a Weaver–Dunn procedure has been carried out, the reconstructed ligament needs to be protected for 6 weeks to allow some healing before formal exercises are begun.

Conclusion

The understanding and subsequent management of shoulder problems in athletes has improved dramatically because of better imaging, shoulder arthroscopy, and deeper knowledge of the basic sciences. The clinician and therapist have a responsibility for making a clinical diagnosis before starting treatment – which in our opinion is the hallmark of the expert.

References

1 Poppen NK, Walker PS. Normal and abnormal motion of the shoulder. *J Bone Joint Surg* 1976;**58B**:195–201.
2 Wallace WA. The dynamic study of shoulder movement. In: Bayley I, Kessel L, eds. *Shoulder surgery.* Berlin: Springer Verlag, 1982, pp. 179–82.
3 Beighton P, Solomon L and Soskolnc CL. Articular mobility in an African population. *Ann Rheum Dis* 1973;**32**:413–28.
4 Thomas SC, Matsen FC. An approach to the repair of avulsion of the glenohumeral ligaments. *J Bone Joint Surg* 1989;**71A**:506–13.
5 Snyder SJ, Karzel RP, DelPizzo W, *et al.* SLAP lesions of the shoulder. *Arthroscopy* 1990;**6**:274–6.
6 Neer CS. Impingement lesions. *Clin Orthop* 1983;**173**:70–7.

7 Jobe CM, Scales J. Evidence for a superior glenoid impingement upon the rotator cuff. Presented at the 5th International Conference on Surgery of the Shoulder, Paris, July 1992.

8 American Academy of Orthopaedic Surgeons. *Joint motion. A method of measuring and recording* Rosemont, Illinois:AAOS, 1965.

9 Basmaijan JV. *Muscles alive*, 2nd edn. Baltimore, MD: Williams and Wilkins, 1967.

10 Perry J. Anatomy and biomechanics of the shoulder in throwing, swimming, gymnastics and tennis. *Clin Sports Med* 1983;2(2):247–70.

11 Simonet WT, Cofield RH. Prognosis in anterior shoulder dislocation. *Am J Sports Med* 1984;**12**:19–24.

12 Burkhead WZ, Rockwood CA. Treatment of instability of the shoulder with an exercise program. *J Bone Joint Surg* 1992;**74A**:890–6.

13 Bankart ASB. The pathology and treatment of recurrent dislocation of the shoulder joint. *Br J Surg* 1938;**26**:23–6.

14 Neer CS, Foster CR. Inferior capsular shift for involuntary inferior and multidirectional instability of the shoulder. *J Bone Joint Surg* 1980;**62A**:897–908.

15 Warren-Smith C, Ward MW. Operation for acromioclavicular dislocation: a review of 29 cases treated by one method. *J Bone Joint Surg* 1987;**69B**:715–18.

18 Injuries in young athletes

NICOLA MAFFULLI

Sport participation is an established feature of Western childhood. In the UK, approximately three quarters of all healthy youngsters between 5 and 15 years participate in organised sport. However, only 11% of these are involved in intensive training. In the USA, up to 50% of boys and 25% of girls between 8 and 16 years take part in organised competitive sport. The increase in competitive sports participation by children and adolescents has resulted in an increase in the number of youngsters requiring treatment for sports-related injuries.

The skeletal system of children is extremely plastic, and shows pronounced adaptive changes to intensive sports training. As sports injuries affect bone and soft tissues, they could damage the growth mechanisms with subsequent life-lasting damage.

Around the period of peak linear growth, adolescents are vulnerable to injuries because of imbalance in strength and flexibility and changes in the biomechanical properties of bone. In immature athletes, as bone stiffness increases and resistance to impacts diminishes, sudden overload may cause

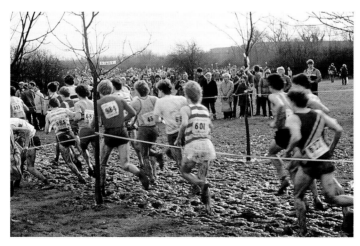

Figure 18.1   There is widespread participation in organised sport among young people in the UK and most Western countries

bones to bow or buckle. Physiological loading has been shown to be beneficial to the young skeleton, but excessive strains may result in serious injury to weight-bearing joint surfaces.

These concerns have led some medical bodies to issue guidelines to regulate sports participation for youngsters. It was feared that a potential epidemic of both acute and overuse sports injuries might break out, but up to now this has not been the case.

This chapter first reviews some epidemiological aspects of sports injuries in athletic youngsters. Subsequently, some of the clinical aspects of sports injuries of the upper and lower limb will be considered. Only the aspects of injuries in children peculiar to this age group will be considered. The reader is referred to the specific chapters on adult athletes for more exhaustive discussion of such injuries.

Incidence of sports injuries

Published studies vary significantly in terms of populations studied, methodology used, and the types and severity of injuries reported. Therefore, the actual incidence of injury in children's sports is very difficult, if not impossible, to determine. In addition, because of the different criteria used to define an injury, comparisons between reports are difficult. Any such comparisons should be interpreted with caution.

Studies in the early 1980s found that between 3% and 11% of school-aged children were injured each year participating in sport. Although boys may sustain twice as many injuries as girls in some series, a similar incidence between genders has also been reported. Boys, however, sustain more severe injuries, possibly because of their greater aggression. In general, the incidence of sports injuries seems to increase with age, approaching the incidence rate of senior players in the older children. Recently, using a mixed longitudinal study design, we found an incidence rate of less than one injury per 1000 hours of training in 453 elite young British athletes. Sports involving contact and jumping have the highest injury risk.

Risk factors

Sports injuries result from a complex interaction of extrinsic factors, such as exposure to different types of sports, sports environment and protective equipment worn, and intrinsic factors, such as physical, physiological, and psychological characteristics of the athletes. A history of having sustained a previous injury is one of the strongest injury predictors.

Although some athletes seem to be more prone to overuse injuries than others, those who train more have a significantly greater number of overuse injuries than those who train less. Overtraining will result in injury in a young athlete as in an adult, however, the former is far less able to say "no" to the coach. The more talented the child, the greater the requirements to compete more and more. Soccer players have been reported as playing over 150 matches in a season. Recognition of this excess has led to some sports legislating to restrict the number of competitions per season.

Imbalances in size and maturity between individuals around the time of puberty affects contact sports and injury risks in particular. Growth spurts lead to imbalances between bone and muscle growth with loss of coordination. Gentle stretching and strengthening work allowing time to return the status quo, together with an explanation to athlete and adult supervisor, is often all that is required.

Young athletes have additional pressures from adults such as parents, teachers, or coaches where inappropriate or excessive training from inexperienced, unqualified, overenthusiastic adult supervisors leads to a significantly increased incidence of injury. Loss of fun is a major factor in stopping sport. Children and young adults use injury as a face-saving excuse to avoid these pressures. The practitioner must be wary of the adult accompanying a child who answers questions directed at the child, uses "we" in replies, and emphasises previous successes and forthcoming competition. Interview the child alone and gain his/her confidence that you have the best interests of the patient at heart. Careful counselling of both child and adult is essential.

Types of injury

Some injuries are essentially the same, although they are sustained in different parts of the body. In this chapter, injuries are presented according to their anatomical location with specific reference to upper and lower limb injuries. Back injuries are not discussed as they have been extensively reviewed elsewhere, as have hand injuries and sports-specific injuries.

Children seek treatment not only for injuries which are unique to physical and skeletal immaturity, but also for injuries that were previously seen almost exclusively in adults. These "unique" injuries represent approximately 15% of all clinically significant sports injuries in children.

Injury patterns are influenced by children's physical characteristics. Joint laxity is associated with ligamentous injury, such as recurrent sprains and dislocations. Tightness is strongly correlated with meniscal injuries and ankle, shoulder, and wrist sprains.

Epiphyseal injuries

These injuries, with no counterpart in adult life, occur at the epiphyseal growth plates. Shearing and avulsion forces are generally responsible,

385

but compression may also play a significant role. The cartilaginous cells of the epiphysis may be damaged, producing premature closure of the epiphyseal plate and growth disturbance bone growth, with subsequent deformity.

Growth plate injuries are broken down according to the Salter–Harris classification into five types. In types 1 and 2, the epiphyseal plate is intact, the prognosis is excellent and, after appropriate reduction and immobilisation, growth continues undisturbed (Figure 18.2). In types 3 and 4, the fracture runs through the joint surface and through the epiphyseal plate. Through accurate closed or surgical reduction, the epiphyseal plate and the articular surface are correctly aligned. Growth can then continue, and restoration of the joint anatomy to congruity prevents secondary osteoarthritis (Figure 18.3). Type 5 injuries are often difficult to detect radiographically at the time of injury, as they are a compression injury of the growth plate, usually with no X-ray changes. Some time after the injury, growth may cease, and deformity or growth disturbance can follow (Figure 18.4).

Upper limb injuries

Acute fractures of the clavicle

This is a common injury in contact sports and in sports involving falls on the outstretched hand or a direct fall on to the shoulder. Reduction is generally not necessary, and the child simply needs a sling to immobilise the arm for 2–3 weeks. Generally, recovery is excellent.

Acute glenohumeral dislocation

Glenohumeral dislocations are rare in youngsters. When they do occur in a shoulder that was previously normal, when the growth plate is still open, a very high (>80%) recurrence rate has been reported.

Fractures of the humerus

The mechanism of injury is usually indirect. Metaphyseal fractures are seen particularly in older children (Figure 18.5). It is rarely necessary to correct the deformity because of the great adaptability of the shoulder joint, and the good post-healing remodelling.

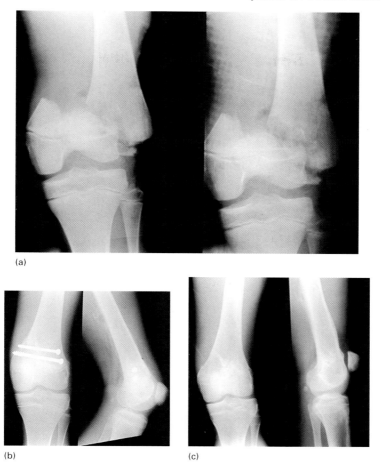

(a)

(b)   (c)

Figure 18.2   (a) Type 2 Salter–Harris epiphyseal injury of the lower femur in a 16-year-old gymnast who injured himself dismounting from the parallel bars. (b) Closed reduction and fixation using percutaneous cannulated screws. (c) Thirty-six months after the injury, and 18 months after removal of the screws. Although he retired from the sport, the knee was fully asymptomatic, and he was coaching part time. There was no limb length discrepancy

Elbow injuries

Elbow injuries in sport are common. Plain radiographs in children are often difficult to interpret, damage to major vessels or nerves may occur, and some children require operative treatment. In adults the elbow is liable to develop post-traumatic stiffness, but in this age group vigorous physical

387

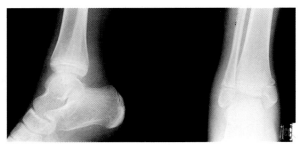

Figure 18.3 (a)

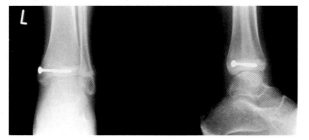

Figure 18.3 (b)

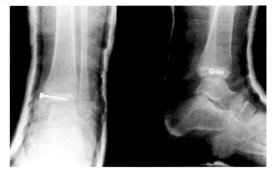

Figure 18.3 (c)

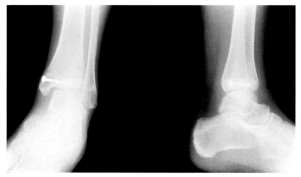

Figure 18.3 (d)

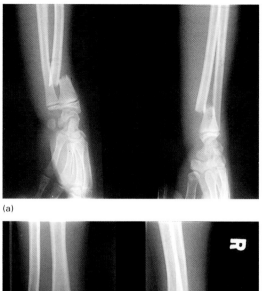

(a)

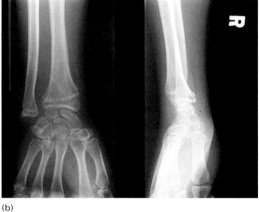

(b)

Figure 18.4   Post-traumatic Madelung deformity in a 14-year-old cyclist. He had fallen off his bicycle two years previously during a time trial. At the time, he had injured both his wrists (a). On the left side, in another centre, a type 2 Salter–Harris epiphyseal injury was identified, and treated with manipulation under anaesthesia and casting. On the right side, no radiographic evident injury was present, and a wrist sprain had been diagnosed. Gradually, he had developed a remarkable wrist deformity which did not hinder his cycling performance. A fellow competitor remarked on the unusual appearance of the wrist, and the patient consulted us (b). A shortening osteotomy of the ulna is planned. Type 5 Salter–Harris epiphyseal injuries are difficult to diagnose at the time of injury. Even if correctly identified, their management often consists of the treatment of deformities secondary to the massive lesion of the growth plate

---

Figure 18.3   (opposite) (a) Type 4 Salter–Harris epiphyseal injury of the lower medial tibial epiphysis in an 11-year-old hockey player. (b) Open reduction and internal fixation using a single intra-epiphyseal screw avoiding the growth plate. (c) Six weeks after the injury, mobilisation was begun. (d) Six months after the injury, there was no apparent residual functional deficit. The boy had returned to his sport

389

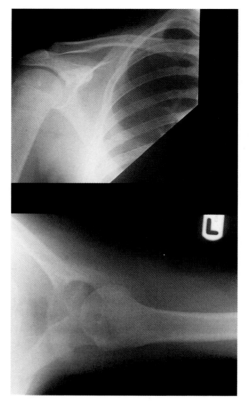

Figure 18.5 Fracture of the upper humeral metaphysis in a 14-year-old judo player. He was immobilised in a broad arm sling and treated with modified rest. Within 8 weeks he was back to gentle training

therapy is generally not needed. Damage to the growth plate can result in subsequent deformity.

The so-called "Little Leaguer's Elbow" is discussed in Chapter 16.

Supracondylar fractures

The distal part of the humerus commonly displaces posteriorly and can involve the growth plate. The arm should be manipulated correcting all the components of the fracture, and held either in flexion with a collar and cuff or in extension in skin traction, depending on the type of fracture. It is imperative to make sure that there is no associated brachial artery injury. If this is the case, surgical exploration with open reduction is mandatory

(Figure 18.6). If the closed reduction is acceptable but unstable, I use percutaneous wiring to maintain reduction.

Dislocation of the elbow

Common in gymnastics, it can be associated with fractures of the medial epicondyle of the humerus, fractures of the neck of the radius, or injury to the median or ulnar nerve. Most of the dislocations in youngsters are posterior or posterolateral. At all ages, they require prompt reduction. Rehabilitation should be gradual, and I discourage return to sporting activities before 8–12 weeks. The child should have regained a full range of movement before resuming full sporting activity.

Forearm and wrist fractures

These fractures are generally due to indirect trauma from a fall on the outstretched hand. All levels of the forearm can be affected, although most fractures occur over the distal third. Some angulation is acceptable in young children, but angular deformity should always be corrected if the child is older than 12. Rotational deformity should always be corrected. When either of these factors cannot be corrected by simple manipulation, open reduction and internal fixation should be undertaken.

Injuries to the distal radial growth epiphysis

Extremely common, this fracture is usually a Salter type 2 injury. Closed reduction and immobilisation are generally sufficient, and results are excellent. A slight dorsal angulation can be accepted, but the young patients must be closely monitored as, in some children, the position is lost and further manipulation is necessary.

Overuse injuries

Traction apophysitis

This condition occurs at the insertion of the triceps into the olecranon epiphysis in gymnastics, diving, wrestling, and hockey. The young athletes complain of local pain and tenderness around the insertion of the triceps tendon, exacerbated by supporting their body weight with the arms. Radiographs may show marked fragmentation of the epiphysis. However, they are difficult to interpret because of normal variants in this region. Treatment consists of a period of rest from upper limb activities, and symptoms usually settle over 3 months. Long term problems are rare.

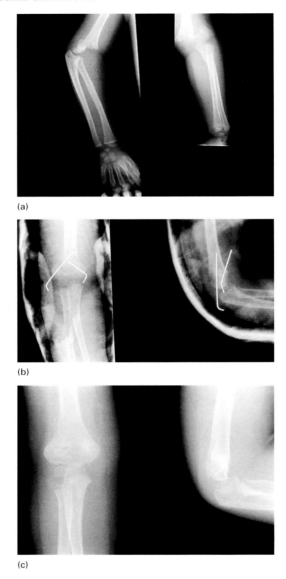

(a)

(b)

(c)

Figure 18.6 (a) Supracondylar fracture of the humerus in a 4-year-old girl. She fell down during a trampolining session. (b) Manipulation under anaesthesia was unsuccessful, and it was necessary to undertake open reduction and Kirschner wiring. (c) One year after the injury. At this stage, the young patient had a deficit of 5 degrees of extension, but no functional limitation

Osteochondritis dissecans

Osteochondritis dissecans (OCD) of the humeral capitellum, and more rarely the trochlea, is well documented, and it can occur in non-sporting children. The dominant arm is affected in Little League baseball pitchers, due to valgus loading of the elbow during pitching, so that the lateral side of the joint is repeatedly compressed (see Chapter 16 for more detail). In gymnasts, compression and rotation during weight-bearing through the arm, and loading of the lateral side of the elbow increased by the physiological valgus of the elbow, affect the joint surface. These youngsters present with elbow pain and some swelling, and are often unable to fully extend the elbow, which is tender over the lateral aspect. Initial signs and symptoms are often minimal. Radiographs are often diagnostic, but early diagnosis may require magnetic resonance imaging (MRI) or computerised tomography (CT). The damaged area of the articular epiphysis can break away to form an intra-articular loose body.

If the condition is recognised early, conservative treatment may be successful, with proscription of weight-bearing on the upper limbs or of stressing the elbow. Loose bodies should be removed surgically or arthroscopically. As the articular surface is damaged and the joint not congruous, early osteoarthrosis can ensue. OCD of the radial head is rarer. Diagnosis and treatment are along the lines of OCD of the humeral capitellum.

Panner's disease (see also Chapter 16)

The entire epiphysis of the humeral capitellum is affected in Panner's disease, with impairment of blood supply of the whole area. Pain, swelling, and limitation of motion of the elbow are evident. The diagnosis is radiological. The lesion will heal, but the mode of healing is important. If it results in a deformity, there will be incongruity of the joint with the risk of later osteoarthrosis.

Epiphyseal growth plate overuse injuries

The epiphyseal growth plate may fail due to repeated microtrauma. Stress fractures through the olecranon epiphysis have been reported in adolescent baseball players, gymnasts, and wrestlers. There is pain in the posterior aspect of the elbow with local tenderness over the olecranon and decreased elbow extension. The growth plate is widened. Healing usually takes place with conservative treatment. Occasionally, the epiphyseal plate fails to fuse, and internal fixation is necessary.

Stress-induced changes in the distal radial epiphysis are well recognised in gymnasts. These children present with wrist pain associated with some swelling and local pain on weight-bearing and rotation of the wrist. Radiographs show widening of the growth plate with failure of the zone of calcification. With rest, the epiphysis recovers. The prognosis is good, although growth can be interrupted. At the end of growth, the child may present a slight shortening of the radius compared with the ulna.

Lower limb injuries

Lesions of the hip joint and pelvis

Traction injuries to the growth plate

Various sites around the hip are weak because of the presence of unfused epiphyses. Large fragments of bone can be avulsed with sudden unexpected loads. The anterior inferior iliac spine tends to fail during football when the kicking foot is suddenly blocked, as happens in a tackle. More often, when the foot hits the ground the anterior inferior iliac spine is pulled off by the reflected head of rectus femoris (Figure 18.7). In similar circumstances, the psoas muscle can avulse the lesser trochanter. The whole apophyseal plate of the ischium can separate through the powerful pull of the hamstrings. This can happen in cross country running when the ditch being jumped is wider than expected, and the leading leg is overstretched. More rarely, the anterior superior iliac spine can be avulsed

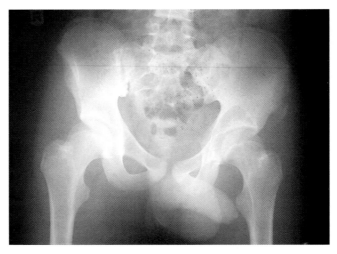

Figure 18.7   Avulsion of the anterior inferior iliac spine in a 17-year-old footballer. At the beginning of a match, started without appropriate warm-up, he had been tackled by an opponent, and experienced sudden pain in his groin. Rest, analgesia, and gentle mobilisation is sufficient after these injuries. Patients generally recover well despite massive new bone production at the avulsion site

by the action of sartorius in a bad gymnastics vault landing. The whole iliac crest apophysis can also be pulled by the abdominal muscles, although displacement is uncommon.

Typically, the young athlete gives a history of severe, immediate, and well localised pain, and the appropriate radiographic views confirm the diagnosis. As the avulsions are deep, cryotherapy is unhelpful, and analgesia is the preferred option for pain relief, with rest and gradual return to activity as pain permits. Immediate surgery is not indicated, and late surgery is exceptionally required despite occasional dramatic radiographic changes.

Perthes disease

One of the hip conditions of late childhood (age 5–10 years) is Legg–Calvé–Perthes disease. If this occurs in a young athlete, a temporary interruption or limitation of sports activities is necessary. In the early phases of Perthes disease, plain radiographs may be normal, but bone scanning may show decreased uptake in the femoral head. MRI does provide better evaluation of involvement in the early stages of Perthes disease than plain radiography, but its cost-effectiveness needs to be assessed.

Perthes disease generally affects the proximal femoral epiphysis between 5 and 10 years of age. It is possible that two or more episodes of raised intra-articular pressure lead to avascular necrosis of part of the head. It presents as an irritable hip with sclerosis of the femoral head. In general, the more complete the lesion, the worse the outcome. On the other hand, the earlier its onset, the better the outcome. Treatment may vary between supervised neglect and aggressive surgery, and the dispute between expert orthopaedic surgeons is far from resolved.

Irritable hip

"Irritable hip" is common in children. It presents with a limp and, at times, non-localised pain. Clinical examination reveals painful restriction of motion of the hip joint, particularly in extension and/or abduction in flexion. In the majority of cases, a specific cause is never identified, and the pain settles after a period of rest and observation. Radiographs, bone scanning, and blood tests are usually normal, and the children can often be rested at home. If the joint space is increased by 2 mm or more, an increased risk of Perthes disease has been reported. Despite its benign nature, investigations are mandatory to exclude the rare cases of infections, tuberculosis, or bone tumour that may present as an irritable hip. A larger joint effusion is generally a sign of sepsis, usually caused by *Staphylococcus aureus*. In this case, the young athlete will generally present with pyrexia, malaise, and severe fatigue. Bone scanning shows increased uptake at both sides of the joint. If pus is aspirated, the hip should be explored surgically, and antibiotics started.

Slipped upper femoral epiphysis

Slipping of the upper femoral epiphysis occurs most commonly in overweight boys with underdeveloped gonads, and in tall thin children during the growth spurt, and typically occurs between 10 and 16 years of age. The child frequently presents after an injury in which the thigh has apparently become suddenly painful. Close questioning often reveals some premonitory discomfort. Knee pain is often the presenting complaint because of the nerve supply of the hip, and many children are referred to an orthopaedic clinic with a painful knee from unknown causes. The physical signs consist of loss of internal rotation or even a fixed external rotation and shortening of the leg, with external rotation of the foot while standing. With the child supine on the couch, internal rotation is restricted or impossible. Such physical signs demand a radiograph of the hip. The deformity is much easier to see in the lateral view. Surgical treatment to prevent further displacement consists of internal fixation of the upper femoral epiphysis in situ without attempting to reduce it unless the slip is very severe. Despite appropriate and prompt treatment, avascular necrosis and chondrolysis may ensue, putting an end to an athletic career, and the hip at risk of secondary osteoarthritis.

Fractures

Fractures of the femoral neck are rare in childhood, and always result from major trauma. Their management is usually open reduction and internal fixation and their prognosis is guarded.

Thigh injuries

Thigh injuries are non-specific to childhood, with the exception of subperiosteal haematoma, a consequence of the more loosely attached periosteum. The story of an injury followed by increasing pain, particularly with sleep disturbance, must alert the physician to a bone tumour or infection. Osteosarcoma (malignant) and osteoid osteoma (benign) are the commonest tumours, and are associated with characteristic changes on radiographs. Benign tumours such as simple bone cysts can present with a fracture through the weakened area. They are treated as a fracture, with many of them healing spontaneously after the injury.

Lesions of and around the knee joint

Ligament injuries

Injuries of the distal thigh merge with those of the knee. Always beware hip pain referred to the knee. In the mature skeleton, valgus and varus stress results in tears of the medial and lateral collateral ligaments, respectively. In the child, the epiphyseal plate is weaker than the ligaments and usually gives way instead. The knee may be unstable, and plain radiographs appear normal, but stress radiographs, taken under anaesthesia if the pain is severe, will reveal the epiphyseal lesion. Treatment consists of immobilisation for 4 weeks, and controlled mobilisation thereafter. These injuries may be very unstable, and some authors have recommended percutaneous or internal fixation.

A similar imbalance between muscle and ligaments on the one hand and epiphyseal strength on the other has been reported to produce the classical anterior cruciate ligament (ACL) lesion in non-athletic children. In these cases, the ligament itself remains intact but a large piece of the proximal tibia is avulsed. The mechanism of injury is a flexion, twisting, or hyperextension injury, with immediate pain and haemarthrosis. Following radiographs, I perform an arthroscopic washout of the joint and use a small cannulated screw to fix the fragment of bone back into place. Some degree of ACL laxity and lack of full extension can occur, even when anatomical reduction has been achieved.

Although children were considered at low risk for mid-substance tear of the ACL, an increasing number of tears of the ACL, often associated with a lesion of the medial collateral ligament, are being reported. MRI can be performed to ascertain whether an ACL tear has indeed occurred. However, clinical examination is still paramount. The few prospective studies performed have shown that sensitivity and specificity of MRI is still relatively low, and arthroscopy should still be considered the gold standard for diagnosis. If the ACL is torn, operative repair should probably be carried out, despite the young age of the patients, to prevent secondary meniscal tears. The procedure would normally give good results with a low subsequent risk of growth abnormalities.

Patella

The patellofemoral joint is often vulnerable, especially in children with patella alta (defined as a patella tendon longer than $1\frac{1}{2}$ times the length of the patella) which does not fully engage in the femoral groove. Twisting of the leg with the knee slightly flexed may cause patellar subluxation or frank dislocation. If the patella remains dislocated, the diagnosis is easy and relocation can sometimes be difficult. On the playing field, relocation by direct pressure on the patella or by passively extending the knee is acceptable

397

management. If the patella spontaneously reduces, the knee is swollen and the medial patellar margin tender due to soft tissue tears. Skyline radiographs are needed to exclude marginal fractures which, if left untreated, can result in loose bodies. Arthroscopy for assessment and arthroscopic or open removal of loose bodies is usually recommended with some surgeons also advocating a medial capsule plication.

Giving way of the knee on twisting should be considered of patellar origin until proved otherwise and should be treated conservatively in the first instance. Although meniscal problems in this age group are unusual, and are generally associated with a discoid meniscus with a painless clonking noise before the tear, meniscal lesions in adolescents need to be considered, and warrant arthroscopy.

The extensor apparatus above the patella is rarely injured in children. In the so-called "sleeve fracture" of the patella, the periosteum is stripped downwards in continuity with the tendon. The diagnosis is usually missed until the bone grows again in the empty pouch and produces the double patella appearance. At this stage, it is too late to operate, but in children the outcome from conservative treatment is usually good.

Joint surface

Within the knee, osteochondral fractures may affect the weight-bearing articular surface of the femur as a consequence of a twisting injury. They present with a haemarthrosis. Radiographs may be helpful, but the diagnosis may only become clear following arthroscopy or MRI. The fragment, usually arising from the lateral side of the medial femoral condyle, must be fixed back, as it can represent a major part of the weight-bearing articular surface.

In osteochondritis dissecans (OCD), intense physical activity and high level sport are frequently encountered. OCD may produce degenerative changes due to the formation of loose bodies or residual deformity of the joint surface. The most commonly affected areas in the lower limb are the lateral aspect of the medial femoral condyle, the femoral head, and the talus but other areas of the articular cartilage of the knee can also be affected. Management of OCD depends on the state of the lesion and on the age of the athlete (Figure 18.8). In the appropriate joints, arthroscopy is the procedure of choice. Non-operative treatment in skeletally immature young athletes may allow resolution in circumscribed stable lesions. Surgical or arthroscopic removal of intra-articular loose bodies resulting from late OCD is mandatory, so as to allow early return to the sport and avoid permanent disability in the young athelete.

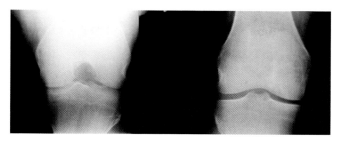

Figure 18.8 Osteochondritis dissecans of the knee in a 19-year-old footballer of club standard. He first developed pain in his knee at age 15, correctly diagnosed as osteochondritis dissecans. Since then, he had played approximately half of the matches in each season, always refusing operation. At 19, due to increasing pain, he decided to undergo an arthroscopy. This is the immediate preoperative film

Traction apophysitis

Sinding–Larsen–Johansson lesion is a syndrome of tenderness and radiographic fragmentation localised at the inferior pole of the patella. The lesion is considered a calcification in an avulsed portion of the patellar tendon, and is self-limiting. Conservative treatment with modification of sporting activity is all that is required.

A mature tibial tubercle forms from ossification centres in the epiphysis. The pulling action by the patellar tendon may cause inflammation and pain, determining the clinical entity known as Osgood–Schlatter's lesion. This is also usually self-limiting and again conservative treatment with temporary restriction from sport is all that is necessary. In rare cases, a short (6 week) period in a cast may be necessary for severe symptoms. Both the Sinding–Larsen–Johansson lesion and the Osgood–Schlatter's lesion occur between 8 and 13 years in girls, and 10 and 15 years in boys. Boys are nearly twice as affected as girls, possibly because of their higher activity levels.

Factors associated with Osgood–Schlatter's disease are:

1. Growth spurt.
2. Overuse, particularly kicking and jumping.
3. Tight quadriceps.

Stress fracture

The tibia and more rarely the femur may be the site of stress fractures. In these cases, pain coming on earlier and earlier after the beginning of activity is pathognomonic. Initial radiographs are normal, but the fracture often becomes evident later. A bone scan is diagnostic, although these images must be distinguished from the tibial stress reaction, a physiological response to heavy use. Treatment consists of reduction of activity to a pain-free level with very gradual subsequent increase.

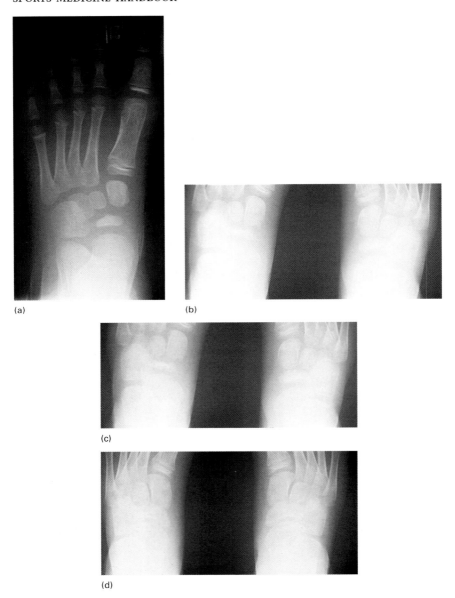

(a)

(b)

(c)

(d)

Figure 18.9   (a) Köhler's disease in a ballet dancer aged 7 years. (b) After 3 months, she started to complain of contralateral foot pain, and a further radiograph revealed bilateral involvement. (c) At age 8.2 years, radiographic progression of the condition. Despite the loss of navicular height, the patient was fully weight-bearing. No dance was allowed. (d) After 4 years there is normal appearance of the bones of the feet, with no pain

Lesions of and around the ankle

The twisting injuries that cause a fracture in adults produce a different pattern of injury in the immature skeleton. In general, ankle fractures in children are minimally displaced. However, when involving the articular surface, they may require open reduction and internal fixation.

Osteochondral fractures in the ankle are much smaller than in the knee, may be difficult to diagnose, and are usually confirmed by a bone scan.

The foot is the site of stress lesions more commonly than usually realised. Sever's lesion presents with well localised activity-related pain at the back of the heel and radiographical fragmentation of the calcaneal apophysis. Some authors consider them stress fractures, but there is often a similar asymptomatic radiograph of the other asymptomatic side. The pain responds to rest, stretching, and a shock absorber under the heel.

Stress fractures of the metatarsals are common, the history is diagnostic and the callus will show on radiographs taken several weeks after the complaint started.

Köhler's disease is similar to Legg–Calvé–Perthes disease, and involves the tarsal navicular which is to became temporarily avascular (Figure 18.9). The condition is generally benign, and is managed by rest and avoidance of jumping and hopping on the involved foot. It takes 2–3 years to return to normal in most cases. Although occasionally there is practically complete restoration of normal bone architecture by maturity, the navicular remains narrowed.

Back lesions

Chronic back pain in children is rare, except in cases of Scheuermann's disease and spondylolysis or spondylolisthesis. More serious conditions should therefore come to mind, such as fractures, infections, and tumours. Adolescent athletes are more prone to disc prolapse, which is best diagnosed by MRI. The high risk sports for acute spinal injuries are American football, diving, gymnastics, and trampolining. Sports injuries account for 18% of paediatric cervical spine fractures.

Although the development of scoliosis (curvature in the coronal plane greater than 10 degrees) is not related to sport, in the sagittal plane excessive physical stress can be a factor in the development of structural kyphosis, or Scheuermann's disease. This is distinct from the functional correctable kyphosis of poor posture known as functional round back. Scheuermann's disease can be diagnosed by a lateral spine radiograph showing three consecutive vertebrae with anterior wedging of 5 degrees or more. In addition, the end plates of the growing vertebra adjacent to the discs are

401

often markedly irregular, and intraosseous herniation of cartilaginous disc material (Schmorl's nodes) may be a predominant feature.

Cervical trauma

Following trauma, fractures of the cervical spine are less common in children than in adults. Most spinal injuries in children below the age of 12 years involve the atlantoaxial or atlanto-occipital joints, although all levels can be affected. Prevertebral soft tissue swelling greatly assists the diagnosis on lateral films. Slight anterior vertebral wedging is normal in children due to incomplete ossification, and up to 2 mm of spondylolysis is acceptable in the upper cervical levels. The normally lax ligaments of children result in a greater prevalence of displacements rather than fractures. Down's syndrome children have such lax atlantoaxial ligaments that it is recommended that sports activity be restricted if a lateral radiograph shows greater than 4.5 mm arch–dens separation. This laxity predisposes to atlantoaxial rotary subluxation with abnormal displacement between the facet joints sometimes presenting as torticollis, but sufficiently serious to make the risk of spinal injury with modest trauma significant. Trampolining and gymnastics should be discontinued if there is evidence of spinal instability. If this is suspected on plain radiographs, CT scanning with the head turned in both directions is required to assess whether this is fixed (a facet joint does not reduce with the head turned towards the direction of C2) or mobile. This is often seen in ballet due to rapid head rotation whilst pirouetting.

Gymnastics, dance, football, weight-lifting, and running are associated with spondylolysis and spondylolisthesis. Spondylolysis is an osseous defect of the pars interarticularis between the superior and inferior facets of the vertebral body. Spondylolisthesis is the slippage of the superior vertebra on the inferior. Both can be related to hyperextension rotation, and axial loading, since there is an increased incidence in gymnasts (11%), ballet dancers, cricket fast bowlers, soccer players, and interior linemen in American football. This structural abnormality is not always symptomatic. Although spondylolisthesis can be due to a congenitally inadequate superior facet, it is usually acquired. Its frequency increases with age through childhood, especially between 5 and 7 years, to reach 6% in adults. It is thought to be a stress fatigue fracture, although occasionally it may be an acute injury. Approximately 70% of spondylolistheses occur at L5–S1 level, and only rarely above L3. They are usually bilateral but occasionally they are unilateral, in which case compensatory hypertrophy of the contralateral pedicle may be seen as increased density on a plain X-ray. CT clearly shows the defect in the posterior arch and also delineates any foraminal encroachment by bone fragments. There is a high rate of healing if sport is temporarily restricted.

402

Lumbar disc

Low back pain in adolescent athletes is rarely due to lumbar disc protrusion. In a study of 70 adolescents undergoing surgery for lumbar disc herniation, 22 were injured during sports activities, and 26 were routinely participating in sports. Not all the patients were suffering from back pain, but they all eventually developed sciatica.

The true incidence of the lesion in sporting youngsters is unknown, and no conclusion can be made. The role of acute trauma as an aetiological factor in the development of disc herniation in young and very young patients has been stressed, but degenerative changes may play a leading role, with trauma acting as a precipitating factor. A single traumatic episode is not sufficient to produce a disc prolapse unless a degenerative condition is present. This could explain the infrequency of the lesion in children, and thence in intensively trained young athletes.

The role of continuous bony microtrauma is not clear. A large group of women examined at least 3 years after retiring from gymnastics showed degenerative changes of the vertebral bodies and of the intervertebral joints in more than half of them.

Conclusions

In general, sports injuries in children and adolescents are limited to mild contusions, sprains, and strains. However, the media often only reports the more severe skeletal injuries sustained, causing much of the concern expressed with regards to the safety of youth sport.

Any sport can cause skeletal injuries, and the specific pattern and location of injuries typical to each sport should be known by health professionals. Training programmes and performance standards should take into account the biological age of the participants, and their physical and psychological immaturity, more than their chronological age. A deep knowledge of the different aspects of training, including duration, intensity, frequency, and recovery, is needed to avoid serious damage to the skeletal system of athletic children. Considerable time is needed for growing athletes to incorporate their own body changes, and it is probably difficult for the young athlete to develop speed, strength, endurance, and resistance at the same time.

Physical injury is an inherent risk in sports participation and, to a certain extent, must be considered an inevitable cost of athletic training and competition. However, coaches and parents can minimise the risk of injury by ensuring the proper selection of sports events, using appropriate equipment, enforcing rules, using safe playing conditions, and providing adequate supervision. Although injuries in young athletes are sustained, it is important to balance the negative effects of sports injuries with the many social, psychological, and health benefits that a serious commitment to sport brings.

Suggested reading

Lysens R, Steverlynck A, van den Auweele Y, *et al.* The predictability of sports injuries. *Sports Med* 1984;**1**:6–10.

Maffulli N. The growing child in sport. *Brit Med Bull* 1992;**48**:561–8.

Maffulli N. *A color atlas and text of sports medicine in childhood and adolescence.* London: Mosby–Wolfe, 1995.

Maffulli N, Baxter-Jones ADG. Common skeletal injuries in young athletes. *Sports Med* 1995;**19**:137–49.

Micheli LJ. Overuse injuries in children's sport; the growth factor. *Orthop Clin North Am* 1983;**14**:337–60.

Orava S, Puranen J. Exertion injuries in adolescent athletes. *Brit J Sports Med* 1978; **12**:4–10.

Rowley S. *The effect of intensive training in young athletes: a review of the research literature.* London: Sports Council, 1986.

Rowland TW. *Exercise and children's health.* Champaign, IL: Human Kinetics Books, 1990.

Rowley S. Psychological effects of intensive training in young athletes. *J Child Psychol Psychiat* 1987;**28**:371–7.

Stanitski CL. Management of sports injuries in children and adolescents. *Orthop Clin North Am* 1988;**19**:689–98.

Stanitski CL. Common injuries in preadolescent and adolescent athletes: recommendations for prevention. *Sports Med* 1989;7:32–41.

Sward L. The thoracolumbar spine in young athletes. Current concepts on the effects of physical training. *Sports Med* 1992;**13**:357–62.

19   The in-shoe orthotic treatment of lower limb injuries

TIMOTHY E KILMARTIN

Introduction

In-shoe orthoses have provided an alternative and seemingly very effective conservative treatment for a number of lower limb sports injuries[1] (Table 19.1). In-shoe biomechanical orthoses may be prescribed when examination

Table 19.1   Lower limb conditions amenable to in-shoe orthotic treatment

Anterior knee pain related to patellar malalignment
Iliotibial band syndrome
Tibialis anterior shin splints
Tibialis posterior shin splints
Achilles tendonitis related to rearfoot malalignment
Recurrent medial and lateral ankle ligament sprains
Plantar fasciitis
Chronic foot strain – medial longitudinal arch pain
Morton's intermetatarsal neuroma
Degenerative joint disease pain associated with hallux rigidus and hallux valgus

indicates abnormal position or function of the joints of the lower limb or foot.

Excessive pronation, in-rolling or flattening of the foot is perhaps the single most important indication for an orthosis. Excessive pronation may be recognised by the following signs:

1. Eversion of the rearfoot. Often referred to as Helbing's sign, the tendo achilles appears to curve as it inserts into the posterosuperior aspect of the calcaneus. This is caused by the everted position of the rearfoot relative to the leg (Figure 19.1).
2. A low medial longitudinal arch.

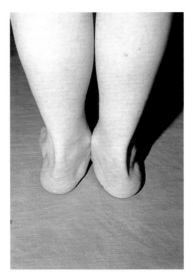

Figure 19.1   The pronated foot; there appears to be bowing of the tendo achillis as it inserts into the rearfoot. Due to abduction of the forefoot there appear to be too many toes

3. A medial bulge caused by subluxation at the talonavicular joint. As the subtalar joint of the foot pronates the talar head will bulge medially beneath the medial malleolus (Figure 19.2).

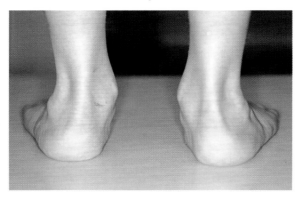

Figure 19.2   A medial bulge may be seen inferior to the medial malleolus; this is due to plantarflexion and adduction of the talus

4. Forefoot abduction manifesting clinically as the "too many toes sign". In the normal foot, as the examiner views the weight-bearing foot from the rearfoot anteriorly, it should be possible only to see the fifth toe. If the forefoot is abducted, however, the fourth and third toes will also be visible. This is a consequence of the rearfoot everting, the talus

subluxating and the forefoot assuming an abducted position relative to the rearfoot (Figure 19.1).

5. Standing the patient with the heel on the ground and knees flexed to 90 degrees gives good correlation with functional pronation when running.

Excessive pronation of the foot may be caused by a number of positional abnormalities of the lower limb and foot (Table 19.2). Orthotic treatment

Table 19.2   (Positional) abnormalities which may cause the foot to excessively pronate

Anteversion or retroversion of the hip
Genu valgum or genu varum of the knee
External tibial torsion
Limited ankle joint dorsiflexion
Rearfoot ankle joint dorsiflexion
Elevated first ray
Hallux rigidus

of these injuries essentially aims to limit the pronation of the foot by inverting the foot, with a wedge to the medial forefoot and medial heel as well as a support to the medial longitudinal arch (Figure 19.3).

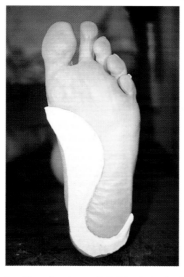

Figure 19.3   The cobra insole will wedge the medial side of the forefoot and heel and support the medial arch of the foot

Pes cavus is also a positional abnormality of the foot. Clinical signs include an inverted rearfoot position, high medial longitudinal arch, and retraction of the lesser digits. Sports injuries associated with pes cavus include iliotibial band syndrome, recurrent inversion sprains, retrocalcaneal bursitis and pump-bump deformity, achilles tendinitis, stress fracture,

407

medial tibial periostitis, severe callosities plantar to the first and fifth metatarsal heads, and corns and callosities dorsal to the interphalangeal joints of the toes. Orthotic treatment of the pes cavus foot aims to force the foot into a more everted position and cushion the plantar surface of the forefoot and heel, while reducing footwear irritation of digital lesions.

Orthoses for sports injuries of the lower limb

Temporary orthosis

In the treatment of any biomechanically related lower limb injury a temporary orthosis should be provided in the first instance. This will allow assessment of whether:

- The injury will actually respond to orthotic treatment.
- An orthosis will be accommodated in the patient's sports shoe.
- Compliance with the orthotic justifies further orthotic prescription.
- The patient can tolerate the orthosis without developing further injuries or side effects.

Compressed felt with an adhesive backing is a very convenient material for making temporary orthoses. Semicompressed or chiropody felt may be used, but bottoms out far too quickly for adequate appraisal of the patient's likely response to orthotic treatment. In all medium to high priced running shoes there is usually an in-sock which provides a good vehicle for a temporary felt orthosis. When felt is used it should be placed on the undersurface of the in-sock. This prolongs the life of the felt as it does not directly absorb sweat. Also placing the felt underneath the shoe's in-sock improves toleration and compliance by reducing the potential for bruising the plantar surface of the foot. If the sports shoe does not have a removable in-sock then fibreboard or card may be used, or alternatively 3 mm thick closed cell rubber materials like Poron*, Cleron†, PPT or Spenco‡ which will also further cushion the undersurface of the foot.

The temporary cobra orthosis

The cobra orthosis (Figure 19.3) is a very useful first line of treatment in the pronated foot. It consists of a heel meniscus bevelled with scissors so it is thicker medially than laterally. The heel meniscus will invert the rearfoot and restrict excessive pronation of the foot. The meniscus section

---

* Available from Footwear Findings, Unit 5, Banscombe Road Trading Estate, Somerton, Somerset TA11 6TB.
† Available from The Foot Shop. The Tanyard, Leigh Road, Street, Somerset BA16 0HD.
‡ Available from Canonbury Products Limited, 2A Ada Street, London E8 4QU.

is extended forward into an arch support which may be the same thickness or thicker than the heel meniscus. The arch support will add to the antipronatory effect by applying a medial wedge just behind the weight-bearing area of the forefoot as well as providing direct support to the medial longitudinal arch. To be effective the cobra should be at least 6 mm thick, though in severely pronated feet it may be necessary to increase the thickness of the arch support to 9 mm.

The cobra orthosis may be manufactured clinically out of felt or closed cell rubber like Cleron or Poron. If rubber is used, double-sided sticky tape should be used to adhere the cobra to the shoe's in-sock.

The reverse cobra orthosis

The reverse cobra orthosis may be used in the treatment of recurrent inversion sprains, sinus tarsi syndrome, and pes cavus. The device consists of a heel meniscus, thicker laterally than medially, which will evert the rearfoot and reduce weight-bearing on the lateral border of the forefoot. When provided for patients with a history of recurrent lateral ankle ligament injuries it provides increased stability, and while inversion injuries may still occur, their severity may be reduced.

When the rearfoot is everted the leg will internally rotate. This will reduce the external tibial position which can be an important factor in patellar malalignment related to high quadriceps angle.[2,3] Eversion of the rearfoot will also reduce compression of the medial compartment of the knee joint and has been shown to be helpful in osteoarthrosis associated with genu varum.[4]

Rearfoot and forefoot wedging

Wedging the rearfoot and forefoot is an attempt to bring the ground up to the foot and prevent the need for compensatory pronation or supination of the foot. The position of the wedge is largely determined by an off-weight-bearing examination of the foot which establishes the presence of rearfoot varus, forefoot varus, forefoot valgus, and plantarflexed or dorsiflexed first metatarsal. The wedge is then placed according to the abnormality detected (Table 19.3).

Arch fillers

Most running shoes contain an arch filler to support the medial longitudinal arch of the foot. In combination with the running shoe's stiffened heel counter, the arch filler may go some way towards resisting excessive pronation of the foot and will certainly increase shoe comfort as the shoe will conform more closely to the contours of the foot.

Table 19.3 Causes of abnormal foot position and how the foot may be wedged with felt to realign it

Condition	Position of wedge	Action
Rearfoot varus	Medial wedge to rearfoot	Prevent rearfoot pronation which will compensate for the inverted position of the rearfoot
Forefoot varus	Medial wedge to forefoot	Prevent rearfoot pronation which will compensate for the inverted position of the forefoot
Forefoot valgus	Lateral wedge to forefoot	Support the everted position of the forefoot
Dorsiflexed first metatarsal	Medial wedge to first metatarsal head	Prevent pronation of the foot as weight is transferred medially to the first metatarsal
Plantarflexed first metatarsal	Lateral wedge to 2345 metatarsal head	Prevent excessive loading under the first metatarsal by using a wedge to distribute load across the whole forefoot

While arch fillers may be absent in cheaper running shoes one can easily be incorporated into the shoe using felt or adhesive backed rubber materials. In running spikes there is little room for an orthosis so an arch filler may be the first line of orthotic treatment for pronation-related injury. Orienteering shoes, bowling shoes, ski boots, and ice skates all lack any sort of arch support or filler. All these footwear types can be made to fit the foot more comfortably by fitting an arch filler to the shoe.

If the shoe contains an in-sock it is preferable to adhere the arch filler to the undersurface of the in-sock to minimise bruising to the arch of the foot. Also if felt is used to make the arch filler, absorption of sweat by the felt can be minimised by placing the material under the in-sock.

Heel raise

Raising the heel slightly can affect foot and ankle function. As the heel rises it will also invert and the rest of the foot will supinate. A heel raise can therefore add to the anti-pronatory effect achieved with other devices such as a cobra orthosis. Raising the heel will also reduce tension on the achilles tendon and the plantar fascia which can be helpful in plantar fasciitis and achilles tendonitis. Pump-bump deformity of the heel may also be palliated by raising the superior lateral corner of the heel just above the top of the shoe counter with a 6 mm heel raise.

Continued use of a heel raise may, however, promote a secondary shortening of the achilles tendon which may in the long term further aggravate achilles tendonitis. It is therefore recommended that gentle calf muscle stretching exercises are used in conjunction with a heel raise.

A variation on a heel raise is a horseshoe heel raise. Used in cases of plantar calcaneal bursitis the "U" shape cut from the centre of the heel pad reflects weight-bearing forces from the central plantar calcaneal area.

Redirecting force from bony or soft tissue lesions of the foot may be achieved with a variety of different devices. In the short term adhesive backed felt may be used to bring relief. In metatarsalgia a pad with a "U" cut-out or wing may be used to deflect pressure from an area of tenderness (Figure 19.4).

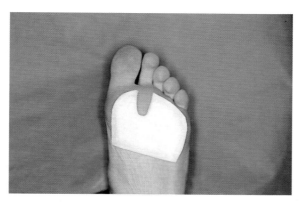

Figure 19.4   A plantar metatarsal pad with a "U" cut-out to the second metatarsal. Tenderness under the second metatarsal often occurs in hallux valgus feet

Digital deformity may also be palliated by the use of felt pads. Rubbing of the shoe on the proximal interphalangeal joint of a lesser toe may be relieved by a felt crescent.

Clawing of the digits with subsequent weight-bearing on the apex of the toe will cause painful corns and callus. This may be relieved by lifting the apex of the toes away from the ground using felt props.

Applying adhesive-backed felt to the skin can only be seen as a short term measure. If successful, more resilient, hygienic devices may be employed.

Permanent orthotic insoles

If temporary felt pads prove successful, a range of closed cell rubber materials can be used to provide a permanent insole. Poron, Cleron, or neoprene rubber are suitable materials, all originally developed for running shoe manufacture. They will provide durable firm cushioning to the foot without causing maceration of the skin, which can be a problem with stuck-on felt.

411

Off-the-shelf orthoses

The apparent success of custom-made orthoses in the treatment of lower limb sports injuries has led to the development of ready made or "off-the-shelf" orthoses designed to invert the foot. The Australian Orthotics Laboratory (AOL)* orthosis (Figure 19.5) inverts the foot with a 4 degree

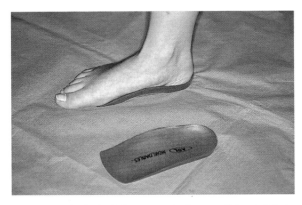

Figure 19.5   The Australian Orthotics Laboratory orthosis – an off-the-shelf device which will invert the rearfoot by 4 degrees

medial wedge to the rearfoot. This standard degree of correction to the rearfoot may not of course be appropriate for all patients but it will at least go some way to controlling excessive pronation of the foot. The AOL orthosis is available in two different material densities, a lighter blue material being used for lighter patients or those who find the denser red orthosis difficult to tolerate.

The Langer multi-balance system† provides an orthotic plate which can be heat moulded to the patient's foot and then 2 and 4 degree wedges can be applied to the forefoot and rearfoot using "snap-on" pieces. This innovation allows for a very accurate orthosis to be made instantly without involving an orthotic laboratory.

As the materials used are extremely light and durable, unlike the AOL device, this orthosis takes up little room within the shoe. It will also allow the athlete to easily vary the degree of orthotic correction according to the symptom relief.

The Tuli's shock absorber was initially developed as a treatment for heel pain. The heel cup construction mimics the arrangement of horizontal and vertical septa in the plantar calcaneal fat pad. The Tuli design is also available as a full insole extending the shock-absorbing qualities to the

---

* Available from Canonbury Products, Unit 7, Boundary Road, Buckingham Road Industrial Estate, Brackley, Northants NN13 7ZS.
† Available from Langer UK, The Green, Cheadle, Stoke on Trent ST10 1RL.

forefoot as well as the heel. It may also be combined with a neoprene ankle support.

Custom-made (bespoke) orthoses

When it is important to ensure maximum control of foot pronation in cases of recalcitrant injury or where there are toleration problems with off-the-shelf devices, a custom-made device may be considered.

A plaster of Paris cast of the foot is taken with the foot in the so-called neutral position when the foot is neither pronated nor supinated. The negative impression of the foot is then sent to a commercial laboratory for filling with liquid plaster of Paris. The thermoplastic orthotic material is then vacuum-pressed against the plaster of Paris model. Wedging of the forefoot and rearfoot sections of the shell (Figure 19.6) is determined by

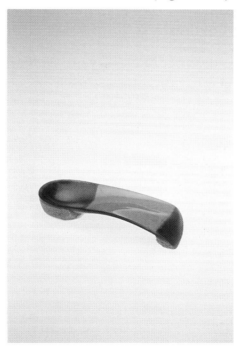

Figure 19.6   A custom-made orthotic device. The rearfoot and forefoot wedging is prescribed according to the individual patient's requirements

measuring the degree of forefoot varus or valgus and rearfoot varus or valgus. The measurements are taken using specialised goniometers with the foot once more in a neutral position.

The effect of this carefully prescribed rearfoot and forefoot wedging is to prevent excessive pronation of the foot by effectively bringing the ground

413

up to the foot rather than allowing the foot to collapse inwards onto the ground.

In order to achieve accurate control of foot position, it is usually necessary to use rigid orthotic materials such as carbon fibre or polypropylene plastic. The thickness of these materials can, however, be varied according to the individual requirements of the athlete or the sport participated in. In general, it is appropriate to use lighter more flexible orthotic material for multidirectional sports like basketball, squash, or tennis. Heavier, more rigid orthotic material is used for single direction running activities where the repetitive nature of the activity is an important predisposition to injury.

Mechanism of orthotic action for lower limb injuries

Anterior knee pain related to patellar malalignment

Poor positioning of the patella relative to the femoral condyles is thought to lead to shearing of the patella against the lateral femoral condyle, fibrillation of the patellar articular cartilage, and pain. Poor patella positioning can be determined by measuring the "Q" or quadriceps angle (see Figure 11.8). The Q angle increases due to internal rotation of the femur. Excessive pronation of the foot causes internal rotation of the leg.[2,3] Reducing the excessively pronated position of the foot with an orthosis will externally rotate the leg and reduce the Q angle. When combined with exercise therapy to strengthen the vastus medialis muscle and avoidance of hill running, especially downhill running which markedly increases the pressure on the posterior surface of the patella, the pain of runners' knee can be alleviated.

Iliotibial band syndrome

This condition is discussed in Chapter 11.

An in-shoe orthosis designed to restrict excessive pronation of the foot will reduce the internal rotation of the tibia and reduce the friction of the iliotibial band against the femur. Because the iliotibial band's primary function is to control flexion and extension of the knee, downhill running will increase the tautness of the band which may increase the friction-related symptoms. Advice on training must therefore accompany orthotic treatment.

414

Medial tibial periostitis

Pain due to periostitis may also develop along the medial border of the tibia as the tibialis posterior tendon or soleus tears off the bone as a result of traction on the origin from the tibia. A line of tenderness along the medial border of the tibia is consistent with this condition.[5]

An in-shoe orthosis which supports the arch of the foot and effectively restricts pronation of the foot will relieve medial tibial periostitis.

Achilles tendinitis related to rearfoot malalignment

In subjects who excessively pronate there will be rapid eversion of the rearfoot just after the heel contacts the ground. This may cause tensile overload of the medial fibres of the achilles tendon which will manifest clinically as tendinitis.[6] Blocking the eversion of the rearfoot with a wedge of material placed under the medial side of the heel will prevent further damage to the tendon fibres.

Recurrent medial and lateral ankle ligament sprains

Chronic instability of the ankle due to recurrent inversion sprains is a most disabling condition for any athlete, no matter what the sport. The problem is often seen in pes cavus feet with marked rearfoot inversion. Preventing further sprains of the ankle may be achieved by providing a reverse cobra orthosis, which will force the rearfoot into a more everted position. Orthoses should be combined with isometric muscle strengthening exercise performed with a rubber power band and proprioception exercises such as hopping on one leg while bouncing a basketball against a wall at head height.

The less common problem of recurrent eversion injuries may be treated using a cobra orthosis (see Figure 19.3), which may prevent further damage to the deltoid ligament of the medial ankle.

Plantar fasciitis

This complex condition is unlikely to respond to just one form of intervention; however, in-shoe orthoses certainly do have a role. An orthosis can be used to cushion the undersurface of the painful heel and also to reduce the traction on the plantar fascia's insertion into the calcaneus. A cobra orthosis made out of closed cell rubber materials like Poron or Cleron will first cushion the heel, second, lift the area of tenderness of the medial calcaneal tubercle away from ground contact, and third, reduce the traction on the plantar fascia which results from the lengthening of the foot as it

415

pronates. The Tuli heel cup is an alternative method for cushioning the plantar heel but this will not address the other causative factors.

Chronic foot strain – medial longitudinal arch pain

Pain in the medial longitudinal arch or a more generalised aching of the whole foot is the result of chronic low grade strain of the joint ligaments. It is particularly common in excessively pronated feet where adduction and plantarflexion of the talus causes the whole foot to elongate while the arch of the foot lowers and the mid tarsal joint subluxates slightly. Wedging the rearfoot into an inverted position while supporting the arch of the foot can bring rapid relief of symptoms as it restores normal joint congruency.

Joint pain associated with hallux rigidus and hallux valgus

These conditions are discussed in Chapter 9.

A simple arch support extended under the first metatarsal will have the effect of restricting first metatarsophalangeal joint motion because for the hallux to rotate over the metatarsal head, the first metatarsal must first plantarflex.[7] Blocking first metatarsal movement will restrict the meta-tarsophalangeal joint's range of movement.[8]

The orthotic treatment plan

While providing orthoses for the sports injured, consideration should also be given to the following factors:

- The athlete's training schedule.
- The surfaces which the athlete is running on.
- The shoes and other equipment being used.
- The athlete's muscle flexibility and strength.

In-shoe orthoses should not be seen as a "single treatment cure" but part of the whole approach. Moreover, it should be understood that orthoses are not an entirely benign intervention. They are expensive and often require replacement. They change the fit of the shoe and can often damage the shoe. They will also make the shoe heavier which could have implications for elite athletes.

When treating an athlete with an injury appropriate for orthotic treatment, an inexpensive temporary device should first be issued to establish likely symptom relief. Only if symptoms have been relieved should the more expensive custom-made devices be prescribed, although the athlete will often obtain even more symptom relief and greater durability with these.

416

The temporary orthosis can be worn for 4 weeks and then reviewed. Once a permanent orthosis has been issued this should be reviewed for any toleration problems or side effects at 2 weeks. The patient should be advised to wear the orthotic as much of the time as possible.

If the permanent orthotic wears out, the patient should be fully reviewed before considering replacement. If the athlete has remained injury-free for some time while not wearing an orthosis it may not be necessary to repeat the orthotic prescription. On the other hand, if the athlete has noticed the recurrence of symptoms it may be necessary to improve the orthosis. In all cases other factors that could be influencing the injury must also be considered.

Orthotic toleration problems

It should be made clear to all patients receiving an orthosis that it will make the shoe tighter as it obviously takes up room in the shoe. Some patients may choose to buy larger shoes. One group that are unlikely to do so are footballers, who often wear very tight fitting boots on the premise that they can "feel the ball" better. In these cases orthoses which are likely to offer the maximum correction can be worn for training while much slimmer devices, offering less correction, can be worn in the match day boots.

The fact that orthoses are often wedged underneath the heel may cause the heel to lift out of the shoe as the patient pushes off from the ground. This problem can be overcome by placing a felt pad under the tongue of the shoe which pushes the heel back into the shoe.

If there are hammer toe deformities, filling the shoe up with an insole is likely to considerably increase dorsal pressure on the digits. In these cases the insole should extend no further than the metatarsal heads.

Custom-made orthoses made from rigid thermoplastic material can sometimes cause bruising of the medial longitudinal arch. This can be overcome by heating up the material with a hot air gun and moulding the orthosis away from the foot.

While an in-shoe orthosis placed under the foot can alter leg and knee function this can occasionally lead to the development of knee pain. In these circumstances the orthosis should be altered to reduce the degree to which the athlete is supinating or pronating the foot.

There are no recorded cases of orthoses causing long term damage to adult athletes. This may be because ill-fitting or inappropriately prescribed orthoses are quickly discarded by the athlete. Alternatively, it could be that as long as an orthosis is comfortable it can be worn without risk whatever the manner of its design.[1]

417

Referral to a podiatrist

Podiatrists receive at least three years of degree level specialist training in the prescription and use of orthoses. To refer to a podiatrist contact the Society of Chiropodists and Podiatrists, 53 Welbeck Street, London WIM 7HE Tel: 0171 486 3381.

References

1 Kilmartin TE, Wallace WA. The scientific basis for the use of functional foot orthoses in the treatment of lower limb sports injuries. A review of the literature. *Br J Sports Med* 1994;**28**:180–4.
2 Rose GK. Correction of the pronated foot. *J Bone Joint Surg* 1958;**40B**:674–83.
3 Rose GK. Correction of the pronated foot. *J Bone Joint Surg* 1962;**44B**:642–7.
4 Sasaki T, Yasuda K. Clinical evaluation of the treatment of osteoarthritic knees using a newly designed wedged insole. *Clin Orthop Rel Res* 1987;**221**:181–7.
5 Mubarak SJ, Hargens AR, Owens MD *et al.* The wick catheter technique for measurement of intramuscular pressure. *J Bone Joint Surg* 1976;**58A**:1016–20.
6 Smart GW, Taunton JE, Clement DB. Achilles tendon disorders in runners – a review. *Med Sci Sports Exerc* 1980;**12**:231–43.
7 Root ML, Orien WP, Weed JH. *Normal and abnormal function of the foot*, Vol. II. Los Angeles: Clinical Biomechanics Corp., 1977.
8 Kilmartin TE, Wallace WA, Hill TW. Measurement of functional orthotic effect on metatarsophalangeal joint extension. *J Am Podiatric Med Assoc* 1991;**81**: 414–17.

20 Use of Braces and Limb and Spinal Protection

W ANGUS WALLACE

Introduction

Braces (now called orthoses) may be used in sport to reduce the risk of injury or to protect damaged structures from re-injury. The prescription of an orthosis requires a careful assessment of the patient and the purpose of the brace should be clearly defined. Braces or orthoses are normally used in sport for one of three reasons:

1. For prophylaxis – that is to prevent an injury.
2. To aid rehabilitation – for instance after an injury, during the recovery period, to protect a weakened part of the body.
3. As a functional brace – to improve function when the limb has a long term weakness or deficiency which will benefit from support.

In all these situations the brace or orthosis attempts to modify the structural or functional characteristics of the musculoskeletal system. The efficiency of an orthosis depends on the doctor or physiotherapist providing an appropriate prescription, the accurate fitting of the brace, and the appropriate use of the brace at the right time. Other important considerations when prescribing a brace are its cosmetic appearance – sportspeople find the aesthetic appearance of a brace very important and will be unlikely to wear it if it is unattractive – and also the structure of the brace, as it must be designed to reduce the possibility of injury to other players.

Braces for prophylaxis against injury

Braces of all types are used to protect the trunk and limbs against injury.

419

Prophylactic spinal bracing

In equestrian sports the spine is at particular risk of injury and spinal braces to protect the spine are now available. In competitive motor racing spinal injury is also a recognised problem, and the trunk is often protected by an appropriate body jacket with design features to protect the thoracic and lumbar spine.

Prophylactic lower limb protection

In soccer one of the most common severe injuries is a fracture of the tibia. Shin pads were initially designed to avoid the pain of contact with another soccer player, but more recently research is focusing on their role in preventing tibial fractures.[1]

Prophylactic ankle bracing

Many sports have a high risk of ankle injury. In skiing, ankle injuries used to be a particular problem. This has been resolved by redesigning the ski boot to act both as footwear and as a brace for the ankle. In field sports, prophylactic bracing and strapping of the ankle has been shown by a number of authors to be effective in protecting the ankle against inversion deformity[2] and in reducing the number of acute injuries.[3,4] An example of a prophylactic ankle brace is the Aircast sports brace shown in Figure 20.1.

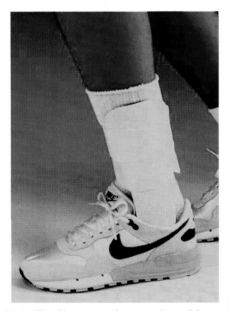

Figure 20.1   The Aircast sports brace can be used for prophylaxis

420

The Cochrane Review by Quinn *et al.*[4] has been summarised as follows:

"This review provides good evidence for the beneficial effect of ankle supports in the form of semi-rigid orthoses or aircast braces to prevent ankle ligament injury during high risk sporting activities (e.g. soccer, basketball etc.). Participants with a history of previous sprain can be advised that wearing such supports may reduce the risk of incurring a future sprain. However, any potential prophylactic effect should be balanced against the baseline risk of the activity, the supply and cost of the particular device, and, for some, the possible or perceived loss of performance.

Further research is indicated principally to investigate other prophylactic interventions and general applicability such as to those without previous ankle sprain".

Prophylactic knee bracing

Many assume that by wearing a knee brace to protect the knee ligaments, then a knee ligament injury will be less likely to occur. However, these devices do not always behave in the way that the manufacturers anticipate. In the US, where the use of prophylactic knee braces is commonplace in American football, studies have been performed in which the number of knee injuries over one season have been recorded. In one study, at the end of the season it was noted that the group who wore no brace suffered fewer knee injuries than those wearing the "prophylactic" knee brace![5] In another study the prophylactic value of the brace depended on the position of the player.[6] In addition, the brace users reported an increased tendency to develop cramps and more calf discomfort. The use of such braces remains controversial with some advising on their use and others opposing them.[5,7] Excellent reviews on this subject have been published by Montgomery and Koziris[8] and Sitler,[6] and in both the value of prophylactic bracing has been questioned. The American Academy of Orthopaedic Surgeons ideals of the prophylactic knee brace are as follows:-

1. It should increase stiffness of the knee to prevent injury from contact and non-contact stresses.
2. It should not interfere with normal joint function.
3. It should not increase injury elsewhere in the lower extremity.
4. It should adapt to the shape of the limb to which it is applied.
5. It should not be harmful to other players.
6. It should be cost effective and durable.
7. It should have a documented efficacy in preventing injuries.

Using these guidelines, it is clear that currently available braces have not yet been proven suitable for prophylaxis.

Braces as treatment for injured joints

Ligamentous injuries amongst sportspeople are common, which is not surprising taking into account the stresses applied to joints and their ligaments during sporting activities. The treatment options available may be either the use of conservative methods or surgical treatment. In addition, most sportspeople are eager to continue their activities and in particular to continue to take part in fitness training even while they are injured. Treatment options such as taping and the use of a brace are very attractive because they allow the athlete to return to some forms of fitness training and even to return to their sporting activity early after the injury. The therapist's role is to advise on the most appropriate form of conservative treatment for the injury, to supervise its application, and to consider whether a cross training programme should be instituted while the injured limb is recovering. This might, for instance, take the form of a soccer player recovering from a collateral knee ligament injury taking up cycling during the rehabilitation phase. This allows the athlete to maintain his aerobic fitness and encourages early recovery of the range of movement and power in the injured limb. The knee brace may also fulfil a second valuable role by "stopping" the player from returning too early to sports which are more hazardous in the presence of a recent injury.

Ankle ligament injuries

Freeman[9] carried out important research on the operative and conservative treatment of severe sprains of the lateral ligament of the ankle. He showed that non-operative treatment could be as effective and often better than surgical treatment and he highlighted the importance of rehabilitation to improve proprioception in the injured joint. Until 1965 it had been believed that after a tearing injury of the ligament, the ligament required immobilisation to allow the apposition of the torn ends until healing had occurred. In recent years it has been shown that in order to achieve optimal length and maximal tensile strength, during repair, the ligament requires limited motion and slight tension during the repair phase. This results in better collagen orientation in the scar tissue. The use of a brace provides protection to the ankle against varus/valgus strains, but allows relative freedom of flexion/extension movements. This has been particularly successfully achieved with the Aircast design of ankle brace as shown in Figure 20.2.

Collateral knee ligament injuries

Severe sprains to the medial collateral ligament of the knee are important in soccer and skiing. Although in the past these have been treated surgically,

422

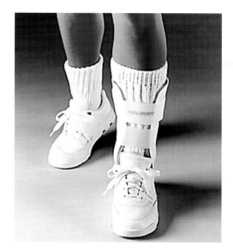

Figure 20.2   An Aircast ankle brace used for the treatment of acute ankle sprains

it has been found that conservative treatment using functional bracing of the knee to protect the knee against a valgus strain but to still allow flexion/extension movements has become the treatment of choice.

Anterior cruciate knee ligament injuries

The management of acute anterior and/or posterior cruciate ligament (ACL/PCL) injuries however is different. In general these injuries are less likely to heal using conservative methods and the role of the brace is to protect the knee against further strains that might extend the soft tissue injury which includes stretching of the capsule and the other ligaments. There remains considerable controversy about whether braces are physically capable of doing this, with strong advocates for and against. Following surgical repair and reconstruction, it was traditional in the 1980s and early 1990s to use a "protective brace" during the 6 month postoperative rehabilitation period. This is no longer the case and many orthopaedic surgeons have now abandoned bracing of the knee after ACL surgery and have focused on closed kinetic chain exercises.

Proprioception and the use of braces

Both in the ankle and in the knee, it is doubtful whether tapes and braces can mechanically withstand the forces that might occur to aggravate a pre-existing injury. As a consequence, some authors have investigated the role of taping and bracing through proprioception – i.e. the brace, directly applied to the limb provides increased proprioceptive feedback which then

423

facilitates protective muscle contraction in certain joint positions or if a deforming force starts to be applied. This has been proposed by Karlsson,[10] Jerosch,[11] and Robbins[12] for the ankle and by Perlau[13] and Jerosch[14] for the knee.

Braces as functional braces to improve function

Sportspeople who have weak ligaments, i.e. the lateral collateral ligament at the ankle and the anterior or posterior cruciate ligament at the knee can have their function improved with a functional brace.

The definition of a functional knee brace is:

"An orthosis designed to facilitate normal tibio–femoral joint kinematics while limiting abnormal displacement and loading which might detrimentally strain an injured ligament, a reconstructed replacement, or a prosthetic replacement or cause abnormal tibio–femoral subluxation in the ligament deficient knee".[15]

Functional bracing of the ankle for a weak lateral collateral ligament

The use of a flexible ankle support can be very successful for some sportspeople with a weak ankle. An elastic or neoprene ankle support probably acts more by reducing any swelling from chronic inflammation and enhancing proprioceptive feedback to the ankle rather than by improving the support of the weakened ligament. Either short ankle supports (Figure 20.3) or longer ankle supports (Figure 20.4) are available and are in common use.

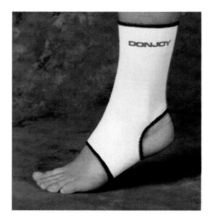

Figure 20.3   A short ankle support – has a similar effect to taping

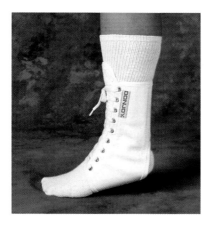

Figure 20.4   A long lace-up ankle support which may have incorporated pressure pads

Functional bracing of the knee for anterior cruciate deficient knees

Functional bracing of the knee can be used in sports such as skiing and jogging for sportspeople who have chronic anterior cruciate deficiency with giving way of the knee. These braces depend on straps and bindings which hold the tibia in a more stable position on the femur, but because the straps have to be applied firmly, they can be uncomfortably tight and consequently they almost inevitably restrict activity a little. An example of one design of a functional knee brace, the Donjoy knee brace, is shown in Figure 20.5.

For the physician or physiotherapist there is no simple way of knowing how much a person will benefit from a knee brace without trying it and they are expensive. The author recommends the following algorithm:

1. Assess the knee carefully and confirm the clinical signs of ACL deficiency.
2. Review the rehabilitation programme – closed kinetic chain exercises, quadriceps strengthening exercises etc. Ensure this has been satisfactorily carried out.
3. Establish that there is a definite on-going disability that requires treatment.
4. **Only then** consider the prescription of a functional knee brace.

The use of braces in sport

A number of sports have laws relating to "players' dress" and these usually, but not always, clarify the acceptability of the use of braces. In the UK the most popular sport with the most body contact is rugby union. The laws

425

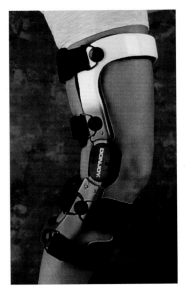

Figure 20.5 The Donjoy Defiance knee brace for ACL deficient knees

for the Rugby Football Union in England were updated in 1998 and the relevant sections are reproduced on page 427 to give an insight into what is permitted today. There are similar laws applying to most other sports and the current regulations in 1999 have been summarised in Table 20.1. In general the use of braces and/or tape only becomes an issue in contact and collision sports.

Table 20.1 The present situation regarding the use of braces of different types in a number of sports*

Sporting activity	Type of brace	Use legal (√) or illegal (×)	Comments
American football (training)	Knee	√	
American football (league)	Knee	√	Padded
Soccer (UK)	Knee	×	
Soccer (UK)	Shoulder	√	
Ice hockey (UK)	Knee	√	
Field hockey (UK)	Knee	×	
Rugby football (UK)	Knee	×	Neoprene braces acceptable
Wrestling	Any	×	Referee's decision
Skiing (downhill)	Knee	√	

* Although the information was correct at the time of publication this should always be checked with the sports governing body if there are any queries.

426

Extracts from the laws of the Rugby Football Union – 1998
Law 4: Players' dress

1. A player's dress consists of jersey, shorts and undergarments, socks and boots.

2. In addition, and subject to (3) below, a player may also wear:
   (a) supports made of elasticated or compressible materials which must be washable;
   (b) shin guards provided that no part of the guard exceeds 0.5 cm, and it is covered by non-rigid fabric and worn under a sock;
   (c) ankle supports which may be of a rigid material other than metal. Such support may only be used if:
       it is worn under a sock
       does not extend higher than one third of the length of the shin;
   (d) mitts (fingerless gloves);
   (e) shoulder pads made of soft and thin materials and which may be incorporated in an undergarment or the jersey provided that:
       the pads shall cover the shoulder and collar bone only
       no part of the pads shall be thicker than 1 cm when uncompressed
       no part of the pads shall have a density of more than 45 kg per cubic metre;
       . . . . . etc;

3. The following are strictly prohibited:
   (a) any item which is contaminated by blood;
   (b) any item which is sharp or abrasive;
   (c) any item containing buckles, clip, rings, hinges, zippers, screw, bolts, or rigid material or projection not otherwise permitted under this law;
       . . . . . etc;
   (g) any item, save where permitted by Law 4 (1) (e), (f), or (h) of which any part is thicker than 0.5 cm;
       . . . . . etc.

Notes: (i) Any player requiring or wishing to wear any dressing, protection, padding or support, or such like material other than that specified within this law should not be permitted to play in a match.

Acknowledgements

I am grateful to Mr Nigel Henderson, medical adviser to the Rugby Football Union for his help and advice and both Aircast and Smith & Nephew for providing illustrations.

References

1 Cattermole HR, Hardy JR, Gregg PJ. The footballer's fracture [published erratum appears in *Br J Sports Med* 1996 Sep;**30(3)**:273]. *Br J Sports Med* 1996; **30(2)**:171–5.

2 Tweedy R, Carson T, Vincenzino B. Leuko and Nessa ankle braces: effectiveness before and after exercise. *Aus J Sci Med Sport* 1994;**26(3–4)**:62–6.

3 Miller EA, Hergenroeder AC. Prophylactic ankle bracing. *Ped Clin North Am* 1990;**37(5)**:1175–85.

4 Quinn K, Parker P, de Bie, Rowe B, Handoll H. Interventions for preventing ankle ligament injuries (Abstract of the Review). *http://www.update-software.com/ccweb/ cochrane/revabstr/ab000018.htm* 1997; Cochrane Collaboration Review.

5 Rovere GD, Haupt A, Yates CS. Prophylactic knee bracing in college football. *Am J Sports Med* 1987;**15(2)**:111–6.

6 Sitler M, Ryan J, Hopkinson W, Wheeler J, Santomier J, Kolb R. The efficacy of a prophylactic knee brace to reduce knee injuries in football. A prospective, randomized study at West Point. *Am J Sports Med* 1990;**18(3)**:310–5.

7 Grace TG, Skipper BJ, Newberry JC, Nelson MA, Sweetser ER. Prophylactic knee braces and injury to the lower extremity. *J Bone Joint Surg – American Volume* 1988;**70(3)**:422–7.

8 Montgomery DL, Koziris PL. The knee brace controversy. *Sports Med* 1989; **8(5)**:260–72.

9 Freeman M, Dean M, Hanham I. The etiology and prevention of functional instability of the foot. *J Bone Joint Surg* 1965;**47–B**:678–85.

10 Karlsson J, Andreasson GO. The effect of external ankle support in chronic lateral ankle joint stability. *Am J Sports Med* 1992;**20**:257–61.

11 Jerosch J, Hoffstetter I, Bork H, Bischof M. The influence of orthoses on the proprioception of the ankle joint. *Knee Surg Sports Traumatol, Arthroscopy* 1995; **3(1)**:39–46.

12 Robbins S, Waked E, Rappel R. Ankle taping improves proprioception before and after exercise in young men. *Br J Sports Med* 1995;**29**:242–47.

13 Perlau R, Frank C, Fick G. The effect of elastic bandages on human knee proprioception in the uninjured population. *Am J Sports Med* 1995;**23(2)**:251–5.

14 Jerosch J, Prymka M. Knee joint proprioception in normal volunteers and patients with anterior cruciate ligament tears, taking special account of the effect of a knee bandage. *Arch Orthop Trauma Surg* 1996;**115(3–4)**:162–6.

15 Beynnon BD, Renstrom PA. The effect of bracing and taping in sports. *Ann Chir Gynae* 1991;**80(2)**:230–8.

21 Taping and strapping in sport

ROSE MACDONALD

The application of tape to injured soft tissues and joints provides support and protection for these structures and minimises pain and swelling in the acute stage. Tape should reinforce the normal supportive structures in their relaxed position and protect the injured tissues from further damage.

Many different techniques are used for injury prevention, treatment, rehabilitation, proprioception, and sport.

Initially, tape is applied to protect the injured structure during the treatment and rehabilitation programme:

- to hold dressings and pads in place;
- to compress recent injury, thus reducing bleeding and swelling;
- to protect from further injury by supporting ligaments, tendons, and muscles;
- to limit unwanted joint movement;
- to allow optimal healing without stressing the injured structures;
- to protect and support the injured structure in a functional position during activity.

Taping is an adjunct to the total injury care programme.

Taping and wrapping products

Good-quality tape should adhere readily and maintain adhesion despite perspiration and activity.

Stretch (elastic) adhesive tape conforms to the contours of the body, allowing normal tissue expansion, and is used in the following circumstances:

- to compress and support soft tissue;
- to provide anchors around muscle, thus allowing for expansion;
- to hold protective pads in place.

Stretch tape will not give mechanical support to ligaments, but may be used in conjunction with rigid tape to give added support. Stretch tape is

429

not normally tearable and must be cut with scissors, but, there are now available very lightweight stretch tapes which may be torn by hand. Stretch tape is available in a variety of widths from 1.5 cm to 10 cm and sometimes even wider. Stretch tape may have:

- one-way stretch – in length or width; and
- two-way stretch – in length and width.

Tip: Stretch tape tends to roll back on itself at the ends, therefore it is wise to allow the last couple of centimetres to recoil before sticking it down.

Non-stretch (rigid) tape has a non-yielding cloth backing and is used for the following:

- to support inert structures, e.g. ligaments, joint capsule;
- to limit joint movement, e.g. check-rein;
- to protect against re-injury;
- to secure ends of stretch tape;
- to reinforce stretch tape;
- to enhance proprioception.

Non-stretch tape may be torn by hand.

Technique: Hold the tape between the thumbs and index fingers, pull the tape tautly and rip quickly in a scissors-like fashion, using the forearms rather than the hands. Do not bend the edges of the tape. It is necessary to practise tearing tape in all directions, both lengthways and crossways, in order to become proficient in the skill.

Hypoallergenic tapes are available, offering an alternative to conventional zinc oxide adhesive tape, to which some athletes are allergic.

Waterproof tape is also available in many widths.

Cohesive bandages are a very useful product and may be used instead of stretch tape. The product sticks to itself and not to the skin, is waterproof, and is reusable. These are most useful when applying spica bandages or as a cover-up for any tape procedure.

Taping for return to activity

When returning to sport after an injury, it is important to remember that the injured area is still at risk, therefore re-injury may be prevented by the judicious use of tape, padding, or supports. By restricting joint and muscle movement to within safe limits – especially hypermobile joints – the athlete may participate with confidence.

430

Taping principles

A thorough assessment is mandatory before taping any structure. The following questions should be answered:

- How did the injury occur?
- What structures were damaged?
- What tissues need protection and support?
- What movements must be restricted?
- Is the injury acute or chronic?
- Is immobilisation necessary at this stage?
- Are you familiar with the anatomy and biomechanics of the parts involved?
- Can you visualise the purpose for which the tape is being applied?
- Are you familiar with the technique?
- Do you have suitable materials at hand?

Note: Should you consider taping a player on the field, ensure that the use of tape does not contravene the rules of the sport, thus making the player ineligible to participate. Therefore *know the sport*. Is there time allowed for taping on the field? Or do you have to remove the player from the field of play in order to apply tape? You must also consider the event in which the athlete is participating, e.g. diving, gymnastics, and dance; ankles must be taped to suit the event.

Taping guidelines

Prepare the area to be taped.

- Wash, dry, and shave the skin in a downward direction.
- Remove oils for good adhesion.
- Cover broken skin lesions before taping.
- Check if the athlete is allergic to the tape, spray etc.
- Apply lubricated padding to friction and pressure areas.
- Apply adhesive spray for better adhesion, e.g. sweaty feet, hands.
- Apply underwrap for sensitive skin.

Tip: If taping the same area frequently, move the anchor point on successive tapings to prevent skin irritation.

Tape application

- Have all the materials at hand.
- Have the athlete and yourself in a comfortable position, e.g. couch at an optimal working height, to avoid fatigue.
- Apply tape to skin which is at room temperature.

431

- Have the athlete pay attention to what you are doing.
- Place the joint in a functional position with minimum stress on the injured stuctures.
- Ensure that the ligaments are in the shortened position.
- Use the correct type, width, and amount of tape for the procedure.
- Apply strips of tape in sequential order.
- Overlap successive strips by half to prevent slippage and gapping.
- Apply each strip with a particular purpose in mind.
- Apply tape smoothly and firmly.
- Flow with the shape of the limb.
- Explain the function of the tape to the athlete and how it should feel.
- On completion check that the technique is functional and comfortable.

The tape should conform with even pressure and must be effective and comfortable. Tape applied directly to the skin gives maximum support.

Tip: For acutely angled areas, rip the end of the tape longitudinally into strips. Small strips are easier to conform, by lapping them over each other:

Avoid:

- excessive traction on the skin – this may lead to skin breakdown;
- gaps and wrinkles – these may cause blisters;
- continuous circumferential taping – single strips produce a more uniform pressure;
- excessive layers of tape – this may impair circulation and neural transmission;
- too tight an application over bony areas – this may cause bone ache.

Tape removal

Never rip tape off, especially from the plantar aspect of the foot. Use a tape cutter or bandage scissors for safe, fast removal, lubricating the tip with petroleum jelly and sliding it parallel to the skin in the natural soft tissue channels. Remove the tape carefully by peeling it back on itself and pushing the skin away from the tape.

Pull the tape carefully along the axis of the limb. Check the skin for damage and apply lotion to restore skin moisture. Tape should not be left on for more than 24 hours, unless using hypoallergenic tape, which may be left on longer.

Tape storage

Tape with zinc oxide adhesive mass is susceptible to temperature change and should be stored in a cool place. Partially used rolls should be kept in an airtight container, or in the fridge. At temperatures over 20 °C the adhesive mass becomes sticky, making the tension stronger and thus more difficult to unwind. Non-stretch tape is also more difficult to tear when warm. Hypoallergenic tapes are not susceptible to temperature change.

Taping techniques

The following diagrams illustrate the most effective and frequently used taping techniques for sport.

Prophylactic ankle taping

Indication: to prevent inversion ankle sprains by providing mechanical and proprioceptive support to the ankle joint during activity.
Position: sitting, with leg over end of couch, foot held at 90 degrees.
Application (Figures 21.1–21.5)

Materials
Adhesive spray
2 gauze
lubricated
squares
Underwrap
3.8 cm tape

A Spray, apply gauze squares, underwrap, and three anchors below the belly of gastrocnemius.

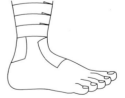

21.1

B Start above the lateral malleolus, draw the tape forward, down the medial side, under the heel, up the lateral side firmly behind the posterior half of the lateral malleolus and attach to anchors.

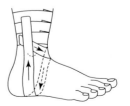

21.2

C Repeat this strip twice, overlapping the previous strip by half aiming for the anterior half of the lateral malleolus . . .

21.3

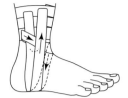

D . . . and, directly over the lateral malleolus before attaching to anchors.

21.4

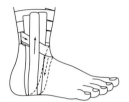

E Reapply the three anchors.

21.5

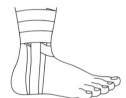

Heel lock (Figures 21.6–21.9)

F Start medially, angle the tape downward on the lateral side aiming for the achilles – pass the tape around the heel, under the foot and pull up and out.

21.6

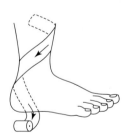

G Continue over the top of the foot, back over the medial malleolus, toward the achilles around the heel – continue . . .

21.7

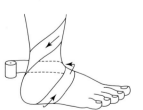

434

H ... under the heel, pulling up and out on the medial side. Continue over the front of the leg and finish high on the lateral side.

21.8

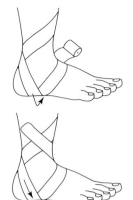

21.9

Easy reminder: Start medially – aim for achilles – around the heel – under the foot – pull up parallel to first strip. Aim for achilles – around the heel – under the foot – pull up and finish.

Heel locks may be applied using stretch tape to practise, but stretch tape is not as supportive as rigid tape.

Ankle taping

The ankle joint is most often sprained because of its anatomical structure. Ligaments take 6–8 weeks to heal and repair after injury. It is therefore necessary to support and protect the injured structures during the treatment/rehabilitation programme, and on return to activity. Stressing the joint too soon after injury will delay the healing and repair process and will increase the likelihood of re-injury. The traditional closed basketweave technique together with reinforcing heel locks has proved to be the best method of protecting the ankle joint during the final stages of repair. It is recommended that the ankle be taped on return to sport.

Closed basketweave: for activity post injury

Indication: ankle inversion sprain.
Function: to support the lateral ligaments without limiting function unnecessarily.
Position: sitting with leg over edge of couch, foot held at 90 degrees and everted.
Application (Figures 21.10–21.13)

Materials
Lubricated gauze squares or heel and lace pads
Adhesive spray
Underwrap
3.8 cm tape

435

A Spray, apply lubricated gauze squares over pressure areas (extensor tendons and achilles tendon), and underwrap.

21.10

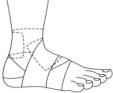

B Apply two anchors to leg about 10 cm above the malleoli, conforming to shape of leg, and to the mid foot. These anchors should overlap the underwrap by 2 cm and adhere directly to the skin. Each tape strip must overlap the previous one by half to prevent slippage and gapping.

Apply a vertical stirrup, starting on the medial side of the anchor. Bring it down behind the medial malleolus, under the heel and up the lateral side with tension. Attach to anchor. (Do not mould to leg.)

Then, apply a horizontal (Gibney) strip, starting on the lateral side of the foot anchor. Draw it back around the heel and attach to the medial side of the foot anchor. These two interlocking strips start the basketweave.

21.11

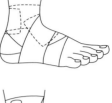

C Apply two more vertical and horizontal strips, alternately. Ensure each strip overlaps the preceding one by half.

21.12

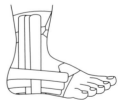

D Apply locking strips to complete the application.

21.13

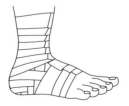

Note: Avoid applying the foot anchors too tightly. Allow for foot splay on weight-bearing!

436

Double Louisiana heel lock (see prophylactic ankle taping)

Open basketweave: for acute sprain (Figure 21.14)

Injured ankles should be taped initially with a compression support to contain swelling, relieve pain, and protect the damaged tissues from further stress. Where there is gross swelling the athlete should remain non-weight-bearing, with the leg elevated and frequent applications of ice. Once the swelling has subsided, **stirrup taping** – open basketweave – may be applied, to support the joint while weight-bearing, and to permit safe range of motion during the rehabilitation programme.

Repeat as for closed basketweave **but** do not close the tape strips in front. This leaves room for swelling.

21.14

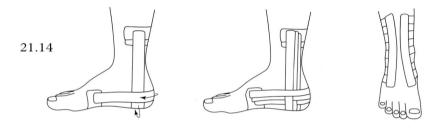

Cover the taped ankle with a compression bandage from toes to knees to contain swelling. Remove the bandage at night.

Tip: A standard Aircast or lace-up ankle support is an excellent alternative for use by those without taping skills.

Heel bruise

Indication: thinning of the fat pad due to over-use and lack of shock-absorbing material in the shoe.

Function: to compress the fat pad from the edges towards the centre.

Position: prone with feet over end of couch.

Application (Figures 21.15–21.18): spray and apply pad.

| **Materials** |
| Heel pad |
| Adhesive spray |
| 2.5 cm tape |

437

A Two anchors of tape – interlocking – around the heel and under the foot – basketweave fashion.

21.15

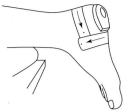

B Repeat strips overlapping the preceding strips by half, anchoring the pad in place.

21.16

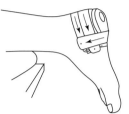

C The last strips must conform to the shape of the heel.

21.17

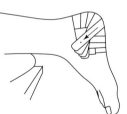

D Reapply the anchors.

21.18

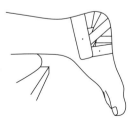

Tip: A plastic heel cup may be used for further compression of the fat pad around the edge of the heel.

Combination taping for plantar fasciitis

Indications: arch strain; plantar fasciitis.
Function: to support the arch, relieve strain on
plantar fascia.
Position: prone with foot over edge of couch.
Application (Figures 21.19–21.23): apply 5 cm
stretch tape to medial side of big toe – just
behind joint line.

Materials
5 cm stretch tape
3.8 cm tape
Heel pad –
optional

A Draw tape along medial side of foot – around
heel and back to where you started.

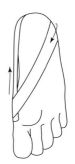

21.19

B Repeat this – starting on the lateral side of the
foot behind the fifth toe joint – around the heel
– back to starting point.

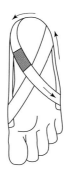

21.20

Note: Pull tape firmly over the plantar fascia attachment to the heel and
slacken off before sticking down.

439

C Fill in the sole of the foot – starting at the ball of the foot – from lateral to medial, overlapping strips by half.

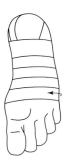

21.21

D Apply 3.8 cm tape along the edge, starting at the little toe – around the heel and finishing at the ball of the big toe.

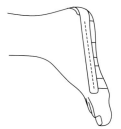

21.22

E Stand the athlete and check for comfort. Have the athlete weight-bearing on the taped foot and apply closing strips over the top of the foot.

21.23

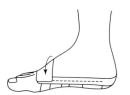

Tip: For activity or sweaty feet apply the closing strip around the whole foot, making sure that the foot is splayed before closing the strip on top.

Low dye taping

Indication: overuse syndromes such as plantar fasciitis, medial arch strain, shin splints – associated with overpronation.
Function: to limit abnormal pronation, reduce strain on the plantar fascia.
Position: leg extended over edge of couch, foot relaxed.
Application (Figures 21.24–21.28): spray the foot.

Materials
Adhesive spray
2.5 cm or 3.8 cm tape (width appropriate for foot size)

A Place tape on the lateral aspect of the fifth metatarsal head, draw the tape firmly along the lateral border of the foot, and around the heel. Depress the first metatarsal head with the index finger, supporting the second to fifth metatarsal heads with the thumb. Draw the tape along the medial border and attach to the first metatarsal head.

21.24

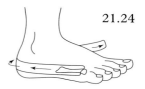

21.25

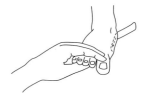

B Repeat this strip once or twice more, overlapping the previous strip by one third.

21.26

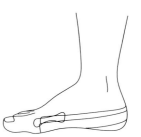

C Tie these strips down with two to three support tapes under the arch, from lateral to medial.

21.27

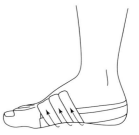

D Stand the athlete and close off the top of the foot with two to three bridging tapes.

21.28

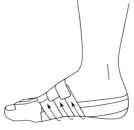

441

Tip: Do not extend the tapes across the joint line as this will "splay" the first and fifth toes. A heel wedge may be placed under the heel.

Taping method for cuboid subluxation

Indication: subluxed cuboid associated with inversion sprain of the ankle.
Function: to maintain cuboid in a stable position after reduction and support the mid foot.
Position: seated with foot over edge of couch.
Application (Figures 21.29–21.31): place 3 mm pad under cuboid on plantar surface of foot.

Materials
5 cm stretch tape
3.8 cm tape
Felt pad

A Using 5 cm stretch tape, start on medial side of foot and draw tape back to heel, angle down around heel on the lateral side, under the arch anchoring the pad in place. Pull tape up on the medial side over the top and finish under the foot.

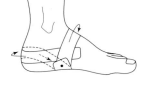

21.29

B Repeat this procedure starting on the lateral side of the foot – around the heel – down under the arch, on the medial side – pull up, and encircle the foot.

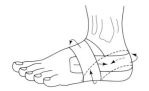

21.30

C Hold in place by applying one or two strips of 3.8 cm tape around the foot.

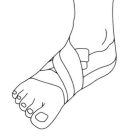

21.31

Tip: Do not apply the tape too lightly over the base of the fifth metatarsal; this may lead to bone ache on weight-bearing.

442

Knee support: Crystal Palace wrap

Indication: jumper's knee; Osgood–Schlatter's disease; patella tendinitis; patella femoral joint pain.

Function: to compress the patella tendon taking stress off the tibial tubercle.

Position: sitting with the knee relaxed and slightly flexed.

Application (Figures 21.32–21.35): cut a strip of stretch tape, approximately 50 cm long, and place a lubricated gauze square pad in the centre.

Materials
Lubricated gauze square
5 cm or 7.5 cm stretch tape
3.8 cm tape

A Slide the tape under the knee with the gauze squares protecting the hamstring tendons. Mould the tape to the femoral condyles.

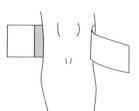

21.32

B Split the lateral strip into two tails. Stretch and twist the tails separately and attach to the medial condyle, passing across the patella tendon in the soft spot between the lower patella pole and the tibial tubercle. Repeat with the second tail.

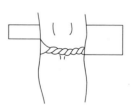

21.33

Note: Do not press the lower patella pole into the fat pad – tip it forward by pressing on the upper patella border with your thumb.

C Stretch the medial strip across the twisted tails. Attach to the lateral condyle.

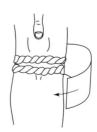

21.34

D Close off with tape strips.

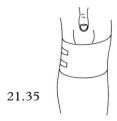

21.35

Tip: Best applied directly to the skin. Shave the skin, if necessary.

McConnell taping for patellofemoral joint pain

This taping method is to be used in conjunction with the McConnell assessment and corrective biomechanical protocol.

McConnell taping is applied daily during the treatment, rehabilitation, and activity programme, therefore the skin should be protected by using a hypoallergenic material to cover the site before the tape application. Hypafix/Fixomul/Meefix is frequently used for this purpose.

A 20 cm wide strip of Hypafix cut on the cross, about 8 cm wide, and laid over the patellofemoral joint acts as a second skin and will "give" as the knee bends, thus the corrective strips of zinc oxide tape may be applied more precisely to hold the patella in place. Should this material be unavailable, a strip of 7.5 cm hypoallergenic stretch tape may be used instead. The skin on the inside of the knee joint is quite sensitive and must be protected from tape drag.

Indication: patellofemoral joint pain; anterior knee pain.
Function: relieve pain; correct faulty patella components based on assessment findings, for example faulty patella glide, tilt, rotation, or fat pad impingement; to unload painful structures.
Position: sitting with knee relaxed and supported on couch.
Application (Figures 21.36–21.41): shave the knee, spray, apply Hypafix.

> **Materials**
> Spray
> 20 cm wide
> Hypafix or 8 cm wide
> 3.8 cm tape

21.36

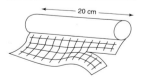

A Correct patella **glide** by placing the tape a thumb's breadth outside the lateral border of the patella. Pull the tape medially, gathering up the soft tissues before sticking the tape to the medial femoral condyle.

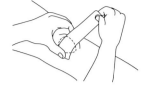

21.37

B Correct lateral patella **tilt** by placing the tape in the centre of the patella and pulling firmly down toward the medial femoral condyle. This will raise the lateral border of the patella. Gather up the medial soft tissues with your fingers before attaching the tape to maintain the tilt.

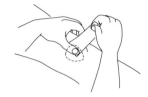

21.38

C Correct **external rotation** by placing the tape on the lower patella pole and pull the tape upward and medially. Rotate the upper patella pole while attaching the tape to the medial femoral condyle. Correct internal rotation by placing the tape in the middle of the upper border of the patella. Pull the tape downward and medially. Rotate the lower pole externally while attaching the tape.

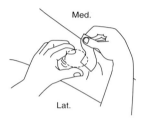

Med.

Lat.

21.39

D Correct **anteroposterior tilt** by placing the tape on the upper patella pole to tip the inferior patella pole anteriorly out of the fat pad. Failure to do this will result in increased pain for the athlete on knee flexion.

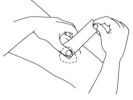

21.40

E To **unload the fat pad:** first correct the anteroposterior tilt as above. Then place the tape below the lower patella pole and pull the tape upward and medially, lifting and compressing the fat pad, attach above the medial femoral condyle. Apply a similar strip on the lateral side by crossing the first strip below the lower patella pole. Repeat the strips alternately – in flexion if necessary.

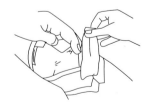

21.41

445

Note: Tape is worn during the day and removed at night to rest the skin.

Hip spica

Indication: groin strain; adductor strain.
Function: to support and protect the hip muscles; to restrict range of motion.
Position: the affected muscle will determine the direction of the wrap; for an adductor strain, internally rotate the leg.
Application (Figures 21.42–21.44)

> **Materials**
> 10–15 cm extra long cohesive bandage
> Lubricated gauze squares
> 3.8 cm tape

A Starting on the outside of the thigh, wind the bandage around the thigh a couple of times from lateral to medial.

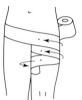

21.42

B Continue across the front of the groin, around the back of the hips and down around the thigh again in a figure of eight pattern.

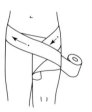

21.43

C Repeat this pattern a couple of times. Close off with a strip of tape.

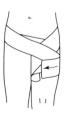

21.44

Note: For a hip flexor strain, wind the spica in the opposite direction with the thigh in neutral position.

446

Tip: When starting the wrap, fold the edge down so that it will be locked in place on the second turn.

Thumb check-rein (a simple figure of eight which may be self-applied)

Indication: sprained thumb/hyperextension.
Function: to stabilise the joint in a functional position and restrict range of motion.
Position: hand pointing toward operator.
Application (Figures 21.45–21.46)

Materials
2.5 or 1.25 cm tape

21.45

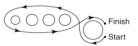

A Apply tape to outside of thumb. Wind tape toward palm – through thumb web – twist tape – stick to back of hand – then to palm of hand – through the web again.

21.46

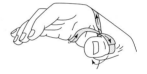

B Twist and stick down to starting point.

Note: Do not wind tape around the thumb as this will restrict circulation.

Tip: When taping an athlete's thumb for the outside environment – for example, rugby/football – stick two strips of tape together, one on top of the other, to ensure it doesn't break in muddy conditions. This is a most useful check-rein for a sprained thumb joint and may be applied over a compression bandage in the acute phase or on its own for activity.

Thumb spica

Indication: sprained thumb.
Function: to compress and support the soft tissue in the acute phase; to support the joint in a functional position.

Materials
2.5 cm stretch tape or 2.5 cm cohesive bandage 2.5 cm tape

447

Position: facing operator, thumb in neutral
 position.
Application (Figures 21.47–21.48): start on the
 centre back of the wrist, moving around the
 wrist to the front (palm) towards the thumb.

A Draw the tape around the base of the thumb
 on the palmar aspect – through the web –
 around the thumb – across the front of the
 wrist to the angle of the hand on the little finger
 side.

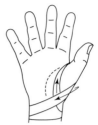

21.47

B Continue around the back of the wrist
 overlapping the tape by half and moving toward
 the tip of the thumb. Continue this figure of
 eight pattern until the sprained joint is
 supported. Finish off with a strip of 2.5 cm
 tape.

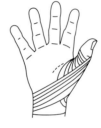

21.48

Note: Slight tension may be applied when crossing the palm to bring the
thumb into a functional position. Do not pull too tightly as circulation and
neural transmission may be impaired.

Tip: For sport – apply a thumb check-rein over the spica to restrict range
of motion and protect the joint from further damage.

Prophylactic wrist taping

Indication: prophylactic wrist support for weak
 wrists.
Function: to protect the wrist from excessive
 flexion/extension; to give extra support to the
 wrist during sport.
Position: facing operator – hand in open position.
Application (Figure 21.49)

Materials
3.8 cm tape

448

A Apply three to four strips of tape around the wrist – overlapping each by half. Finish just below the wrist crease. Do not apply too tightly.

21.49

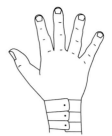

Note: Check for function. Is there enough support? If not, reapply one or two more strips.

Wrist and hand taping

Indication: hyperextension/hyperflexion injury.
Function: to support wrist and hand; to restrict range of motion; to act as a splint.
Position: facing operator – hand in open position.
Application (Figures 21.50–21.54)

Materials
3.8 cm tape
5 cm cohesive bandage

A Apply two anchors around lower third of forearm 10 cm above wrist, and around the palm of the hand.

21.50

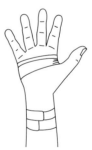

Note: If the athlete is using this hand to hold a racquet/golf club, this second anchor should be applied diagonally to allow for palm-on contact with the equipment.

21.51

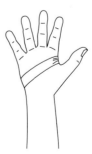

B With the hand flexed 30–40 degrees, measure the distance between arm and hand anchors. Tear off five strips of tape this length and construct a check-rein on the couch surface (see diagram).

21.52

C Apply this check-rein to the anchors on the forearm and hand.

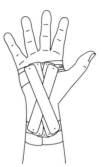

21.53

Note: The wrist should not be able to extend beyond neutral – allow for skin mobility.

D Reapply original anchors and cover the tape with a cohesive bandage.

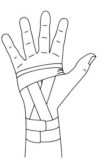

21.54

Tip: Change the placement of this check-rein in order to:

- restrict hyperflexion – place on back of wrist;
- restrict pronation – place diagonally across the palm to fifth finger side;
- restrict supination – place diagonally across palm to thumb side of hand.

The check-rein may also be placed on either side of the wrist to restrict bending the wrist from side to side.

450

Basic shoulder spica

Because of the extensive range of motion in the shoulder joint a spica bandage is more appropriate than tape to control movement. Tape tends to lift off during activity, especially when the athlete sweats. A pad may be applied over the acromioclavicular joint and be held in place securely with a spica.

Indication: acromioclavicular (AC) or gleno-humeral (GH) joint sprain.
Function: to support and protect the shoulder joint in the acute phase; as a functional support during rehabilitation and activity.
Position: arm internally rotated with back of hand on hip.
Application (Figures 21.55–21.58): protect under the arms with lubricated gauze squares. Place pad over the a/c joint.

> **Materials**
> 8–10 cm extra long cohesive bandage
> Lubricated gauze squares
> 3.8 cm tape

A Starting on the outside off the upper arm, wind the bandage around the arm a couple of times.

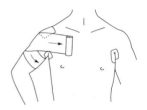

21.55

B Draw across the chest under the opposite arm and diagonally upward across the back over the shoulder with tension to secure the paid in place . . .

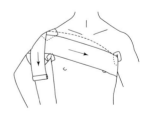

21.56

C . . . down under and around the arm – across the chest, etc.

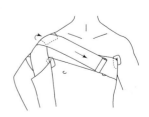

21.57

451

D Repeat this three to four times. Lock the end in place with a piece of tape.

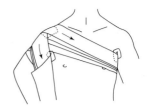

21.58

Note: This figure of eight will prevent excessive abduction and external rotation of the arm.

Tip: To secure the wrap at the start, fold down the corner and overlap it on the second turn.

Further Reading

Austin K, Gwynn-Brett K, Marshall S. *Taping techniques.* London: Mosby, 1994.

Macdonald R. *Taping/strapping.* Milton Keynes: BDF Medical, 1988.

Macdonald R, ed. *Taping techniques: principles and practice.* Oxford: Butterworth–Heinemann, 1993.

Macdonald RP. Taping techniques. Physio Tools for Windows. BH MARS (Butterworth–Heinemann Medical Artwork Retrieval System), 1996.

Perrin DH. *Athletic taping and bracing.* Champaign, IL: Human Kinetics, 1995.

Acknowledgements

The following illustrations are reproduced by permission of Butterworth–Heinemann from *Taping techniques: principles and practice*, edited by Rose Macdonald, 1993. Figures 21.1–21.5, from p. 38; Figures 21.6–21.9 from p. 44; Figures 21.15–21.18 from p. 66; Figures 21.19–21.23 from p. 78; Figures 21.32–21.35 from p. 92; Figures 21.42–21.44 from p. 149; Figures 21.45 and 21.46 from p. 136; Figure 21.49 from p. 126. Figures 21.37–21.41 are reproduced from course notes with kind permission from Jenny McConnell.

22 Principles of rehabilitation

D GLENN HUNTER

Rehabilitation can be defined as "restoration to a pre-existing state of normal use and function following impairment of that function".[1] The difference between rehabilitation applied to an athlete and a non-athlete lies in the definition of what constitutes normal use and function. In general, athletes subject their bodies, or an area of their bodies, to a greater level of stress than the non-athlete. Hence the rehabilitation process is usually longer with much less scope for error; for example a small decrease in positional sense may have a minimal effect on the function of a non-athlete, but have serious consequences for an athlete.

The main aim of the rehabilitation process is to return the athlete to a level where their body and the injured area can cope with the stresses of their particular activity in the shortest and safest possible time. Achievement of this aim centres around an understanding of the SAID principle – Specific Adaptation to Imposed Demands.[2] This principle applied to the rehabilitation process means that any treatment should be based on the specific functional demands that will be placed on a person when they return to their previous level of function, thus a thorough understanding of the stresses of the athlete's particular sport is essential to the formulation of a successful rehabilitation programme.

This chapter will discuss the general principles of rehabilitation applied to the athlete from the time of injury to return to normal function.

Application of the SAID principle will be encountered throughout the chapter, with the underlying theme being that the soft tissues and bones of the body adapt to the manner in which they are stressed.[3]

Rehabilitation principle 1

The difference between the rehabilitation of the athlete and non-athlete lies in the level to which the rehabilitation process must take the injured tissues and the athlete's body, in order to cope with the imposed demands of the athlete's sport.

The rehabilitation process

The rehabilitation process consists of three phases:

1. Initial assessment of the patient.
2. Treatment of the primary and secondary consequences of the injury.
3. Functional testing and return to "normal" activity.

The focus of many rehabilitation texts is the treatment phase. However, the initial assessment and functional testing are critical to the success of any rehabilitation programme. Each of these phases will be considered in turn, and the key principles of rehabilitation will be highlighted in each phase.

Phase 1: initial assessment of the patient

A detailed assessment is essential prior to the commencement of a rehabilitation programme to determine the following:

- The suitability of the patient for conservative treatment.
- The prognosis.
- Subjective and objective measurers to gauge improvement.

The assessment should focus on the following three areas:

1. Analysis of the mechanics of injury.
2. Accurate diagnosis.
3. Evaluation of the prognosis and goal-setting.

Analysis of the mechanics of injury

The ultimate aim of the rehabilitation process is to prevent recurrence of the injury once the athlete is pronounced "fit". To achieve this aim, the mechanics of the injury must be identified and analysed, to highlight any factors which may sabotage the rehabilitation process. These factors should be corrected during the rehabilitation process prior to return to "normal" activity. It is useful to consider the forces that cause injury as either extrinsic or intrinsic in nature.

Extrinsic forces

These are forces that are applied to the body from an external source and result in acute injury, for example a blow to the thigh from an opponent's knee. As the application of the force lies outside the receiving athlete's

454

control, recurrence of these injuries can be difficult to prevent, but emphasis usually focuses on correcting the following:

- The use of protective devices.
- Correct footwear.
- Adherence to the rules of the sport.
- Correct pairing in terms of size and ability in contact sports.

Intrinsic forces

These forces are generated internally by the athlete and can result in either acute injury, for example a quadriceps tear when kicking a ball, or an injury of insidious onset due to microtrauma, for example patella tendinopathy. Careful exploration of the mechanics of intrinsic injuries, in particular those of insidious onset, can be most fruitful in preventing their recurrence.

It is useful to consider the aetiology of intrinsic injuries in two ways.

1 *The suitability of the anatomical and biomechanical structures of the athlete's body to cope with the imposed demands of the activity.* The essential feature of this classification is that the stresses of the particular activity are within "normal" parameters, but the athlete falls to cope with these stresses because of anatomical or biomechanical abnormalities.

During development, structural abnormalities or faulty movement patterns may have developed which predispose the athlete to injury in certain sports. These abnormalities may be congenital or due to previous trauma or incomplete rehabilitation. Factors that have been linked to injury include:

- Joint hypermobility – congenital or traumatic.[4]
- Muscle imbalance.[5]
- Decreased flexibility.[6]
- Biomechanical factors such as leg length difference or excessive pronation or supination.[7]

Once the abnormality has been identified, correction should be attempted during the rehabilitation process; for example, the use of orthotics to control excessive pronation or supination may help to reduce the intrinsic forces predisposing the athlete to injury.[8]

2 *The stresses imposed on the athlete due to training and equipment errors.* In this classification, the anatomical and biomechanical structures fall within "normal" limits but errors in training, equipment, and technique predispose the athlete to injury.

Training errors relate to the intensity, frequency, duration, and periodisation of training and competition. Equipment errors relate to the type of surface, the specifications of each piece of equipment, and the technique of use. Correction during the later stages of the rehabilitation process should be performed where appropriate.

455

Determining the mechanics of injury often requires a multidisciplinary approach, where the athlete, coach, and various sports medicine specialists form the link between the mechanics of injury and the pathology produced.

Rehabilitation principle 2

Use a multidisciplinary approach to determine the mechanics of injury in relation to intrinsic and extrinsic forces and correct these factors during the rehabilitation process.

Accurate diagnosis

The diagnosis should be specific enough to yield the following information:

1. The anatomical structures affected by the injury. This allows consideration to be given to the function of the tissue in relation to the specific demands of the athlete's sport, and in turn to incorporate these demands in the design of a rehabilitation programme.
2. The specific location of the pathology in the anatomical area affected, for example the proximal third of the lateral aspect of the achilles tendon. This specificity is occasionally difficult to achieve, particularly where the lesion is not palpable, but its importance lies in the principle that rehabilitation techniques must be specific to the affected area and not just to the anatomical structure affected.
3. The severity of the pathology and stage of the healing process.
4. Associated pathologies or previous treatment that may place restrictions on the rehabilitation process; for example an athlete who is suffering from retropatellar symptoms may require alterations to a standard anterior cruciate ligament reconstruction rehabilitation programme.
5. Identify subjective and objective signs, both clinical and functional, by which to evaluate the effectiveness of the rehabilitation programme.

Rehabilitation principle 3

An accurate diagnosis is essential to:

- Determine the suitability of the patient for rehabilitation
- Determine the specific site of tissue damage
- Determine the function of the damaged tissue in relation to the sporting activity
- Determine subjective and objective measures to evaluate the effectiveness of the rehabilitation programme

---

456

Evaluation of the prognosis and goal-setting

The functional demands of the athlete's sport are combined with the pathology and the hopes and aspirations of the athlete to determine a realistic prognosis and treatment approach. The following questions should be addressed:

1. Are the functional stresses of the athlete's current level of activity compatible with the pathology?

If the answer is "No" then consider the following:

- Is operative or conservative treatment likely to improve the prognosis?
- Is a reduction in training or competition required, if so to what degree? For example, many of the traction apophysitides experienced in the young athlete respond simply to a reduction in the frequency of training and competition.
- Would external support from a brace or tape allow the athlete to train and compete?
- Would an alteration of technique or team position allow the athlete to train or compete?

If rehabilitation is the chosen treatment approach, the following should be established:

- A realistic time scale for return to "normal" activity. This is the most often requested information from the athlete. The advice given should err on the conservative side and the coach and athlete should be educated as to all the stages of the rehabilitation process and associated variables that will affect the time scale.
- Realistic short and long term goals. The goals should be measurable in terms of clinical or functional tests, for example jogging once 15 degrees of dorsiflexion of the ankle has been achieved. Short and long term goals gradually improve the confidence the injured athlete has in the affected area and will help to decrease the psychological effects of the injury.

Rehabilitation principle 4

Establish short and long term goals for the rehabilitation process which are measurable in terms of subjective and objective clinical and functional tests.

Phase 2: treatment of the primary and secondary consequences of the injury

The rehabilitation programme focuses on the primary and secondary consequences of the injury. The primary consequence refers to the pathology occurring at the site of tissue damage and the emphasis of the rehabilitation programme is to facilitate the healing process in order to achieve a functional outcome.

The secondary consequences of injury relate to all the factors that are affected secondary to the primary site of tissue damage. These factors may be listed as:

1. Decreased range of motion.
2. Decreased strength, power, endurance, and muscle control.
3. Altered proprioception and coordination.
4. Decreased sport-specific skills.
5. Decreased cardiovascular "fitness".
6. Psychological changes.

In order to restore the primary and secondary consequences of injury to "normal" limits, each parameter has to be progressively challenged by imposing demands on it which resemble the demands occurring in the athlete's sport. It is important that the imposed demands are progressively introduced and are at the correct intensity to stimulate improvement. The underlying guide to the level of the imposed demands is that they must not affect the healing of the primary site of tissue damage.

Because the imposed demands must be applied progressively it is useful to think of the rehabilitation process as passing through a series of stages, each one more functionally challenging (Table 22.1).

Table 22.1 Stages of the rehabilitation process

Early stage
Minimal functional activity – often non-weight-bearing

Intermediate stage
Increasing functional activity – partial or full weight-bearing

Late stage
All functional activity – full weight-bearing

Sport-specific stage
Sport-specific exercises

In many cases the rehabilitation programme involves treating the primary and secondary consequences at the same time. However, in some cases rehabilitation begins by focusing on the secondary consequences, and then addressing the primary consequences at a later stage, for example when a limb is immobilised following surgery.

458

Although the treatment of the primary and secondary consequences of injury may be considered separately in the design of the rehabilitation programme, they become integrated towards the later stages of rehabilitation, as the programme involves more functional activities.

Rehabilitation principle 4

The rehabilitation process can be divided into those measures that specifically treat the primary site of tissue damage, and those that affect the secondary consequences of the injury. Both these areas unite in the functional stage of rehabilitation.

Primary consequences of tissue damage

The treatment applied to the primary site of tissue damage aims at facilitating the healing process, and in particular its ability to cope with the demands of the athlete's sport once healed. The choice of treatment is influenced by the stage of the healing process, the severity of the injury, and specific restrictions placed on the tissue following surgical procedures. This section will illustrate the treatment principles by considering treatment applied to the primary site of tissue damage following mild to moderate soft tissue injury.

With few exceptions, the soft tissues of the body have to cope predominantly with the force of tension, and do this by possessing an inherent but varying degree of tensile strength.[9] Following injury, the tensile strength of the tissue is reduced, and a major role of the healing process lies in the restoration of the tensile strength of the healing tissue to "normal values".[10] Figure 22.1 illustrates the stages of the healing process in relation to their role in the restoration of tensile strength over time.

The role of rehabilitation in aiding this process can be considered in relation to the three phases of the healing process.

Lag phase

This phase lasts for approximately 4–6 days, and during this phase the tensile strength of the wound does not increase.[11] The lag phase can be considered as two phases; the initial inflammatory phase, from the time of injury to approximately 24–48 hours post injury, and the fibrin phase from 24–48 hours until approximately 4–5 days post injury.

The aims of treatment during the lag phase are:

1. To control the degree of inflammation.
2. To protect the area from further injury.
3. To facilitate the onset of the regenerative phase.

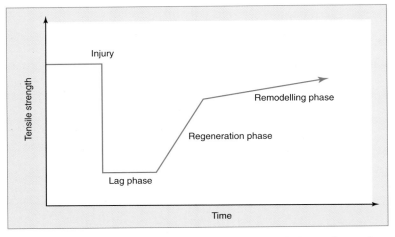

Figure 22.1 The stages of the healing process in relation to their role in restoring tensile strength over time

These aims are achieved as follows.

Controlling the inflammatory phase: day 0 to 24–48 hours

This is achieved by the use of protection, rest, ice, compression, and elevation – remembered by the acronym PRICE.

Protection The affected area should be immobilised to limit all motion at the affected site of tissue damage.

Rest Includes both rest of the injured area due to the immobilisation, and rest of the athlete to reduce cardiac output and hence the degree of blood flow to the affected area reducing the potential for haemorrhage.

Ice Ice is thought to reduce the degree of pain, swelling, and duration of disability following injury by the following effects:[12]

- Decreasing the inflammatory reaction.
- Decreasing the amount of oedema.
- Decreasing the degree of haemorrhage.
- Producing analgesia.
- Decreasing muscle spasm.
- Decreasing the local tissue metabolism.

460

Ice can be applied in various forms, but crushed ice placed in a wet towel or a plastic bag, with a thin layer of oil to protect the skin, will usually suffice.

Controversy exists as to the length of time for which ice should be applied post injury. Current treatment approaches are based on models relating to vasodilation and constriction theories,[13] or relating to the prevention of secondary cellular damage due to tissue hypoxia following injury.[14] The range of individual responses to ice are highly variable and therefore treatment should be based on treatment principles rather than pre-arranged doses. The author suggests that ice should be applied for 10–15 minutes every 2 waking hours for the first 48 hours post injury for superficial lesions, and for 20–30 minutes every 2 waking hours for deeper lesions.

The effectiveness of ice on the inflammatory reaction may be increased by using it in combination with compression.[15]

Compression Compression applied to the site of tissue damage will increase the hydrostatic gradients from the tissue to the circulation thus helping to force fluid into the vessels by increasing the interstitial hydrostatic pressure. The compression must be specific to the affected area, and the use of foam

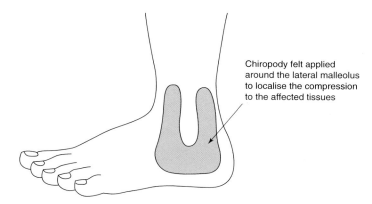

Chiropody felt applied around the lateral malleolus to localise the compression to the affected tissues

Figure 22.2   Foam pads or chiropody felt are useful to localise the compression to the affected area

pads or chiropody felt is useful in achieving this specificity (Figure 22.2). It is important to reapply the compression between ice treatments.

Elevation This will increase lymph flow away from the area and reduce the intracapillary pressure to the affected area, reducing the tendency for oedema.

Protecting the area from further injury

During the first 24–48 hours, motion of the affected area should be restricted to avoid increasing the inflammatory reaction. Following this period, motion should be allowed but not in a direction or range that will tension the affected area as the tensile strength of the area has not increased and consists of a weak fibrin scaffold.[16] For example, dorsiflexion and limited plantarflexion would be allowed following a mild to moderate anterior talofibular ligament injury of the ankle, but not plantarflexion and inversion. Taping and braces are useful adjuncts in achieving this aim.

Facilitating the onset of the regeneration phase

After the initial inflammatory reaction has ceased, the aim of treatment is to increase the blood supply to the affected area to hasten the onset of fibroblast proliferation. Various electrotherapeutic modalities are available and claim to facilitate this process. Of all the modalities available, ultrasound appears to have the strongest research base and involves exposing the injured tissues to high frequency mechanical vibrations, which range from 0.5 to 3 MHz, to stimulate the repair of soft tissues and to relieve pain. Ultrasound has been shown to shorten the inflammatory phase due to its effects on modifying the permeability of calcium ions of the plasma membrane of growth factor secreting cells such as macrophages, which

---

Key rehabilitation principle 5

Treatment in the lag phase consists of:

- **P**rotection, **R**est, **I**ce, **C**ompression and **E**levation = PRICE
- No motion for the first 24–48 hours
- Electrotherapy after 24–48 hours
- Motion allowed after 24–48 hours but not in a direction that tensions the damaged tissue
- Tape or brace to control motion

---

leads to the stimulation of the activity of other cells involved in the reparative process.[17]

Regeneration phase

This phase ranges from approximately the fifth day to 10–12 weeks post injury and is the period of the greatest increase in the tensile strength of the wound.[18] The degree of increase in tensile strength is influenced by the amount, direction, and cross links between collagen fibres, and these factors are influenced by tension applied to the wound.[19]

The aim of the rehabilitation process is progressively to tension the site of tissue damage in order to orientate the collagen fibres along the lines of functional stress and to increase the amount of collagen in the wound. Tension can be applied either passively or actively and the principles of application are as follows:

- Ensure that no hypermobility exists.
- Heat prior to stretch.
- Tension the wound to the point of slight discomfort.
- Sustain the stretch for 30 seconds.
- Repeat the stretch three times every 4 hours.
- Progress the stretching from passive, to active, to functional movements.

Table 22.2 gives an example of progression of treatment for a mild sprain of the proximal attachment of the medial ligament of the knee joint.

Table 22.2   Tension applied during the regeneration phase

Example of progressive tension applied to a mild sprain of the proximal attachment of the medial ligament of the knee joint

Early stage
Patient supine – knee flexed to 15–20 degrees, valgus and external rotation stress applied passively to the medial ligament to the point of minimal discomfort

Progression
Apply tension as above, but with the knee moving through a full range of motion

Progression section
- Straight line running
- "S" shape and figure of eight running
- Side stepping and "cross over" running
- Multidirectional shuttle running with increasing speed
- Gradual introduction of sport-specific activity, e.g. for a footballer
- Kicking – progressing from kicking side foot with a soft ball over short distances to a hard ball over increased distance. Progress from a stationary to a moving ball
- Tackling against a wall, to tackling the physiotherapist, to tackling in controlled game situations, to tackling in full competition

---

Key rehabilitation principle 6

Treatment in the regeneration phase consists of progressively tensioning the wound to increase and orientate the collagen fibres. The tension should be applied along functional lines of stress for the particular tissue affected.

Remodelling phase

During this phase intra- and extramolecular cross linkage occurs between the collagen fibres which leads to a tendency for scar tissue contracture.[20]

463

The aim of treatment in this phase is to continue to tension the healing tissue to promote collagen fibre orientation and to prevent scar tissue contracture.

The principles of application of the stretch are as for the regeneration phase.

Rehabilitation principle 7

Treatment in the remodelling phase consists of tensioning the wound to further orientate the collagen fibres and prevent wound contracture. The tension should be applied along functional lines of stress for the particular tissue affected.

Progression of treatment applied to the primary site of tissue damage

Any therapeutic movement that is used to tension the site of tissue dysfunction should be applied carefully and progressively due to the tissue's initial vulnerability post injury. This progression usually takes the form of initial passive stretching followed by more functional activity. Table 22.3 gives an example of this progression for a mild to moderate sprain of the calcaneofibular ligament of the ankle joint.

Table 22.3 Example of progressive treatment of the primary site of tissue damage

Injury
Mild sprain of the calcaneofibular ligament of the ankle joint

Treatment
1 Passive movement – patient supine, ankle in plantargrade, inversion of the subtalar joint
2 As for 1 but with passive dorsiflexion and plantarflexion
3 Walking on slightly uneven ground – slope away from affected side
4 Jogging on slightly uneven ground
5 Side stepping – slow speed
6 Side stepping – increase speed
7 Multidirectional activities – increasing speed

In some cases, the severity of injury or surgical treatment will dictate when tension can be applied to the wound. In cases where hypermobility is to be prevented, tension should not be applied for a considerable time period; for example after anterior dislocation of the glenohumeral joint abduction and external rotation should be avoided.[21]

In some cases the primary site of tissue damage occurs in a tissue which functionally is not subjected to tensile forces, for example bursae. Here the treatment aim is to decrease the inflammatory reaction and protect the area from further injury.

464

Orthotics and tape are valuable in some cases to reduce the stresses on the primary site of tissue damage during the rehabilitation process; for example taping distal to the lateral epicondyle of the elbow in the treatment of lateral epicondylitis to relieve tension in the affected area, the use of tape to alter patella tracking, or a heel raise in the treatment of achilles tendinopathy.

Rehabilitation principle 8

Treatment of the primary site of tissue damage relates to:

- Restoring the ability of the tissue to withstand tensile stresses – tension the area
- Decreasing the inflammation in tissues not normally subjected to tension

---

Secondary consequences

All the secondary consequences should be addressed in the rehabilitation programme with the aim being to restore their values to "normal" limits. Care must to taken to ensure that no activity aggravates the primary site of tissue damage. In some cases the rehabilitation process may focus only on the secondary factors because it is difficult to influence the healing process directly. For example, in a patient with chondromalacia patellae treatment may consist of stretching "tight" soft tissues and strength and co-ordination activities for the vastus medialis obliquus.

Rehabilitation principle 9

Rehabilitate all the secondary consequences of injury without aggravating the site of tissue damage

---

Each of the secondary factors will be considered in turn.

Decreased range of motion

Following injury, the joint or surrounding soft tissues have a tendency to decreased range of motion, this occurs particularly after a period of immobilisation. Progressive mobilisation techniques are required to increase the range of motion, with the general principles of application being as follows:

1. Apply heat prior to mobilising.

465

2. Use a slow sustained stretch to the area – sustained at the point of minimal discomfort for 30–60 seconds.
3. Repeat the exercise three times, and this sequence 2–4 hourly throughout the day.
4. Continually reassess to ensure that the primary site of tissue damage has not been aggravated.

In some cases manual therapy techniques are necessary to restore accessory joint motion.[22]

Decreased range of motion of a specific tissue can be the cause of the primary site of tissue damage, for example, illiotibial band tightness related to anterior knee pain[23] or posterior tightness of the glenohumeral joint related to shoulder impingement.[24] Specific stretches should be used to correct this decrease in soft tissue mobility.

Decreased strength, power, endurance, and muscle control

A decrease in muscular strength, power, and endurance commonly occurs post injury due to reflex inhibition.[25] It is important to eliminate the cause of the reflex inhibition during rehabilitation as this will retard muscular development. In practice, this means reducing joint effusion and not exercising in the presence of pain.[26]

Restoration of strength, power, and endurance requires the application of progressive resistance loads to the muscular tissue while the muscle performs different types of physiological contractions. Many exercise regimens can be designed by combining the following three components:

1. Type of exercise.
2. Type of muscular contraction.
3. Type of resistance.

Type of exercise

1. Endurance exercise: light resistance but many repetitions; usually the initial phase of rehabilitation due to the small resistance used.

2. Strength exercises: heavy weights lifted for 8–10 repetitions; a useful regimen for strength development is the DAPRE regimen;[27] a working weight is selected and is used for the DAPRE technique as illustrated in Tables 22.4 and 22.5. The aim of this technique is to determine the optimum time needed to increase resistance, or the optimum resistance that should be added.

466

Table 22.4 Determining the working weight and number of repetitions to be used in the DAPRE regimen

Set	Portion of working weight used	Number of repetitions
1	1/2	10
2	3/4	6
3	Full	Maximum[a]
4	Adjusted	Maximum[b]

[a] Number of repetitions performed in set three determines the adjusted working weight for the fourth set (see guidelines in Table 22.5).
[b] Number of repetitions performed in set four determines the adjusted working weight for the next day (see guidelines in Table 22.5).

Table 22.5 Determining the adjusted working weight to be used for the DAPRE technique

Number of repetitions performed during set	Adjustment to working weight for:	
	Fourth set[a]	Next day[b]
0–2	Decrease 5–10 lb	Repeat set
3–4	Decrease 0–5 lb	Stay the same
5–7	Stay the same	Increase 5–10 lb
8–12	Increase 5–10 lb	Increase 5–15 lb
13 to ...	Increase 10–15 lb	Increase 10–20 lb

[a] Number of repetitions performed in set three is used to determine the adjusted working weight for the fourth set (see Table 22.4).
[b] Number of repetitions used in set four is used to determine the adjusted working weight for the next day (see Table 22.4).

3. Power exercises: the resistance is lifted in a certain time period – work over time; introduced towards the later stages of the rehabilitation process;

Type of muscular contraction

1. Isometric – involves no joint movement. The strength appears to be specific to the joint angle. Used in the initial stages of rehabilitation as there is minimal chance of increasing irritability.
2. Dynamic exercise, i.e. concentric or eccentric exercise.

Type of resistance

1. Free weights.
2. Elastic resistance – has the advantage of allowing functional movement patterns, but the exact force cannot be measured.
3. Body weight – function and proprioception is enhanced.
4. Manual resistance.
5. Isokinetics.

467

Although restoration of muscular strength power and endurance are important, coordination of muscular activity is equally important. This is achieved by the use of functional exercise, and also by the use of biofeedback; for example, to retrain the infraspinatus in patients with anterior instability of the glenohumeral joint.

Altered proprioception Proprioception refers to the neural inputs that originate from mechanoreceptors located around a joint which measure changes and rates of changes of position rather than static positions. Proprioception can be increased by subjecting the area to progressively more complex movement tasks.

Altered coordination As rehabilitation progresses, activities become more complex, with the ultimate aim being to reproduce the coordinated actions required for the athlete's sport.

Decreased sport-specific skills As the primary site of tissue damage heals, more sport-specific drills can be introduced into the rehabilitation programme, for example, walking through squash drills on court.

Decreased cardiovascular fitness As much activity to maintain CV fitness should be performed as possible during the rehabilitation programme, but without aggravating the primary site of tissue damage. These activities can take the form of weight-training circuits, static bike circuits, and jogging in water.

Psychological changes A well structured rehabilitation programme with specific goals can help the athlete to cope with the emotional reaction to injury.[28]

The linkage of the primary and secondary consequences of injury and functional rehabilitation

Initially the activities used in the rehabilitation programme are usually non-functional in nature and are aimed at developing sufficient capabilities of the primary and secondary consequences of injury to cope with the demands of more functional activities. The early introduction of functional activities facilitates the development of proprioception and coordinated movement, and begins to stress the healing tissue and the secondary consequences of injury in a functional pattern.

468

Phase 3: functional testing and return to "normal" activity

At the end of the rehabilitation process the decision has to be made when to allow the athlete to return to training and competition. The decision is made on the basis of two evaluations.

1 *Clinical evaluation.* This involves the application of clinical tests to determine the state of the primary and secondary consequences of injury, and is usually performed in the surgery/clinic room.
2 *Functional testing.* This takes the form of a field test and should be performed on the appropriate surface and with the equipment that the athlete uses for their sport. The test involves a series of functional activities that progressively stress the injured area, leaving the activity that stresses the affected area the most until last. An example of a functional test following a mild to moderate hamstring lesion in a hockey player is given in Table 22.6.

Table 22.6 Example of a progressive functional test

1	Warm-up
2	Jogging – 1/4 pace forwards for 30 m
3	As for 2, but jogging sideways
4	As for 2, but backwards
5	As for 2, 3, and 4 but at 1/2 to 3/4 pace
6	Running 3/4 pace in straight line and cut to left/right
7	Running backwards, turn to left/right and sprint
8	Walk forwards and sprint on command
9	Standing start and sprint on command
10	Short, multidirectional sprints in star formation
11	Jumping and landing on both legs
12	Jumping and landing on affected leg
13	Running drills with hockey stick and ball
14	One on one game situations
15	Stop and start sprinting with stick and ball

At the beginning of each phase of the functional test the athlete is questioned regarding the onset of any symptoms, and the test terminated should symptoms appear. If the athlete completes the whole test asymptomatically, they should be re-evaluated clinically and if no subjective or objectives signs have appeared they should be pronounced functional enough to return to either gradual or full training.

The most difficult decision following a functional test occurs when the athlete feels only mild symptoms during the test and the athlete has an imminent major competition. In this situation the athlete needs to be warned of the potential risks of competing and the decision to compete should be made on the basis of the location and severity of the injury, the potential risks of stressing the area in the competition, and whether any measures such as taping will decrease the risk of injury.

Summary

Rehabilitation is an essential part of the treatment of all injuries to athletes. A well structured and skillfully applied rehabilitation programme will facilitate the return to sport of the injured athlete in the shortest and safest possible time. Without rehabilitation, the injured tissues will not be progressively introduced to the specific stress of the athlete's sport and therefore be more vulnerable to injury. The general principles of the rehabilitation process described in this chapter are summarised in Figure 22.3.

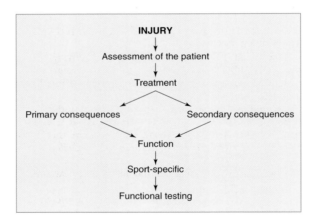

Figure 22.3   Summary of the rehabilitation process

References

1 *Churchill's illustrated medical dictionary.* Edinburgh: Churchill Livingstone, 1989.
2 Kegerreis S. The construction and implementation of functional progression as a component of athletic rehabilitation. *J Orthop Sports Phys Ther* 1983;5:14–19.
3 Woo S L-Y, Buckwalter JA. Injury and repair of the musculo-skeletal soft tissues. *American Academy of Orthopaedic Surgeons Symposium,* 1987.
4 Hawkins RJ, Kennedy JC. Impingement syndrome in athletes. *Am J Sports Med* 1990;8:151–8.
5 Grace TG, Sweetser ER, Nelson MA, Ydens LR, Skipper BJ. Isokinetic muscle imbalance and knee joint injury. *J Bone Joint Surg* 1984;66A:734–40.

6 Muckle DS. Associated factors in recurrent groin and hamstring injuries. *Br J Sports Med* 1982;**16**:37–9.
7 Detmer DE. Chronic shin splints: classification and management of medial tibial stress syndrome. *Sports Med* 1986;**3**:436–46.
8 Newell SG. Functional neutral orthoses and shoe modification. In: Lehman JF, ed. *Orthotics, Clinics in PM&R. Philadelphia: WB Saunders*, 1992;**3.1**:193–222.
9 Akeson WH. The response of ligaments to stress modulation and overview of the ligament healing response. In: Daniel D *et al*, eds. *Knee ligaments: structure and function, injury and repair*. New York: Raven Press, 1990, pp. 315–27.
10 Forrester JC, Zederfeldt BH, Hayes TL, Hunt TK. Wolff's law in relation to the healing skin wound. *J Trauma* 1970;**10**:770–9.
11 Wahl SM, Wong H, McCartney-Francis N. Role of growth factors in inflammation and repair. *J Cell Biochem*1989;**40**:193–9.
12 McMaster WC, Liddle S, Waugh TR. Laboratory evaluation of various cold therapy modalities. *Am J Sports Med* 1978;**6**:291.
13 Benson TB, Copp WP, The effects of therapeutic forms of heat and ice on the pain threshold of the normal shoulder. *Pharmacol Rehabil* 1974;**13**:101.
14 Knight K. *Cryotherapy in sports medicine*. Champaign, IL: Human Kinetics, 1995.
15 Sloan JP, Giddings P, Hain R. Effects of cold and compression on oedema. *Phys Sports Med* 1988;**16**:116.
16 Barlow Y, Willoughby J. Pathophysiology of soft tissue repair. *Br Med Bull* 1992; **48**:689–711.
17 Dyson M. Role of ultrasound in wound healing. In: Kloth LC, Feeder J, McCullough J, eds. *Wound healing: alternatives in management (Contemporary perspectives in rehabilitation*, series editor S Woolff). Philadelphia: FA Davis. 1990, pp. 229–85.
18 Peacock EE. *Wound repair*, 3rd edn. London: WB Saunders, 1984.
19 Loitz BJ, Zernicke RF, Vailas AC, Kody MH, Meals RA. Effects of short term immobilisation versus continuous passive motion on the biomechanical and biochemical properties of the rabbit tendon. *Clin Orthop Rel Res* 1989;**224**: 265–71.
20 Evans P. The healing process at a cellular level: a review. *Physiotherapy* 1980; **66**:256–9.
21 Aronen JG, Regan K. Decreasing the incidence of recurrence of first time anterior shoulder dislocation with rehabilitation. *Am J Sports Med* 1984;**12**:282.
22 Maittand G. *Peripheral manipulation*, 3rd edn. Oxford: Butterworth–Heinemann, 1991.
23 Puniello MS. Iliotibial band tightness and medial patellar glide in patients with patello-femoral dysfunction. *J Orthop Sports Phys Ther* 1993;**17**:144–8.
24 Litchfield R, Hawkins R, Dillman CJ, Atkins J. Rehabilitation of the overhead athlete. *J Orthop Sports Phys Ther* 1993;**18**:433–41.
25 Stokes M, Young A. The contribution of reflex inhibition to arthrogenous muscle weakness. *Clin Sci* 1984;**67**:7.
26 Young A, Stokes M. Reflex inhibition of muscle activity and morphological consequences of inactivity. In: Saltin B, ed. *International series of sport sciences*, vol. 10: *Biochemistry of exercise VI*. Champaign, IL: Human Kinetics, 1986.
27 Knight KJ. Guide-lines for rehabilitation of sports injuries. In: Harvey JS, ed. Rehabilitation of the injured athlete. *Clinics in Sports Medicine*, vol. 4, no. 3. Philadelphia: WB Saunders, 1985.
28 Nideffer RM. The injured athlete: psychological factors in treatment. *Orthop Clin North Am* 1983;**14**:373–85.

Further reading

Albert M. *Eccentric muscle training in sports and orthopaedics*. Edinburgh: Churchill Livingstone, 1991.
Tippett SR, Voight ML. *Functional progressions for sport rehabilitation*. Champaign, IL: Human Kinetics, 1995.

Index

contract–relax agonist–contract 30
contusions, thigh 198–9
coracoclavicular ligament repair 381
"corked thigh" 198–9
coronary heart disease and anabolic
  steroids 79
corticosteroids 56, 57
  asthma 60
  eczema 62
  hay fever/allergies 61
  inflammatory bowel disease 63
  injury/pain management 57–8
    Achilles tendinitis/
      paratendinitis 177
    back pain (low) 267
    bursitis in knee 225
    lateral epicondylitis 336
    plantar fasciitis 181
    subacromial impingement 379
  respiratory infections 62
cosmetics effects, anabolic steroids 80
costovertebral joint injury 270
cramps, heat 143
cranial damage/fracture 275, 286
creatine 58–9, 87–8, 128
Crohn's disease 63
cruciate ligament injuries
  anterior 206–11
    bracing (functional) 425
    bracing (therapeutic) 423
    child 397
    medial ligament injury combined
      with 213, 214–15
  posterior 211–13
    bracing 423
crush injury, fingertip 299, 310
Crystal Palace wrap 433–4
cuboid subluxation, taping 442
cycle theories 74–5
cyclists
  helmets 292, 293
  nerve compression 319

dairy foods 95, 117, 119
Dangle's angle 179
DAPRE regimen 466, 467
dead arm syndrome 379

dehydration 123–4, 126 *see also* fluid
  intake
  hot climates, affecting
    performance 124, 141
  post-event 127
deltoid ligament *see* medial ligament
deltoid muscle
  stretch 47–8, 49–51
  supraspinatus and, imbalance 366
  tests 369
de Quervain's disease 308
dermatitis (eczema) 62
diagnosis, accurate 456
diarrhoea
  traveller's, prophylaxis 147
  treatment 62
diet *see* nutrition
digit(s) *see* fingers; toes
digital nerve block 301
disability *see* ABC(D); neurological
  status
disc(s), intervertebral
  anatomy/biomechanics 250–1
  pathology 253, 270
    adolescents 403
    treatment 268
dislocation
  elbow 349
    child 391
  finger 300
  hip 246
  patella 203–4
    child 397–8
  shoulder 358
    acromioclavicular joint 363,
      380–1
    child 386
    glenohumeral joint *see*
      glenohumeral joint
    habitual 359
    treatment 377–8, 378–9, 380–1
    voluntary 358, 360
  wrist joint 326
diuretics 55, 58, 77, 88
doctor
  notification of prescribed drug
    by 61, 68
  team *see* team doctor

481